Praise for
"The Main Ingredients
of Health & Happiness"
by Susan Smith Jones, Ph.D.

Susan's book contains information on how to achieve health and happiness. I find, however, that most people aren't inspired enough to seek information. So I invite you all to wake up to life and all its potential, read her book, become informed and live a healed life.
—**Bernie S. Siegel, M.D.**, author of Love, Medicine and Miracles

The Main Ingredients of Health and Happiness *offers the tools you'll need to enrich every aspect of your life."*
—**John Gray, Ph.D.** author of
Men are from Mars, Women are from Venus

If you're ready to improve your diet, reduce stress in your life, or exercise your way to radiant health, this book is loaded with secrets to improve your quality of life.
—**Gerald Jampolsky, M.D.**, author of Love is Letting Go of Fear

The Main Ingredients of Health and Happiness *is filled with useful information that is presented in ways that are both easy to understand and fun to read.*
—**Dean Ornish, M.D.**, author of Eat More, Weigh Less

The Main Ingredients *is a wellspring of wise and heart-centered information by an author who has devoted her life to well-being. I have the deepest respect for Susan Smith Jones as a model of Spirit-guided, well-balanced living. This book is sure to be a welcome companion to anyone seeking to live their highest potential.*
—**Alan Cohen**, author of I Had It All The Time

Susan Smith Jones writes clearly and cogently about the enormous power of changing our diets and learning how to live in balance. I grew up on a diet of roast beef and pork chops, but learning to eat a healthier diet was one of the major changes in my life. Susan Smith Jones will help many other people enjoy the same benefits.
    —**Neal D. Barnard, M.D.**, author of *Eat Right, Live Longer*

Too frequently we forget that we are mind, body and spirit. **The Main Ingredients** *helps us put those three facets together into a synergistic force.*
    —**Tommy Hawkins**, Vice President, Los Angeles Dodgers

The Main Ingredients of Health and Happiness *is a light that can lead us out of the moras of ill health. This book inspires and empowers the reader to "seize the day" while providing a well conceived blueprint for creating a life filled with health, happiness and peace . . . an excellent book.*
    —**Gabriel Cousens, M.D.**, *author of* Conscious Eating

Susan Smith Jones has created an uplifting book dedicated to everyone's health and happiness. It should be on your bookshelf. It is on mine.
    —**Earl L. Mindell, Ph.D.**, author of *Earl Mindell's Vitamin Bible*

I would recommend Susan Smith Jones' workshops to anyone. However, if one cannot meet in person this fabulous example of balanced spiritual and practical living, the next best thing is this book. All Susan's books are great, but this one may well be her best ever!
    —**John A.V. Strickland**, Senior Minister, Unity Church of Hawaii

Body, mind and spirit—Susan Smith Jones harmonizes the trio in this delightful journey into health on every level of our being.
    —**Victoria Moran**, author of *Get the Fat Out*

This is a beautiful, clear, uplifting book. A guide to living joyfully, passionately, heartfully, and peacefully, it is also a fine example of the heart-centeredness that brings grace to life. Outstanding.
    —**John Robbins,** author of *Diet for a New America*

the Main Ingredients

of Health & Happiness

To Eleanor,

Celebrate Life!

♡ Susan Jones

The health suggestions and recommendations in this book are based on the training, research and personal experiences of the author. Because each person and each situation is unique, and because some risk is involved, neither the author nor the publisher are responsible for possible adverse consequences.

Also by Susan Smith Jones

Choose to Live Each Day Fully
Choose to Be Healthy
Choose to Live Peacefully

Copyright © 1995 Susan Smith Jones

All rights reserved. No part of this book may be reproduced or transmitted to any form or by any means, electronic or mechanical, including photocopying, recording, or by any information and retrieval system, without permission in writing from the publisher.

ISBN 1-883220-38-6

Published by DAWN Publications

14618 Tyler Foote Road
Nevada City, CA 95959
916.292.3482

Printed in USA

10 9 8 7 6 5 4 3 2 1
First Edition

Designed by Nancy Raynes
Cover design by LeeAnn Brook
Color photograph by Richard Thompson
Index by Brackney Indexing Service

Contents

Foreword

I have known Dr. Susan Smith Jones for more than ten years. She is a Smith also, but that's not the reason I always appreciate seeing her radiant face in health magazines. She says all the things I have wanted to say but said them sooner, clearer, and more cogently than I have.

She has been faced with the same dilemma that faces most writers on health. You just get a book out and then some research comes along that forces you to write another book. She also knows that people must be able to read to get the writer's message. And then comes the hard part: to get the reader motivated to do something positive about their health, like eat more fruits and vegetables, walk around the block occasionally, and at least, stop smoking and drinking.

This latest book of Susan's is the embodiment of everything known today that should make a human body—despite the poisons in our environment, and some rotten genetic forces—last into a happy and healthy old age, and go quietly in our sleep. We all want this house of clay to last until close to a century has gone by, and then go all at once. I hate these diseases that pick off one system at a time: your eyes go, then the joints stiffen, the bladder is unreliable, and then sleep is a daytime phenomenon instead of a happy eight hours at night.

My wife was immobile for a couple of months recently with a sciatic-like problem, so I bought and fixed the meals. My menus were enough to motivate her to get well. I tried to push us both into more raw foods, and less meat. Actually I found it easy to shop; I just stayed around the periphery of the supermarket, and did not enter the aisles where the packaged and processed foods have been waiting for months for the customers. Oh, sure, we got some yogurt "ice cream." I found that if there are no cookies in the cookie jar, I cannot eat them. A piece of whole grain toast is almost as good. We have also tried Johanna Budwig's recipe for some kind of health: a tablespoon of flaxseed oil mixed with a half cup of low-fat cottage cheese. We can get used to health.

I think I know why the people of my generation have lived long and reasonably healthy lives, even before Susan got on the scene. We were not exposed to so many pollutants, herbicides, and toxic chemicals. We also did not have the "advantage" of modern food marketing techniques that process and deplete natural foods so that they can stay on the grocers' shelves forever. Bugs cannot survive on them; now we know that humans cannot either. Since World War II the rates of most diseases have increased: cancer, asthma and allergies, Attention Deficit Disorder, arthritis, and autoimmune diseases like lupus. People are getting degenerative diseases earlier in life instead of at the end of their lives.

Now Susan knows all these things, but how can we get our population to follow her leadership and make themselves healthy? Adolescents think they are immune and immortal, middle-aged people feel their insurance will get them through, and the elderly figure "What's the use, I'm too old to start now." Wrong! Susan can show the way if people will follow the simple outlines in this book.

I would suggest that you, the reader, take one chapter at a time to read, study, ponder, and follow her recommendations and incorporate those ideas into your lifestyle. Don't try to do too much at once. One step at a time is the idea.

When people ask me what to do about their bowels, their phlegm, their headaches, their cravings, and their disturbed sleep, my first question is, "What is your favorite food?" If people love a food so much they would kill for it, it represents an allergic-addictive situation. There is something in that food that they need, like the magnesium in chocolate, or the calcium in milk. Susan knows about all those things and can give insight into your particular eating and lifestyle mismanagement. Insight gives motivation.

The best thing about Susan is her cheerful ambience. She knows how to turn someone on to her style and methods, even though you may be reluctant to take that first step. Once you are into her ways, and you feel better, you will thank your lucky stars that you have this book as your guide.

It is interesting that she has placed the chapter on "Acts of Kindness" towards the end of the book. I have found that surly, grumpy people are so self-centered they will never, like Scrooge, say "Hello" or even give a smile or a nod to some other human being. My feeling is that those misanthropes have not eaten well or exercised for days or weeks. Once they get to Chapter 18, they should have figured out why they are such jerks, and changed their ways.

I have an easy phone number to dial, but it is similar to a number for airline information and a bank. When people call and get me, I ask what they had for breakfast. Most of them have not had anything or it was coffee and a doughnut. I insist that they at least eat a handful of almonds or some greens, or fruit, or a piece of whole grain bread, wait twenty minutes and then dial again. No one gets my number again by mistake. See how it works?

You see how simple is her message? You could have figured it out for yourself. Try to think of yourself as your ancestors two million years ago, running through field and forest, eating as you go, cooking little, laughing a lot, and sleeping with one eye open. You might be eaten by some wild thing, but at least you know your body is good enough to eat.

Happy foraging—in the store and in this book.

Lendon H. Smith, M.D.
author of *Feed Your Body Right*

This book is lovingly dedicated:

*To my mom, June B. Smith,
the most loving, forgiving and tenderhearted person I know.
You are my very best friend and greatest inspiration.*

*To Paramhansa Yogananda,
who has taught me
through his shining example and teachings
how beautiful life can be
when we choose to put God first.*

*"The greatest romance is with the Infinite. You have no idea
how beautiful life can be. When you suddenly find God everywhere,
when He comes and talks to you and guides you,
the romance of divine love has begun."*

—Paramhansa Yogananda
Man's Eternal Quest

Introduction

CHERISH YOUR VISIONS
cherish your ideals;
cherish the music that stirs in your heart,
the beauty that forms in your mind,
the loveliness that drapes your purest thoughts,
for out of them will grow all delightful conditions,
all heavenly environments;
of these, if you but remain true to them,
your world will at last be built.
—James Allen

There is a single magic, a single power, a single salvation, and a single happiness, and that is called loving. **—Hermann Hesse**

What a joy it is to have this opportunity to share my thoughts, experiences, and research on being healthy, happy and fully alive in *The Main Ingredients of Health & Happiness*. Thank you for spending time with me through my writing. I want you to feel like we are sitting across from each other and I'm talking to you personally through this book. I already know that we have lots in common since you've chosen to read a book on health and being the best you can be.

Twenty-four years ago I fractured my back in an automobile accident. The doctor told me that I should get used to a life of pain, inactivity, and difficulty, as I would never be able to carry anything heavier than a light purse. I was quite upset when I heard the doctor's prognosis. For me it was what I refer to as a "wake-up call" where the universe got my attention in a big way. All I could see was a closed door. I was filled with depression, self-pity, confusion and feelings of being victimized. After a couple of weeks, I went to a favorite spot overlooking Santa Monica Bay where I often would go when in need of inspiration. I had a heart-to-heart talk with myself.

On the one hand, I was convinced that life was meant to be a magnificent adventure. To me a full adventurous life meant living joyfully, passionately, healthfully and peacefully. Yet the life the doctor had described didn't align with my beliefs and desires. I just couldn't accept it. I knew I had a choice to make and I made it. Helen Keller once wrote: "When one door closes, another opens; but often we look so long at the closed door that we do not see the one which has opened for us." Although I didn't know how I could change my physical condition, I recognized that there was a Higher Power within me that had the answers. So I simply made *a deep commitment to let go, live from inner guidance, and accept only vibrant, radiant health.*

The tool that makes life a truly wonderful adventure is our power of choice. It's up to us to create a meaningful life. We are all made in God's image and have the potential to make our lives extraordinary. We are all magnificent spiritual beings having a human experience here on spaceship earth. If you don't like your current circumstances and want to live a more peaceful, healthy and happy life, you can change it. You can choose to be radiantly healthy and filled with joy and thanksgiving. You can choose to be at peace with life. You have the power and ability to make your dreams a reality, to manifest your heart's best desires.

This is true because life constantly flows in the direction of one's choices. Knowing that helps keep me on course. No longer do I look to people, things, or circumstances as my source of happiness and fulfillment. The value in my life is what I bring to it. Henry David Thoreau knew this when he said, "There is no value in life except what you choose to place upon it, and no happiness in any place except what you bring to it yourself."

Of course, it hasn't always been an easy road. I have made many mistakes, or what I prefer to think of as simply learning what doesn't work for me. Nonetheless, in retrospect, I can see that the car accident was a valuable experience, for it was out of hitting that real low spot that my life turned around. As a result, I chose to embark on a great adventure of learning and growing and discovering how to live my highest vision.

After my experience by Santa Monica Bay, a stream of events began that assisted me in healing my condition: finding the perfect books and tapes, hearing certain lectures, meeting people who told me about healing and salutary foods, visualization, and meditation—much of which sounded kind of weird to me at the time.

During the months following the accident, and to this day, I have made several changes in my lifestyle, behavior, thoughts and attitude. I've learned to bring more consciousness to my living, to pay attention to life and observe patterns, to use the ones that support me in new ways, and to change the ones that don't. I now choose to live more deeply, to find the intention beneath my intention and to always talk things over with God before making any decisions.

I've also discovered the tremendous power of commitment, belief and faith. Faith means belief in an inner knowing, appearances notwithstanding. Commitments link me, both mind and heart, to people, aspirations, and goals. When I give myself wholeheartedly to a relationship, my work, or some plan, I do well. However, when my first commitment is to be God-centered, I bring a greater measure of love, understanding, and imagination to all my other commitments. When I am God-centered I do my best in a new or long-standing relationship. When I am God-centered, I bring love and compassion to every interaction with others, and inspiration to every activity I undertake.

I have the following poem by Goethe on my refrigerator door so I can read it often. It inspires and beautifully expresses the impact commitment can have on your life.

> *Until one is committed there is hesitancy,*
> *the chance to draw back, always ineffectiveness.*
> *Concerning all acts of initiative and creation there is one*
> *elementary truth*
> *the ignorance of which kills countless ideas and splendid plans:*
> *that the moment one definitely commits oneself*
> *then Providence moves too.*
> *All sorts of things occur to help one*
> *that would never otherwise have occurred.*

A whole stream of events issues from the decision,
raising in one's favor all manner of unforeseen incidents
and meetings and material assistance,
which no man could have dreamed would come his way.
Whatever you can do or dream, begin it!
Boldness has genius, power, and magic in it.
                                        —**Goethe**

After examining me at my six-month checkup following the accident, the doctor just shook his head in bewilderment and said, "This just can't be. There is no sign of a fracture, and you seem to be in perfect health, free of pain. There must be some mistake. It's just miraculous."

Perhaps it was. Yet, I've since discovered that miracles are a natural part of committing to being healthy, happy and peaceful. This magnificent universe is alive and mysterious, ultimately benevolent and orderly. Intention and consciousness, discovery and synchronicity are magical. Yet since we cannot see synchronicity or experience it directly with our senses, we become skeptical of it. Western culture teaches that events which intuition tells us are special are really only random happenstance, coincidences. We've been taught not to believe something until we see it with our own eyes, even though the most important things in life are intangible.

I believe in the magic of life, the ultimate source of creativity and love which I call God. I know I can never be separated from God. This divine presence is for me like returning home to a parent who loves me unconditionally. It is my connection to synchronicity, and to miracles. The point of connection is through love, and through the conscious, unconscious and superconscious mind. It responds to our power to choose. Believe in your connection with the Divine and its power to create synchronicity.

When you choose to live an inspiring life, you make a difference in everyone's life with whom you come in contact. Every day the world presents you with miracles waiting for your awareness. Hidden beneath the "wrapping" of every experience is a new opportunity to know the joy, the wonder of growth and love. *Carpe diem:* Seize the day. What makes certain people seize life? Why are some people open to growth, to unfolding, to deepening and living more fully? Some people have an enormous capacity for maintaining a steady equilibrium, for accepting what they cannot change, for facing what they can, and moving on. You can choose to live that way by loving life and aligning your thoughts with God's.

One of the most important lessons I've learned is that if I'm facing a challenge—whether it's pertaining to health, relationships, finances, or whatever—all I need to do is to turn my focus from the challenge to God, and let the Divinity reveal the hidden gift within it. We're given the circumstances we require for our awakening. Every situation, seen rightly, contains the seeds of freedom. You can be sure that it's there, just waiting for you to look at it from the right perspective. *A Course in Miracles* says, "When any situation arises which tempts you to become disturbed, say: 'There is another way of looking at this.'"

My auto accident taught me that dark nights of the soul can reveal the true purpose of suffering—namely that out of our pain we can rise, expand, grow, conquer, achieve new and even better things. Like the butterfly that is strengthened by its desperate struggle to break out of a constricting cocoon, we too can emerge stronger, wiser, and more resilient because of the dark, difficult times in our lives. In those times we learn to simplify life, clarify values, sort out priorities, and discover which friends are true and which are not.

By rising out of my distress I've also come to realize that the purpose of my existence is to become truly loving. That's how we find the way back to the divine source. *Nothing will change your life more quickly for the better than the consistent feeling of love.* Everything in your life—making decisions, raising children, your lifestyle, your career, your friends, your contribution to society—will become a more coherent whole when you love life fully. Loving all aspects of your life, regardless of challenges you may be facing, opens doors and lets in light, energy and joy. Love yourself out of sheer gratitude for existence. Love the mystery of life and the process of creating what you want. When you love, you become transformed spiritually. *A Course in Miracles* says, "Every loving thought is true. Everything else is an appeal for healing and help, regardless of the form it takes."

The more you love, the more you come to realize you don't need to force things. The *Tao-Te-Ching*, the classic manual on the art of living, is referred to simply as *The Book of the Way*. The author, Lao-Tsu, was a sage whose large-heartedness, humor, and wisdom grace every page. He teaches that the true way is "to do by not doing," a paradigm for nonaction, the purest and most effective form of action. He wrote, "The way to do is to be." For a long time, this has been one of my favorite maxims. You don't need to force things. Let go and let God. Or, as the Buddha put it at the end of a long life dedicated to teaching mindfulness and peaceful living, "Be a light unto yourself."

Ultimately, your choices are what separate you from everyone else. They are the only road to becoming truly independent. Choose what you want and how you want to live. Accept and expect the best. Learn to trust your ability to make decisions. The greatest lessons often come from the ones that prove to be wrong. Taking risks is our chance to find out what works for us, what we can do well. We must learn to choose what we want and to not worry about the rest, knowing it's all in God's hands. If we're the best we can be, we learn to respect what we can become in the future. Choosing— it's the only way.

In my time of crisis, I didn't just choose health. There's more to health than a strong body, toned muscles, clear mind, and disease-free and pain-free existence. I chose to be the best I could be— physically, mentally, emotionally and spiritually. That's what this book is about: tapping into your inner truth and power and choosing to be the best you can be. It's about living your truth and reclaiming your spirituality. And it's also about taking loving care of yourself, honoring the Divinity within you, and bringing spirituality into your everyday life.

Why not become the best that we can be? *The Main Ingredients of Health & Happiness* will help show you the way. We all owe it to ourselves to choose health and happiness; no one is going to do it for us. You may find that I suggest things that are entirely new to you such as meditation, visualization, healing music, solitude, certain foods and supplements or a way of living that's different from your lifestyle now. When applicable, refer to the Resource Directory for more information. Don't simply take my word for it. You have all the answers within you. Always consult your inner guidance on every decision and choice in your life. Deep within our hearts, each of us knows the truth.

Like you, I have a lot of things I want to accomplish in this life, and I have no interest in being slowed down in any way by health problems. Because I want to be the best I can be, I want to embrace the best life has to offer. So can you. I believe in you and your ability to be the best you can be, and I salute your great adventure.

Namaste.*

Susan S. Jones

Susan S. Jones

"If one advances confidently in the direction of his dreams, and endeavors to live the life which he has imagined, he will meet with a success unexpected in common hours. . . . If you have built castles in the air, your work need not be lost; that is where they should be. Now put foundations under them." **—Henry David Thoreau**

* "I celebrate the place in you where we are all one."

ONE

A Balanced Life
Key Ingredient of Health

Y ou are not being called upon to change yourself. You are being asked to be more of what you already are. The invitation is bold, the stakes are high, and the outcome is certain. Dare to live your destiny now. —**Alan Cohen**

Man is made or unmade by himself. By the right choice he ascends. As a being of power, intelligence, and love, and lord of his own thoughts, he holds the key to every situation. —**James Allen**

For most people, being radiantly healthy is simply a matter of choice. But it is not merely a matter of choosing to exercise regularly and eat wholesome, nutritious foods. The latest research discloses that what we think, believe and expect in life powerfully influences our well-being, our immune system and our lives, and that it affects not only our own lives but the condition of the entire planet.

The idea that we have control over our wellness and that we can choose to be healthy and functioning fully is now a new science that's rapidly gaining popularity. From around the world, immunologists, psychiatrists, endocrinologists, neuroscientists, microbiologists, and psychologists—who rarely step out of their own fields—are coming together to unite their expertise in this new field called psychoneuroimmunology. This new science deals with the mind's effect on the immune system's incredibly complex network of organs, vessels, and white blood cells.

Research indicates that the immune system, brain, and other vital body systems communicate, connect with, and influence one another. That means that your body will be in a better position to cope with factors that can cause disease and heal itself if you are not under stress. In other words, if your brain allows your stress level to get out of control, it suppresses the immune system. Well-managed stress, however, may help keep your immune system healthy. We can't totally avoid pressure in this world but we can choose a healthy balance.

Psychoneuroimmunology researchers have looked extensively into the body/mind connection and how each of us can become masters of our lives. The fruits of this approach are already being harvested in comprehensive programs of mind/body medicine at Harvard University, the University of Massachusetts, Stanford University, the University of Miami, and the University of California at San Francisco and Los Angeles. There people with such life-threatening and debilitating illnesses as cancer, AIDS, coronary heart disease, and chronic pain are learning to change their habits and attitudes—what they eat, when they exercise and how they think. A number of landmark studies have shown that these men and women are functioning far more effectively, feeling better and, in some particularly striking instances, living longer.

Particularly impressive is the work of Dr. O. Carl Simonton in Pacific Palisades, California, and the incredible advances he has made with cancer patients using visualization. He reports that only about ten percent of the people who come to him are willing to do the work he recommends. The remainder would rather get the operation, the injection—anything to keep the reality "out there" rather than looking within and taking charge.

There are those who receive a lot of "value" out of being victims. They get to blame everybody else for their problems. They hold on to resentment and are unforgiving. As research discloses, people have a difficult time processing emotions. Some scientific evidence suggests that much of the sickness we experience comes at least in part from the inability to express anger, guilt, and fear. Researchers have even gone so far as to say that our level of stress and how we deal with it is a main contributing factor to our level of health.

The Biology of Emotions

A "whole-person approach" is the foundation to recovery from all ailments and diseases. Dr. Simonton's method calls on the patient to alter emotions, attitudes and expectations. Very important to the process are daily exercises in relaxation and imaging techniques, and physical activity intended to reduce the stresses that Simonton says play a role in disease.

At its most basic, mental therapy—known in some circles as the "mind-body connection"—uses emotions to prod certain brain chemicals into stimulating the body's defense systems. By the same token, the repression of certain emotions can depress the body's ability to maintain a healthy immune function.

"If you get angry and that emotion doesn't get discharged, the resulting hormonal products and smaller particles such as neurotransmitters and endorphins don't get used," says Dr. Caroline Sperling, a clinical psychologist and director of the Cancer Counseling Institute in Bethesda, Maryland. "The residue remains and can become toxic in our bodies." The opposite is also true. "When you release those emotions effectively, you get real well-being and adrenal charging so that the immune system stays strong and the body stays healthy," adds Sperling.

According to Dr. Joan Borysenko, author of *Minding the Body, Mending the Mind,* and co-founder and former director of the Mind/Body Clinic at New England Deaconess Hospital in Boston, these messages are transported instantaneously between the brain and a newly discovered site called a neuroreceptor on the white blood cells. So when someone is happy or thinks a happy thought, the white blood cells—which are the body's primary defense system—receive that message immediately. Conversely, when someone is depressed, that same message is transmitted directly to the white blood cells through the nervous system. All this happens very quickly. Everything which is registered in our minds is registered in our bodies. The discovery of the neuroreceptor site on the white blood cell is an exciting breakthrough.

Following the footsteps of Dr. Simonton, Dr. Paul Rosch, president of the American Institute of Stress in New York, agrees that there is some very exciting work going on in the field, particularly in the area of visual imagery and cancer. "It has been determined that negative emotions have a high link to certain types of malignancies, and support for that comes from the observation that there are receptor sites on T-cell lymphocytes (white blood cells) for certain brain chemicals, which suggests that there is a conversation going back and forth between the immune system and the brain," says Rosch.

Sperling concurs. "Imagery works like a computer to program into the hypothalamus the directions you want. It helps open up the parasympathetic nervous system so your body gets healthy. In other words, you're giving messages to your body, which translates them into neurotransmitters . . . to get the immune system to work better and the hormone system to calm down a little and stop creating abnormal cells."

Along these same lines, Dr. Deepak Chopra spoke on a national television talk show about this mind-body connection and how the mind and body are inseparable. He explained that the mind is in every cell of the body and that each thought causes a release of neuropeptides that are transmitted to all the cells in the body. Thoughts of love, he said, cause the release of interleukin and interferon which help heal the body. Anxious thoughts cause the release of cortisone and adrenaline which suppress the immune system. Peaceful, calming thoughts release chemicals in the body similar to Valium which help the body to relax.

Similarly, Norman Cousins throughout his insightful book, *Head First: The Biology of Hope*, presents evidence that hope, faith, love, will to live, purpose, laughter and festivity help combat disease. Cousins writes, "The greatest force in the human body is the natural drive of the body to heal itself—but that force is not independent of the belief system, which can translate expectations into physiological change. Nothing is more wondrous about the 15 million neurons in the human brain than their ability to convert thoughts, hopes, ideas and attitudes into chemical substances. Everything begins, therefore, with belief. What we believe is the most powerful option of all."

A clue to the magnitude of impact that knowledge of this inner healing/belief system may have is evident in the phenomenon of the placebo effect. Medical researchers are well aware that a certain percentage of participants in medical studies who are treated with placebo drugs or procedures (i.e., treatments of no known medical value) will improve because they believe they have received a potent treatment. In the past, researchers tended to dismiss the placebo effect as a distraction, a confounding psychological variable that interfered with the real aims of the research. Yet the fact that belief can override the non-physiological actions of placebo medicines demonstrates the remarkable capability of this inner healing force.

While the messages from the brain through the nervous system are instantaneous, there is also another transport system that's slower and more steady. Through our endocrine system, our thoughts trigger what's known as the hypothalamic-pituitary-adrenal axis, which gradually influences our body to respond to our emotional responses. Borysenko writes about the studies on neuropeptides, a group of hormonal messengers (neurotransmitters) secreted by the brain, immune system and digestive system. Endorphins, for example, which are commonly associated with the "runners' high" experienced by joggers, are one among several dozen neuropeptides researchers have identified. These substances represent a rich pharmacy of natural drugs that the body produces in response to various internal and external stresses.

Borysenko explains: "When you react to your boss as if he is a saber-toothed tiger, your body secretes chemicals that prepare you to die rather than helping you to live. These drugs are then pumped out into the blood stream and eventually bind to the surface of all the cells in the body the way that a key fits into a lock. They then affect the function of the cells. So, if you are fearful, for example, it is not just an emotion. It is that every cell in your body has now received a biochemical signal about fear broadcast by the neuropeptide system, and has changed its metabolism in some way."

As exciting as these insights are, Borysenko adds an important caveat when she cautions not to exaggerate the connection between personality and disease. "It is not as if everyone who is hostile and cynical will have heart disease or that everyone who acts like a doormat will develop cancer," she explains. "Personality is only one of many variables that can affect health."

Put another way, British cardiologist Dr. Peter Nixon explains that increased stress and arousal causes numerous changes in body functioning that eventually interfere with immune function, protein synthesis, and cardiac functioning. Repetitive stress also uses up the body's reserves, leading to increased stress on other physiological functions. This, in turn, can result in heart disease, cancer, or depression.

These ideas about the body-mind connection are not new. Plato said that the physician who treats just the body and does not address the mind is not treating the whole patient. In ancient Rome, Galen, in 140 A.D., said that it is depressed women who get breast cancer. Our reaction to stressful situations plays an integral part in our health and illnesses.

Clearly, health represents a complex and dynamic interplay of attitudes, emotions and physiology that affect our state of mind and sense of well-being. The amount of exercise in our lives, the foods we eat, a hug from a loved one, can all have a decided influence on our moods. In turn, anxious or worried thoughts can cause such physiological effects as tense muscles or elevated blood pressure. Emotional depression can translate into fatigue. And having fun with people we enjoy can create energy.

It is within our power to take charge of our lives, our thoughts and emotions, and our beliefs and attitudes. It is within our power to become the best we can be—physically, mentally, emotionally and spiritually.

"Each patient carries his own doctor inside him."
—Dr. Albert Schweitzer

20 Steps to a Balanced Life

Here are some ways to live a balanced life—to be the best you can be, healthier and happier than ever before.

1. Keep fit and live a wellness lifestyle. Develop a well-rounded fitness program that includes lifting weights or body-building, aerobics, and stretching. Make it a top priority in your life and stay committed. There is nothing that will do more good for you in terms of being vibrantly healthy, energetic and youthful than a regular fitness program. To create the body of your dreams, participate in a regular, well-rounded fitness program. (See Chapter 11 on Exercise.)

Besides exercising regularly, make sure to get enough sleep, water, and wholesome foods. Eat your foods close to the way nature produced them. Get plenty of fresh air, healthy amounts of sunshine and take saunas, too. Avoid dependence on caffeine, nicotine, alcohol, and drugs that interfere with your immune functioning. Be a good role model for your family. The only person's health and fitness you can change is your own. If you want to be an influence on the health and fitness of those you love, take care of yourself. The compelling influence of personal example will ripple outward.

Only when you approach health and fitness from a holistic perspective can you expect to achieve optimal well-being. You must include body, mind, and spirit. Here's a great question to ask yourself from Satchel Paige. "How old would you be if you didn't know how old you are?" The more healthy and fit you are, the younger you feel. (See Chapter 2 on Nutrition.)

2. Learn to elicit a relaxation response. This means becoming deeply relaxed in mind and body. Our nervous systems are bombarded by excessive environmental stimulation. Learn deep relaxation techniques such as meditation, yoga and breathing exercises so that stress levels are under control. Every hour, take a deep breathing break instead of a coffee break. For two to three minutes every hour, breathe slowly and deeply. This practice will do wonders to relieve stress, foster calmness, clear your mind, and help you to see your life from a higher, more positive perspective.

3. Watch out for stress associated with prolonged feelings of anger and depression. Beware of unexpressed feelings—especially negative ones. People who do not express feelings get sick more often, stay sick longer, and die sooner than expressive people. Nonexpression of emotion and denial of hostility or anger are two of the factors most related to unfavorable prognosis in cancer patients. Unexpressed negative feelings feed on themselves—for instance, anger can turn against the self and emerge as depression or severe anxiety. (See Questions and Answers.)

Negative emotions also trigger the release of substances that can suppress immune function. Solve your problems in a way that lets you clear up your negative feelings as thoroughly and quickly as possible. Remember that feelings aren't good or bad; they just are. Sharing feelings with a trusted friend or other support person is healing. Have positive expectations about everything in your life, including your wellness.

There is a classic study of people about to have surgery. The first group of patients dreaded surgery and attempted to avoid it. The second group, which had the same medical problems, regarded the surgery as an opportunity to rid themselves of their illnesses. After surgery, those who had positive expectations had better post-operative experiences. Similar outcomes have been repeatedly documented.

If a person is able to integrate a loss into a broader meaning of life, and feel some loss, grief and depression, those feelings will be relatively temporary. But if a person responds to loss with a prolonged state of depression, the body will also be in a prolonged state of depression, making that person vulnerable and susceptible to many things. When a person sees himself as a participant in life rather than as a victim of undesirable circumstances he or she will experience a more wholesome and less stressful life.

4. Be aware of your thoughts. Thoughts determine your experiences. Each of us has the freedom to accept and embrace whatever thoughts we choose. We possess within the silence of our being the ability to think, create and become whatever we want to become. So don't think negatively; instead, only think about things you want to be part of your life. (See Chapter 16.)

5. Feel the fear and let it go. In *The Knight In Rusty Armor* by Robert Risher, the knight in the story considers it his sole and noble mission to be the best knight there is. When not saving damsels or slaying dragons, he is trying on his armor and admiring its brilliance. As the story progresses, the knight grows to love his armor not only because it shows everyone who he is, but also—and most importantly—because it keeps him from feeling anything. Furthermore, he wears the armor for so long he forgets how things feel without it. Then when he tries to remove it, he can't—it won't come off. He asks the advice of Merlin, the magician, who helps him realize that the only way to rid himself of the armor is to rust it away. To do so, he must feel something so deeply that he cries, thereby rusting the armor and causing it to fall away, part by part.

No matter how brave or strong we are, we all wear a type of invisible armor to protect us from some aspect of life. Fear is a significant, powerful force that we feel on many levels—physically, mentally, and emotionally. Whatever our fears, they are neither good nor bad—they just are. All we risk by uncovering them is becoming healthier and more fully human and tasting another part of life and love.

6. Visualize your goals and dreams daily. James Allen wrote these words three quarters of a century ago, and they are still true today: "You think in secret and it comes to pass. Environment is but your looking glass." And it was Albert Einstein who so aptly said, "Imagination is more important than knowledge." Every day we should spend a few minutes visualizing with our mind's eye not only our goals but also how we would like our lives to be. In addition to visualizing, assume the feeling of the wish fulfilled. (See Chapter 16.)

7. Find time each day to be alone. Find some time each day to enjoy the peace of your own company. It is by spending time alone, breathing deeply and quieting everyday thoughts, that you can do the most for your health, happiness and peace of mind. Silence nourishes your soul and heals your heart. It restores peace and takes you back home. It is always sacred. Solitude is necessary for deep silence. The word *alone* is derived from the Middle English phrase *"all one."* When you are alone, you are with the best company possible—you and God. It's in silence that I see most clearly exactly what is out of balance in my life. And it's in silence that I feel the all-providing power that is the Source of all creation. Mother Theresa writes, "We need to find God, and He cannot be found in noise and restlessness. God is the friend of silence." (See Chapter 17.)

8. Practice some kind of meditation daily. This goes hand-in-hand with spending time alone each day. Research by Dr. Herbert Benson of Harvard University, author of *The Relaxation Response,* has shown that meditation not only improves immune function, but is associated with a host of other beneficial physiological effects such as altered brain states, decreased heart rate, lower blood pressure, a relaxed body and a more youthful appearance.

By spending time each day in meditation, listening to your inner guidance or intuition, you realize you are never alone. Too often we look outside ourselves for our worth and forget that nothing will ever be enough until we are enough. Meditation nourishes faith and connects us to our Source, which I call God. In the marvelous and inspiring book, *Discovering the Laws of Life,* John Marks Templeton says, "The most important thing in human life is to seek and do the will of God. A person who does this is living by faith. He or she doesn't have to look around trying to find faith; it springs from within." (See Chapter 19.)

9. Simplify life. Contrary to popular belief, we are not mere victims of our environment. When we go faster and continually push harder without keeping life in perspective, we grow more and more insensitive to our needs and the needs of those around us. Slow down. Find joy in simple pleasures. Breathe deeply, smell the flowers, talk to the animals, sing with the birds, be with friends, greet the sun, scratch behind your kitty's ear, make someone smile, marvel at the miracle you are, tell someone you love them, and laugh out loud and often.

10. Develop a sense of humor. A healthy degree of emotional detachment and hearty laughter every day can stimulate the immune system. Don't take life so seriously. Strive to move gracefully among all the activities of daily life without being ensnared by either outer things or inner desires.

Research shows that humor aids most—and probably all—major systems of the body, says Dr. William F. Fry, a psychiatrist at the Stanford University School of Medicine in California. A good laugh, he says, gives the heart muscles a good workout; improves circulation; fills the lungs with oxygen-rich air; clears the respiratory passages; stimulates alertness hormones that stimulate various tissues; alters the brain by diminishing tension in the central nervous system; counteracts fear, anger and depression, all of which are linked to physical illness; and helps relieve pain.

11. Nurture and develop your intuition. Intuition is sometimes called a sixth sense, a hunch, a gut feeling, going on instinct or just knowing deep inside. Psychologists call it intuition—an obscure mental function that provides us with information so that we know without knowing how we know. Intuition can be nurtured in a variety of ways—through contemplation, gazing out a window, relaxing or by taking walks in nature. The best way is to be still and listen. The more we act on our intuitive hunches, the stronger and more readily available they become.

12. Embrace an attitude of gratitude. An attitude of gratitude creates blessings. Be grateful for everything that's going on in your life, no matter the circumstances, for it's this kind of attitude that will help foster happiness and peace of mind and assist you to live more fully. There is power in difficulty and challenge—it forces you to tap reserves of courage, hope, faith, surrender and love you weren't aware you possessed. My friend Dan Millman has written many wonderful books about rising above difficult times. "Tragedies serve as an express elevator to Spirit," he says. In my life, I clearly see that pain and heartache accelerate the learning and growing process and foster personal power and peace. We don't have to have problems to grow. We can grow in spiritual maturity as we turn to God. But it seems to me that only a faith and belief in God and His goodness can give us the understanding and strength to be grateful in the midst of challenge. In *A Course in Miracles*, it says: "Love cannot be far behind a grateful heart and thankful mind. . . . These are the true conditions for your homecoming."

13. Become more childlike. Young children seem to know how to celebrate life, live fully, and create magical moments. They see the everyday world as full of wonder and mystery, and with this perception, they infuse the most ordinary things with magic. Children know how to open the door to the kingdom of wonder. Take their example. Be more flexible, practice forgiveness, leave time for spontaneity in daily activities, don't plan your calendar minute-to-minute, and let go of being critical and judgmental. Let your inner child come out and play.

14. Live in the present. Living *in* the moment is different from living *for* the moment. Don't compare the present with the past. Children live in the timelessness of the present. To be fully present each moment, we must free ourselves from the past. To achieve this freedom, we must heal our past. If we don't, the past will repeat itself and keep us trapped in it. When we're trapped in the past, we're not here now; we're not fully present and we can't pay attention to what's happening all around us. We must stop living our lives mechanically and unconsciously and start paying attention to the present moment. Every step you take is upon holy ground. Every moment is imbued with wonder and miracles. Thich Nhat Hanh, world-renowned Vietnamese Zen Master, has written an enlightening book called *Peace Is Every Step.* In it, he says: "Life can be found only in the present moment. The past is gone, the future is not yet here, and if we do not go back to ourselves in the present moment, we cannot be in touch with life."

15. Share your love and kindness. Being loving and kind improves health. We all need love—and I'm not just talking about romantic attraction. That warm, loving feeling you get from hugging a child, counseling a friend, being a good listener or even treating yourself to a luxurious bubble bath boosts the immune system. Petting a dog or watching fish in a tank lowers your blood pressure. In one study, people watching a film of Mother Theresa tenderly caring for sick children experienced the same heightened immune response as people who had recently fallen in love.

Whether we are at work or at play, with friends or with strangers, a friendly smile and a kind word can go a long way toward brightening someone's day. Every day, we also have opportunities to express our responsibility to our environment. Take care of your home, planet Earth. Act in caring, loving ways for your own sake and for the future sake of your children and of all children.

Led by divine guidance, welcome every opportunity to express love and kindness. (See Chapter 18.)

16. Live with integrity. To live with integrity means that who you appear to be is who you really are. Your inner realities—your beliefs, your commitments, your values—are all reflected in how you live your life on the outside. The more you live with synchronicity in what you believe, think, feel, say and do, the more peace and happiness you will invite into your life. It takes a lot of energy to live without integrity. It is emotionally and intellectually exhausting when who you are on the inside and how you behave on the outside are not aligned or congruent with one another. It's enervating to be dishonest.

Honesty and integrity go hand-in-hand. It was Thomas Jefferson who said, "Honesty is the first chapter in the book of wisdom."

To be honest is to be genuine, authentic and real. To be dishonest is to be partly forged, fake or fictitious. In the sagacious and enlightening book, *The Book of Virtues,* by William J. Bennett, he writes: "Honesty expresses both self-respect and respect for others. Dishonesty fully respects neither oneself nor others. Honesty imbues lives with openness, reliability, and candor; it expresses a disposition to live in the light. Dishonesty seeks shade, cover, or concealment. It is a disposition to live partly in the dark." Honesty is best cultivated by being honest. The more you choose to be real and honest, the more it becomes a habit.

17. Reverence for life. Live your life with joy and reverence. Greet each day with joy and enthusiasm regardless of circumstances. Be thankful for everything that touches your path—the warm sun on your face, the food that you eat, your family and friends, for nature all around you, and for the air that you breathe. Living with reverence brings happiness and fulfillment and makes every moment sacred. Take notice and enjoy the everyday miracles that make up your life. And behold the divine in everyone and everything.

18. Develop high self-esteem and self-love. High self-esteem is important for your well-being, as well as for the well-being of your children. You are the most powerful influence on your children. Your children learn from watching you live. When you are the best, you are a positive model for them to emulate. "Nothing has a stronger influence psychologically on their environment, and especially on their children, than the unlived life of the parents," says C.G. Jung. Heal your emotional wounds of the past. Release your emotional baggage and treat yourself with respect and kindness. Your life is a reflection of how you feel about and treat yourself.

Be true to yourself. This means following your heart. We just need to have enough confidence in ourselves to follow our inner guidance. Being true to yourself is to be in a state of grace. To find out if you are being true to yourself, ask yourself these two questions: 1. If I weren't getting paid for what I'm doing, would I continue to do it? 2. If I only had one year to live, would I continue to do what I'm doing? If the answer is "no," carefully consider what you can do to make different choices that will change your answer to "yes."

19. Live in God's loving presence. The whirlwind of life may suggest that you are at the mercy of other people or random circumstances, but you're not. With practice, you can withstand any turbulence by keeping your thoughts centered on God.

God's loving presence is with us at all times. No matter where we go or what activities are before us, God's presence is right there in the midst of each person and event. The light of God shines where the darkness of doubt once existed. This guidance illumines the paths we walk and shows us the best way to go.

What is the single most important relationship we can have? Our relationship with God. We are always in God and God's life nourishes us and provides for us. Our peace is founded on God's eternal presence and love. No problem is too big or too small, no question too unimportant to place in His hands. Turn to Him for everything. Give everything to God. Ask that only God's purposes be served in every situation. Ask Him to show you the love and innocence within all people. Be honest and humble. Honor your holiness. Participate in a divine love affair with God. His loving presence is who you are. I love this Sufi saying: "I searched for God and all I found was myself. I searched for myself and all I found was God."

20. Live peacefully. What would be a greater goal in life than peace of mind? What asset could be of more value to us than unshakable calmness and tranquillity? What better evidence of spiritual strength could we have than a peaceful mind and heart?

Peace of mind comes from accepting what you can't control and taking responsibility for what you can. It grows out of faith in your higher power and your spiritual nature. It comes when you let go of guilt, fear and doubt. It is the result of forgiving yourself and others for all human imperfections. When you let go of the delusion that something will someday make you happy, you can concentrate on the peace and contentment of the present moment. Inner peace is always found in the here and now. It waits quietly for you to discover it.

A healthy lifestyle is more than eating right and exercising regularly. Make a commitment to yourself to enrich each day physically, mentally, emotionally, and spiritually. By choosing to put this balance into your life, you'll reap the rewards of living . . . healthfully and happily.

"If I would have known that I was going to live this long, I would have taken better care of myself." —**Mickey Mantle**

TWO

Wholesome Nutrition
The Upcoming Dietary Revolution

Diseases are opportunities for the victims to discover what went wrong. If people make basic, safe adjustments in their nutrient intake, they can start functioning normally, usually without the use of medications. —**Dr. Lendon H. Smith**

Your body is composed of over 60 trillion cells. Think of each cell as a little engine. Some of these engines work in unison, some work independently, and they all work twenty-four hours a day. In order for engines to work right, they require specific fuels. If the engine is given the wrong fuel blend, it won't perform to maximum capacity. If the fuel is of a poor grade, the engine may sputter and hesitate, creating a loss of power. If the engine is given no fuel, it will stop.

Much of the fuel for our cells comes directly from the things we eat. The food we eat contains nutrients. These nutrients come in the form of vitamins, minerals, water, carbohydrates, fats, proteins and enzymes. Just as a car requires different forms of energy for the brakes, transmission, and battery to run smoothly, the cells of the body require different amounts and types of nutrients depending on their location and function in the body. These nutrients allow us to sustain life by providing our body's cells with the basic materials needed to carry on.

Each nutrient differs in form, function, and amount needed; however, each one is vital. Nutrients are involved in every body process, whether it be combating infection or repairing tissue or thinking. Nutrients have different functions such as to provide energy or promote tissue repair, but their common goal is to keep us going. To eat is one of the most basic and powerful of human drives. Although eating has been woven into many cultural and religious practices, essentially we eat to survive.

A fundamental problem with most of us is that our bodies simply do not get what we need from our "modern diet." Consistent absence of the proper nutrients eventually causes great harm to the body by impairing its normal functions. Even if you are not sick, you may not necessarily be healthy. It simply may be that you are not yet exhibiting any overt symptoms of illness. Unlike a car engine which immediately malfunctions if you put water into the gasoline tank, the human body has tremendous resilience and often camouflages the repercussions of unhealthy fuel choices. By understanding the principles of holistic nutrition, and knowing what nutrients and foods we need, you can improve the state of your health, stave off disease, and maintain a harmonious balance in the way nature intended.

There is a huge industry in the "developed" countries working to convince us that it doesn't matter what we eat. Fast food chains are trying to convince us that what we eat has no effect on our health. We are told that any combination of heated, treated, processed, chemicalized "foods" will meet our nutritional needs so long as we take plenty of vitamin pills, heartburn medicine, headache and other remedies.

"Call it science. Call it the state of the art of medicine. I now believe," writes Dr. Lendon H. Smith in his excellent book, *Feed Your Body Right,* "what I learned in medical school in the early 1940s was a calculated effort by the pharmaceutical industry to get fledgling medical doctors to use drugs, their drugs. We were taught to make a diagnosis, clear and simple. Once a label was attached to the patient, a drug was attached to the disease label. It was neat and clean. If we could not remember the name of the drug, the pharmaceutical representative (drug rep) who came to our offices one or twice a month reminded us. Ads in the medical journals kept the name alive in our memory storage banks."

Last year over a million people left the same suicide note:

Shopping List
Sausage, Whole Milk, Cake, Hot Dogs, Margarine, Eggs, Mayo, Potato Chips, Sour Cream, Hamburger, Pastries, Ham, Cookies, Bacon, Cheese, Chicken, Ice Cream, Donuts, Luncheon Meats

Heart-Healthy Lifestyles Pay Off

It's tough these days to pick up a newspaper without reading yet another article about some strange factor, like baldness or short stature, that might cause a heart attack—factors that we often can't do anything about. That's why a major study published in the *British Medical Journal* is so redeeming. All those headline-catching items, investigators from Finland have found, aren't worth a moment of worry. In tracking the lives of 14,257 men and 14,786 women for 20 years, the researchers concluded that the reductions in mortality rates from heart disease that Finland has experienced over the past two decades were brought about primarily by changes in three main coronary risk factors: cholesterol levels, blood pressure and smoking.

Finland had a vested interest in finding the keys to coronary prevention. In the early 1970s middle-aged Finnish men had the highest mortality rates from cardiovascular disease in the world. *They also consumed some of the highest amounts per capita of full-fat dairy products.*

Early on, government officials took action, instituting health education programs and tracking the results of various preventive measures. The researchers recruited a random sample of close to 30,000 Finnish men and women ages 30-59, and, in surveys conducted in 1972, 1977, 1982, 1987, and 1992, kept close track of their medical history, current health, socioeconomic factors, and lifestyle habits. Specially trained nurses measured height, weight and blood pressure, and took blood specimens to determine cholesterol concentrations. Nonsmokers were defined as those who had never smoked regularly as well as those who had smoked regularly but had quit at least six months before the start of the survey.

During this same two-decade period, the rate of heart disease in Finland had begun to drop dramatically. It was the perfect opportunity, the investigators knew, to see just how much the country's reductions in risk factors had influenced that decline. They predicted that, among their 30,000 subjects, a nonsmoking lifestyle and decreases in cholesterol and blood pressure levels would be associated with decreases in mortality from heart disease of 44 percent in men and 40 percent in women. It turns out, to their delight, that their estimates were conservative. The observed decline was 55 percent in men and 68 percent in women.

"Most of the decline in mortality from heart disease," the authors concluded, "can be explained by changes in the three main coronary risk factors."

Atherosclerotic vascular disease is a buildup of fat in the blood vessels. The associated heart attacks and strokes caused by this fat buildup prematurely cause half of all deaths each year. Cancer of the breast, colon, prostate, lung and other organs cause another 25 percent of deaths each year. Diabetes, cirrhosis of the liver, and emphysema also kill many people prematurely.

All these conditions have one thing in common: they are caused or greatly influenced by what we put or don't put into our mouths. Of all the things human beings put in their mouths, says Dr. Alan Goldhamer, co-director of the Center for Conservative Therapy in Penngrove, California, tobacco, alcohol, caffeine, recreational and prescription drugs are perhaps the most harmful. Attempts by people to modify their internal chemistry through powerful chemical agents and quick fixes is an ever-widening tragedy. More and more people are suffering and dying from the consequences of using and abusing chemicals. Headaches are not caused by an aspirin deficiency. There are better ways of modifying moods than with pills, potions and elixirs.

The Impact of Animal Protein

"Nothing will benefit human health and increase the chances for survival of life on earth as much as the evolution to a vegetarian diet."

—**Albert Einstein**

Perhaps the second most destructive habit Goldhamer sees is the use of animal products. Meat, fish, fowl, eggs and dairy products all have much in common. In addition to economic, environmental, humanitarian—and, for many, spiritual—reasons, there are well-documented health reasons that support the adoption of a vegetarian diet.

In their search for evidence on how food affects health, researchers have often considered Asian countries because, statistically, their longevity surpasses other more developed countries. While they do not have a perfect diet, they do a much better job of holding cancer, heart disease, and many other serious conditions at bay than do Western countries.

One of the most ambitious nutrition research projects ever undertaken is the China Oxford Cornell Project (called the Grand Prix of epidemiology). Conducted by Dr. Colin Campbell of Cornell University and his colleagues, Drs. Chen Junshi and Li Junyao of Beijing, China, and Dr. Richard Peto of Oxford University, the Project looked in detail at China as a natural laboratory. Diets vary significantly from one part of the country to another, yet people in China tend to stay in the same place all their lives, allowing observable relationships between diet and health to emerge. Beginning in 1983, the team collected information about the typical foods of 65 Chinese provinces. They studied records of health and illness, took blood samples and made other tests. In 1991, they published an 896-page monograph filled with data from this and subsequent and even larger studies which they continue to analyze.

The Project's hypothesis was that a diet substantially enriched with good quality plant foods prevents a variety of chronic degenerative diseases, and that the more the diet contains plant-source foods, the lower the disease risk. "In a sense," explains Dr.

Campbell, "one might say that we are testing whether a diet which contains no animal products and is low in fat, is better than, say, an average vegetarian diet which usually contains dairy and egg products and nutrient compositions which are not too different from non-vegetarian diets. Our study suggests that the closer one approaches a total plant food diet, the greater the health benefit."

Their first finding was that, overall, Chinese diets are extraordinarily healthy by Western standards. Rice and other grains, vegetables, and legumes are consumed in much greater quantity than in the United States. While Americans get around 40 percent of their calories from fat, the Chinese get much less—ranging from six to 24 percent—and their health is much better.

The study placed much emphasis on protein (how much and what kinds) and its influence on heart disease, cancer and other diseases. There is a tremendous difference between the two countries in source of protein. The average protein intake from animal sources in the United States is 70 percent. In China, only seven percent comes from animal sources. But in spite of the generally low levels of protein intake from animal sources in China, those Chinese who add just a little bit of animal protein to their diet register increases in cholesterol levels, heart disease, and cancer. This suggests that it doesn't take much animal protein to start changing cholesterol levels and consequently increase the risk of heart disease and cancer, explains Campbell.

"There is strong evidence in the scientific literature that when a reduction in fat is compared to a reduction in protein intake, the protein effect on blood cholesterol is more significant than the effect of saturated fat," says Campbell. Animal protein is a hypercholesterolemic (increases cholesterol) agent. He adds, "We can reduce cholesterol levels either by reducing animal protein intake or exchanging it for plant protein. Some of the plant proteins, particularly soy [see Chapter 7 on Soybeans], have an impressive ability to reduce cholesterol. I really think that protein—both the kind and the amount—is more significant as far as cholesterol levels are concerned than is saturated fat, and certainly more significant than dietary cholesterol itself."

Animal protein is about as well correlated with overall cancer rates across different countries as is total fat. Of course, animal protein is tightly coupled with the intake of saturated fat, so a lot of these associations between saturated fat and various cancers could just as easily be accounted for by animal protein. "The consumption of animal protein has a profound effect on enzymes that are involved in the metabolism of cholesterol and related chemicals and this occurs very quickly—within hours after the consumption of the meal," explains Campbell.

Protein is so highly regarded by everyone, including investigators themselves, that there is a tremendous bias against considering its implication in disease. "It is easy to see that fat is greasy and nasty," says Campbell, "so most people more readily accept the idea that fat might have something to do with the emergence of disease. They do not want to imagine that animal protein does the same things as excess fat intake. But it turns out that animal protein, when consumed, exhibits a variety of undesirable health effects. Whether it is the immune system, various enzyme systems, the uptake of carcinogens into the cells, or hormonal activities, animal protein generally only causes mischief. High fat intake still can be a problem, and we should not be consuming such high-fat diets. But I suggest that animal protein is more problematic in this whole diet/disease relationship than is total fat."

Many Americans are switching from beef to skinless chicken breasts and other animal-based foods, simply to reduce their intake of fat. However, the evidence suggests that this makes little or no sense. It may reduce fat intake a bit, but even lean cuts of meat or poultry still contain around 20 to 40 percent of total calories as fat, or even more. This is not going to get us very far. We might get our fat intake down a bit, but our protein intake is not going to change; if anything, its already high level may go even higher. As Campbell says, "One really has to change the total diet."

If you want to see big changes in your health, you must make big changes in your life. Token changes don't work. Only dramatic reduction or elimination of all animal products merits your consideration. In the short run, if you are accustomed to a high-salt, high-fat, high animal protein diet, you might not like healthier foods at first. But with a little patience, you will find that after two or three months, perhaps longer, you adapt to new tastes. And then you discover new tastes that you never realized were there before.

Since heart disease is the leading cause of death in this country, it is appropriate to also describe a landmark study in heart disease, the "Lifestyle Heart Trial," conceived by Dr. Dean Ornish of the University of California, San Francisco. This interventional study, conducted on patients with documented coronary artery disease, split participants into two groups, a control group and an intervention group. All of the patients in the study had cardiac tests before beginning the study. These tests were repeated a year later to document the effect of the intervention.

The control group was placed on the American Heart Association recommended diet, which is similar to the diet recommended by the American Diabetic Association for diabetics. This diet includes limited red meat, chicken, fish and substitutes margarine for butter, resulting in a reduction from the American norm of about 40 percent of calories from fat down to 30 percent, and reducing cholesterol to less than 300 mg daily (the norm is higher). These patients also were advised to exercise and to stop smoking. To the surprise of many, the majority of participants in this control group that was following the American Heart Association recommendations showed worsening of their cardiac status on the one-year follow up.

The intervention group did dramatically better. These patients were placed on a low-fat vegetarian diet, with less than 10 percent of calories from fat. To achieve this, they ate—without restriction in quantity—plant foods, such as fresh fruits, vegetables, legumes and grains, with a limited amount of egg whites and non-fat milk or yogurt. They also engaged in light exercise and stress management. After one year, researchers found reversal in atherosclerotic plaque in 82 percent of this intervention group, all of whom were coronary disease patients.

The Lifestyle Heart Trial is just one of several impressive studies that show that standard dietary recommendations, utilizing 30 percent of calories from fat, allow the progression of heart disease and that heart disease is reversible with vegetarian diets. Studies such as this one were initiated after numerous population-based studies showed that cardiovascular deaths were virtually non-existent in rural populations consuming vegetarian diets, and that deaths from heart disease increased gradually as populations gradually increased their consumption of animal-based foods.

If the problems associated with animal proteins aren't enough to convince you to eliminate animal products, read on. In addition to parasites, bacterial infestation, toxic poisons, carcinogenic agents, and free radicals, animal products all suffer from the problem of biological concentration. Animals consume large quantities of grain, grass, and other foods that are, to a greater or lesser extent, contaminated with herbicides, pesticides, and other agents. In addition, animals often are fed antibiotics and treated with other drugs and toxic agents. These poisons concentrate in the fat of the animal and are present in the animal's milk and flesh. This biological concentration of poisons poses significant threats to the health of humans who consume animal products.

In spite of the millions of dollars the meat and dairy industry spend on advertising to try to make you believe otherwise, it is excess protein, not inadequate protein, that is the threat to health. Animal products are extremely high in protein. Excess protein, especially the high sulfur-containing amino acids found in animal products, has been strongly implicated as a causal agent in many disease processes, including kidney disease, various forms of cancer, a host of autoimmune and hypersensitivity disease processes and osteoporosis.

Osteoporosis is a condition common to postmenopausal women. Bones become weak and fracture easily. Campbell found in his study that osteoporosis is not caused by a calcium deficiency, and calcium supplementation does not prevent it. In osteoporosis there is a loss of the bone matrix that holds calcium. A diet high in animal protein can help cause osteoporosis by creating toxic nitrogenous wastes that must be neutralized by calcium drawn from the body's reserves, creating a negative calcium balance where more calcium is lost in the urine than is taken in. Thus, no matter how much calcium is taken, if the individual is on a high animal protein diet, the calcium balance remains negative. To prevent osteoporosis, a low animal protein diet and regular weight-bearing exercises are essential. It's a misconception that you have to eat dairy products to prevent osteoporosis. Dairy products are implicated in many diseases, including autoimmune disorders, heart disease, arthritis, and cancer.

The Non-Dairy Alternatives

I choose not to eat dairy. When I announce this at my workshops, hands inevitably go up to ask, "What do I use in place of milk?" I either use a soy beverage called Westsoy, made by Westbrae (see Resources) or I make fresh nut milk.

Nut milks are also an excellent replacement for dairy products. You can use a variety of nuts and seeds to make milks, ice cream, dips, and dressings. Here's a simple recipe:

- *Almond Milk*

    3 1/4 cups warm water
    1/3 cup organic raw almonds
    1 Tbs. Omega-Life fortified flax seed meal (see Resources)
    1 tsp. lecithin granules
    2 Tbs. sweetener (optional - I use pure maple syrup)

    In a two-quart saucepan, heat approximately 3 1/4 cups of pure water to almost boiling. Turn stove off and allow to sit. Place the nuts in a grinder (or blender). Grind to a fine powder. Transfer the mixture to a blender. To your blender add flax seed, lecithin granules, and sweetener. Then add 3/4 cup of the warm water and blend on medium speed to a smooth, pudding-like puree. Add the remaining water and blend on high speed until creamy. Use only three cups water per recipe for extra creamy nutmilks.

    Pour the contents of the blender through a fine mesh strainer into a bowl or pitcher. Serve immediately or refrigerate for up to seventy-two hours. It's delicious when you blend in fresh fruit or a frozen banana.

This is a basic recipe that's simple to use. The nut milk I usually make has a few more things in it that I'll mention. To the above mixture, I also blend in 1 Tbs. Spectrum Naturals Organic Flax Seed Oil, 1 tsp. Spectrum Naturals Wheat Germ Oil, 1 tsp. Y.S. Bee Farms Super All Bee Power, and 2 Tbs. Mori-Nu Lite Tofu. After it's all blended, I don't even bother to strain it. However, before using it, you need to make sure it's stirred well. Here's an excellent book I recommend, containing more than 40 delicious nut and seed milks recipes: *Not Milk . . .Nut Milks!* by Candia Lea Cole.

It's ironic that the chief argument used to promote the use of animal products—the purported need for large quantities of protein—is one of the greatest reasons for avoiding them. If animal products are included in the diet in significant quantities, it is virtually impossible to design a healthful diet that is consistent with the overwhelming evidence in the scientific literature on nutrition.

Changing to a Healthy Diet

I'm often asked, "If I have to avoid drugs, including alcohol, coffee, cola and chocolate; and avoid animal products including meat, fish, fowl, eggs and dairy products; and refined carbohydrates—what's left?" The answer is: a diet derived from whole natural foods—fresh fruits, vegetables, whole grains, legumes and the variable addition of nuts and seeds.

Sometimes, however, when changing from an animal-based diet to a plant-based diet, you'll experience headaches, indigestion and other uncomfortable symptoms. Have no fear—what you are experiencing is actually encouraging! People who initially experience severe symptoms when changing over to a healthy diet usually find that these symptoms resolve within the first two weeks. From that point on, they generally feel better and are more energetic than they have felt in years. The fact that changing your diet exacerbated your headaches illustrates how necessary it was for you to improve your diet.

Keep these points in mind:

1. When you remove something harmful from your system, withdrawal symptoms can occur, especially headaches. People who discontinue the use of heroin, alcohol, cigarettes, caffeine, etc., also temporarily experience unpleasant symptoms, especially head-

aches. Having these diet-related headaches appear, then resolve, is a very common experience for people who are recovering from chronic periodic headaches. The "exacerbated" headache brought on temporarily by dietary change is a withdrawal symptom, and is a necessary step toward recovery.

2. The average American consumes a low-fiber diet, and the digestive tract of the typical person is unaccustomed to the higher fiber and water content of stools as a result of an improved diet. These stools contain more weight, allowing them to pass through the digestive tract at a faster rate. The peristaltic waves that propel the food have to adjust for the new type of stool. It can take two weeks or longer for this adjustment to take place. During the transition time, you might experience diarrhea, bloating, gas or other digestive discomforts.

3. When you switch to a lowered protein, low-fat diet, the body starts to eliminate retained proteinaceous wastes. Fat cells also are broken down, and the toxins stored in the fat cells are released into the bloodstream. In this manner, the body is able to "clean house" more effectively. It's not uncommon to feel enervated and lethargic. The above symptoms are the temporary result of this "detoxification." Do not let any temporary discomfort lead you to abandon your new eating habits. You cannot accomplish healing overnight. It will be helpful to eat slowly and chew the vegetables very well, or temporarily eat a few leaves of lettuce with each meal rather than one big raw salad at dinner. If you are experiencing indigestion and cramping, do not eat asparagus or the cruciferous vegetables (cabbage, cauliflower, broccoli or Brussels sprouts) for the first two weeks as they may produce bloating and gas. Fruit juices and other sweet drinks also can increase gas, so these also should be avoided temporarily if you are experiencing this problem.

4. Be informed. Educate yourself as much as you can on nutrition and an optimum diet. There are numerous excellent books available.

Feed Your Body Right by Dr. Lendon H. Smith will help you understand your individual body chemistry for proper nutrition without guesswork.

Food for Life: How the New Four Food Groups Can Save Your Life by Dr. Neal Barnard will show you how to harness your inner power with a three-week program (including recipes) designed for weight control, cholesterol-reduction, cancer prevention, and all-round vitality.

I also highly recommend *The Love-Powered Diet* and *Get the Fat Out* by Victoria Moran. *The Love-Powered-Diet* shows you how to tap the transformative power of love that can revolutionize your relationship with food forever. She reveals how you can get back the gift of choice about what to eat, and learn to make choices that express love to your body, to all livingkind, and to the earth itself. Her book, *Get the Fat Out,* offers 501 simple ways to cut the fat in any diet.

Diet for a New America by John Robbins is another one of my favorites. It reveals how your food choices affect your health, happiness and the future of life on earth.

Some of my other favorites include:

- *Conscious Eating* by Dr. Gabriel Cousens,
- *The McDougall Program* by Dr. John McDougall,
- *Think Before You Eat* by Diane Olive,
- *Dr. Dean Ornish's Program for Reversing Heart Disease* and *Eat More, Weigh Less* by Dr. Dean Ornish,
- *Staying Healthy With Nutrition* and *A Diet for All Seasons* by Dr. Elson Haas,
- *The Essene Way—Biogenic Living* by Edmond Bordeaux Szekely,
- *Alternative Medicine* by Burton Goldberg Group,
- *Dietary Wellness* by Phyllis A. Balch, C.N.C. and James F. Balch, M.D.,
- *The American Vegetarian Cookbook* by Marilyn Diamond,
- *The Quintessence of Natural Living* by Keki R. Sidhwa, D.O.,
- *Natural Hygiene: The Pristine Way of Life* by Herbert Shelton.

Some excellent books on raising healthy children include *Hyper Kids Workbook* by Dr. Lendon H. Smith, *Good Food Today Great Kids Tomorrow* by Dr. Jay Gordon, *Great Food for Great Kids Recipes* by Meyera Robbins, *Pregnancy, Children, and the Vegan Diet* by Dr. Michael Klaper, and *Raising Your Family Naturally* by Joy Gross.

The long-term rewards of improvement to your diet—increased vitality, improved sleep, more energy, regular and soft bowel movements, lower cholesterol and a healthy heart, lower cancer risk, and stronger bones—are well worth any temporary discomfort. A longer and healthier life, free from compulsive, addictive behavior and the occurrence of degenerative diseases can only be realized by avoiding the dietary causes of illness and adopting a plant-based diet.

Why do we find it so difficult to eat what we should eat and avoid what we shouldn't? To eat well, we have to understand the factors that drive us to eat wrongly. Very often we eat for the wrong reason. One reason is genetics—we are programmed to eat concentrated foods when they are available. That is an important survival trait. In a natural setting, there are no ice cream cone trees, hot dog vines or candy bushes. But today, surrounded by unlimited access to concentrated foods, we must overcome instincts with intellect.

We might eat because we are emotionally distraught. Instead, take a walk, listen to relaxing music or do some deep breathing. We might feel fatigued and eat for stimulation. But when we are tired, we should sleep. Fear of being different is another factor that drives us to make poor food choices. "Friends" can create a lot of pressure with comments like, "You're no fun anymore," "You're so thin," "Don't you think you're carrying this a little too far," "I made it just for you," or "A little won't hurt." Thank them for their concern and stay committed to your health program. Often a short explanation is all that is necessary. You don't need to justify yourself or your health habits.

Your body is a wonderful feedback machine. It is continually giving you messages about what's working and what's not. Pay attention to the signs and symptoms, the emotions and stressors. I really like what Dr. Lendon H. Smith has to say about this in his book *Feed Your Body Right*. "The more we investigate the origin of symptoms, signs, and diseases, the more we find that nutrition—and specifically, the chemical imbalances in the blood and tissues—is at the bottom of what ails us. The triggering event that precipitates an actual disease may be an emotional upset or a physical injury. Something has stressed our body chemistry beyond its ability to compensate; our ability to buffer the changes accompanying stressors has been comprised by our lifestyle, which includes our diet. We are all at risk—some more, some less."

The Upcoming Dietary Revolution

Health is the result of healthful living. This is the philosophy known as Natural Hygiene (see American Natural Hygiene Society in the Resources). Natural Hygiene is about health promotion and I've practiced this way of living for over 20 years, although I do take a few nutritional supplements as described in this book which strict hygienists do not advocate. Hygienists believe that the body heals itself if you give it a chance. The method is to remove the factors that interfere with healing and provide the requirements for health. That is what you do whether you are trying to get healthy or stay healthy. The emphasis may be slightly different for different conditions, and it might need to be fine-tuned for different individuals.

One of the phenomenal things about the hygienic approach is that it teaches people about the power of their own vitality. Acute symptoms are the direct expression of this vitality, and the most expedient means to recovery. Hygienists fully realize the integration of the body, and how to really allow the body to function at its highest potential.

Science keeps supporting hygiene. A growing body of scientific studies on the disease-preventing and healing properties of food confirms the value of a vegetarian diet and even validates the nutritional teachings of the spiritual leader Paramhansa Yogananda, as well.

In 1929 Yogananda gave a talk in Washington D.C. about renewing and transforming your body, mind and spirit. He said: "We must also understand about food values. Meat is detrimental to your system; but so is an improperly cooked vegetable dinner of killed vitamins. Resurrect your mind from the bad habits of wrong eating. Start with carrots. Don't forget them. They are hard and nice—you have not to chew bones to get strength. When you chew carrots they give power to the teeth. Carrots contain valuable vitamins. Wash them, but do not do anything else to them. I ordered some raw carrots at a place I was visiting, and when they were brought in they didn't have any heads or feet. The tops and bottoms are rich in vitamins."

He went on to say, "A lemon a day; an apple a day; an orange a day; half a glass of orange juice with two tablespoonsful of ground nuts (preferably almonds); and eight leaves of raw spinach. . . . Grapefruit, too, is very good. Then a little piece of banana—about one-fourth. Then unsulphured figs and raisins. . . . Eat these things every day. I do not mean that you shall live only on this regimen; you may eat more or less. But if you remember these basic rules— an abundance of fresh fruits and vegetables, not denatured by improper cooking or storage, and nuts, and some whole grains— you will not be making any transgression on nature. . . . Nature will not listen to your excuses of your years of transgression against her health rules. If you eat sensibly, then if you are in the habit of breaking some laws occasionally, it will not so much hurt you." He added, "Since you have to eat, why not eat rightly?" Good question!

Scientists are actually proving that some of the old folklore medicine is absolutely true, according to a program called "Every-day Healing Food," broadcast on the American Public Radio (APR). "Medical science is now discovering an entire hidden world of disease-fighting substances that nature quietly deposited in every-day produce," APR said. "Foods like garlic, onion, carrots, broccoli, beans, and citrus fruits contain an amazing network of natural ingredients that may help you prevent heart attack, cancer, and other serious illnesses."

Because a broad consensus of medical authorities recognizes the disease-preventing properties in fruits and vegetables, this knowledge is revolutionizing the way we think about food and health.

In 1992 the National Cancer Institute (NCI) published a review of 156 specific studies on how foods safeguard us from disease. They were done in a variety of countries, used a variety of methods, and looked at a variety of fruits and vegetables. Of these studies, 82 percent showed that fruits and vegetables have a "protective effect" against cancer. "Overall, the evidence of an association between fruit and vegetable consumption and cancer prevention is exceptionally strong and consistent," the NCI report said.

To gain this protection, "you should eat at least five servings of different fruits and vegetables every day," said Dr. Jerianne Heimendinger at the NCI. "A medium apple would be one serving, whereas a large apple or a large salad would be two servings," she explained.

Dr. Paul Talalay of Johns Hopkins University School of Medicine said on the APR broadcast that scientists have become interested in the potential of food to fight cancer and other illnesses at a time when the success of medical efforts at treatment generally has not been encouraging. Despite extraordinary advances in our understanding of the cancer process and breakthroughs in the treatment of some specific forms of the disease, Dr. Talalay said that the overall incidence of cancer and the mortality rate of victims have not changed significantly in the last twenty years.

Dr. Talalay heads a team that studied a compound called sulforaphane in the much-maligned broccoli. This compound significantly reduces the development of mammary cancer in lab animals. Sulforaphane activates a process that, in effect, kicks carcinogens out of cells. The results, which Dr. Talalay described as "dramatic," were reported in the Proceedings of the National Academy of Sciences.

The food substances that have scientists excited are called phytochemicals ("phyto" comes from the Greek word for plant). Plants produce these chemicals to protect themselves against such hostile elements as fungi, insects, and too much sunshine. By a benevolent act of nature, however, phytochemicals also seem to protect us. "We just borrow the compound that they use for their diseases and use it to treat our own diseases," said a U.S. Department of Agriculture researcher, Dr. James Duke, on APR.

"At almost every one of the steps along the pathway leading to cancer there are one or more compounds in vegetables or fruit that will slow up or reverse the process," said Dr. John Potter of the University of Minnesota.

Here's some good news for tomato lovers. Dr. Joseph Hotchkiss and other scientists at Cornell University reported last year that two of the tomato's estimated 10,000 phytochemicals stop the formation of cancer-causing substances. You don't like tomatoes? Well, these same phytochemicals also exist in green pepper, pineapples, strawberries, and carrots, which should give almost everyone something to chew on.

There's more help from our food friends. Besides the sulforaphane in turnips, they also have a phytochemical that inhibits or "disarms" cancer, as does cabbage. Another phytochemical called ellagic acid, found in strawberries, grapes, and raspberries, performs a similar service. When harmful substances enter the body through food, drink, smoke, or air, certain cell enzymes feed on them. These enzymes are messy eaters, however, and leave small fragments. The fragments can cause mutations in critical genes, and sometimes initiate an explosive growth of cancer cells. Before this occurs, ellagic acid feeds itself to these enzymes and neutralizes them, a self-sacrifice that works to our benefit.

Dr. Duke confided on the APR broadcast that he smoked three packs of cigarettes a day for thirty years. Although he has stopped smoking, Dr. Dukes' long indulgence left him more at risk to develop cancer. As a result of his food research, he now eats two carrots daily. These contain enough beta-carotene to halve his chances of getting lung cancer, he asserted.

All this adds up to very hopeful news for those concerned about life-threatening chronic diseases. As Jean Carper, author of *Food, Your Miracle Medicine,* put it:

"We see that our modern drugs are not going to solve those chronic diseases, because they have to be prevented rather than cured. Food seems to me one of the absolute best preventive medicines we could have."

Enzymes & Fiber for Health

The old saying "You are what you eat" is only half true. We are actually no more than we can digest. The key is effective assimilation of what we eat, through good digestion. Optimal digestion depends on more than just eating the right foods. The key to good digestion is the class of complex chemical substances known as enzymes.

Three types of enzymes have been identified: digestive enzymes (which digest our food), food enzymes (available only in fresh, live food) and metabolic enzymes (which science has discovered no means of replenishing). When we eat cooked food over a period of many years, we eventually deplete our digestive enzymes and have to rob our pool of metabolic enzymes to assist the digestion process. As the metabolic enzymes are depleted, deterioration of the body sets in. The aging process begins.

Food enzymes are necessary in order to break large food components into smaller ones which the body can absorb. Each enzyme has a specific job and can only break down certain components. The three main components that we consume are fats, proteins and carbohydrates.

Most nutritionally aware people take care to get a daily ration of fruits and vegetables, grains and legumes. But unless they are eaten raw, the fresh-food nutrients may not be effectively absorbed by the body. Once a piece of food is steamed, baked, fried, boiled, broiled, barbecued, toasted, roasted, sautéed, poached, grilled or microwaved, it is in many ways as good as dead. The fresh, raw food's "life force," its vital energy, is lost. If you take a handful of raw sunflower seeds, bury them in the earth, and water them, chances are good they will sprout. If boiled first, they will rot in the ground. The difference between raw and cooked is the difference between life and death.

The reason a cooked seed won't sprout is because the enzymes have been destroyed by the heat of cooking. "Enzymes are substances that make life possible," explains one of the world's leading experts in enzyme research, Dr. Edward Howell in *Enzyme Nutrition, The Food Enzyme Concept.* "They are needed for every chemical reaction that takes place in the human body. No mineral, vitamin, or hormone can do any work without enzymes.

"Our bodies, all of our organs, tissues, and cells, are run by metabolic enzymes. They are the manual workers that build the body from proteins, carbohydrates, and fats, just as construction workers build our homes. You have all the raw materials with which to build, but without the workers (enzymes) you cannot even begin," he says.

Among many important enzymes so far identified, three start out as major league players in the assimilation of food. The body needs protease for the digestion of proteins, amylase for breaking down carbohydrates and starch, and lipase for digesting fats. These and other enzymes can be gotten from raw foods, in which naturally present enzymes tend to correlate with the nutritional factors of the food itself. Raw fatty foods such as oils and nuts, for example, contain lipase. But if these same fatty foods are cooked, the lipase and other enzymes are destroyed, placing extra demands on the body (especially the pancreas) to produce more enzymes in order to facilitate digestion.

The human body will produce its own enzymes, but only in a limited quantity over the course of a lifetime. When the enzyme potential is depleted beyond a certain point, according to research documented in Howell's book, a given life is effectively over. Researchers in Chicago have found that enzyme levels in the saliva of young adults are 30 times higher than in persons over 69 years of age. Research in Germany has found that the urine of young people contains nearly twice the amount of the starch-digesting enzyme amylase than the urine of old people. An individual's enzyme potential, maintains Howell, not only determines the length of that person's life but is directly related to good health and resistance to disease.

A diet of mostly cooked foods is a disservice to the body. The pancreas must borrow enzymes from other parts of the body to properly digest cooked food. Inadequately digested food can putrefy in the intestines, creating gas and toxins and further impeding nutrient assimilation.

Enter Acidophilase (made by Wakunaga of America and available in health food stores), an enzyme supplement I take on a regular basis. Acidophilase contains the above three key food enzymes in combination with the friendly intestinal bacteria, B. bifidum, and L. acidophilus. Taking this enzyme supplement, especially with cooked meals, can effectively satisfy the body's requirement for the digestive enzymes needed for maximum metabolic function. The precise mix of enzymes can ease demands on the digestive system while releasing the maximum nutritional value of food.

It's also important to get enough fiber in the diet. While not a source of fuel, fiber is an essential component of an effective health program, especially if you want to lose weight. You should try to get about 30 to 50 grams of fiber per day. That's not really difficult if your diet contains plenty of fruit, vegetables, grain and legume products.

The typical American diet derives 40 to 60 percent of its calories from fats, 30 percent from carbohydrates (mainly refined sugars), and 20 percent from protein. Its fiber content is a mere ten grams. Obviously, this is a diet tailor-made to produce obesity and ill health since a health-promoting diet is exactly the reverse.

Dietary fiber helps digestion and elimination. It adds bulk to your diet and provides a feeling of fullness that may help you be more moderate in your food intake. Fiber also increases the amount of necessary chewing, thus slowing the eating process. When you eat too quickly, without chewing well, it places extra stress on the digestive system. Fiber stimulates the release of intestinal hormones that, along with its bulk, satisfies your appetite by giving a feeling of fullness. Fiber is also helpful in disease prevention. Diets rich in fiber appear to decrease risks of constipation, coronary heart disease, hemorrhoids, diverticulitis, and colon cancer. (See Chapter 3 for more on fiber.)

Dietary fiber consists of both insoluble types, which are not digested in the gut, and soluble types which are. Soluble forms of fiber include pectins, gums, and certain hemicelluloses, and are found especially in oats, barley, dried beans, and other legume foods. Soluble fibers help lower blood cholesterol by trapping it in the gut and preventing its absorption. These fibers are often useful in the treatment of heart disease and diabetes.

Insoluble forms of fiber include complex carbohydrates such as cellulose, lignins and some hemicelluloses, and are found in wheat bran, whole grain breads and cereals, and the skins of fruits and vegetables. Insoluble fibers are useful in promoting elimination.

Rates of colon cancer risk are quite low in populations that subsist on diets high in insoluble dietary fiber, perhaps because of the ways in which it speeds the passage of carcinogens through the intestine and/or changes the metabolism of bacteria residing in the gut.

The Standard American Diet (SAD) consists of a high intake of refined carbohydrates such as pastries, cakes, cookies, candy, fries, and so on; foods which are often stripped of vitamins and minerals, but are full of simple sugars, salt, fats and chemicals; animal products which are excessively high in protein and loaded with cholesterol, saturated fats and hormones; and an extremely low intake of fiber, complex carbohydrates, fresh fruits and vegetables.

Not surprisingly, a natural weight loss diet turns out to be the same as the one which promotes health. Whether your goal is long life, lots of energy and/or a lean youthful body, your diet should be high in dietary fiber (30 to 50 grams) and complex carbohydrate foods (60 to 70 percent), sufficient in protein (10 to 15 percent), and low in fat (10-20 percent). Whole grains and legumes, along with lots of fresh fruits and vegetables, will provide you with generous amount of vitamins, minerals, soluble and insoluble fibers, fuel for sustained energy, and more than adequate amounts of protein and essential fats.

Antioxidant Aids

We have been hearing a lot in the early 90's about the importance of eating foods rich in antioxidants to reduce the risk of certain diseases. Beta-carotene, vitamin C, vitamin E and selenium belong to a group of vitamins called dietary antioxidants. The scientific evidence is undeniable. One of their roles includes the prevention of a certain undesirable chemical event in the body called a "free radical reaction," which may be associated with several disease processes. (See Chapter 5 on Flax Seed for more information.) Some studies have shown that daily consumption of vegetables and fruits rich in antioxidants (or high blood levels of these vitamins) is associated with a decreased risk of some forms of cancer and heart disease. Antioxidants have been shown to be effective in fighting disease, slowing the aging process and supporting the body's natural defenses which are often weakened by environmental pollution, poor diet and stress. However, it's difficult to pinpoint exactly which component(s) of these foods account the most for their beneficial effects. For example, fruits and vegetables high in beta-carotene and vitamins C and E also tend to be high in fiber and some minerals, and low in fat. These qualities may also affect risk in the same or different ways.

You may want to consider supplementing your diet with a good antioxidant combination. I take Anti-Oxidant Plus (see Red Rose Collection in the Resource Directory). It combines a natural source of beta-carotene processed from the carotene rich sea algae, *Dunaliella salina,* with other key anti-oxidant vitamins and minerals. This synergistic formula of nutrients is set in a whole food and herbal base of wheat sprouts, milk thistle, Siberian ginseng, gingko biloba, and schizandra and is enhanced with the inclusion of the latest generation of anti-oxidants known to science including L-glutathione, co-enzyme Q10, and green tea extract.

I also take a multivitamin mineral supplement called Foundation. This food-based, whole food supplement delivers nutrients in forms as close as possible to the good foods you eat throughout the day. Whole food supplements are superior because they're easier on the stomach and studies indicate that, like food, their nutrients may be better absorbed, retained, and utilized by the body than standard USP vitamins. For more information, please refer to Red Rose Collection in the Resource Directory.

C Power

If you were stranded on a desert island with only one vitamin to choose, which one would you pick? Without question, it should be vitamin C. There is no vitamin more fundamental for health and disease prevention. In fact, many researchers believe that vitamin C's role in the body goes far beyond that of a nutrient. The evidence comes from studies of animals and the health benefits people derive from taking high doses of vitamin C. For example, most animals produce their own vitamin C—literally hundreds of times the amount people routinely obtain from food. In addition, scientific studies on people show that a high intake of vitamin C extends life span, fights infections, lowers blood pressure and cholesterol, as well as reducing the likelihood of dying from heart disease and cancer. According to Linus Pauling, "Vitamin C is different because, at one time, all animals made their own vitamin C in their livers. All of this extra vitamin C must be important—otherwise, the majority of animals wouldn't be producing so much of it."

So, why don't people make their own vitamin C? One theory holds that a genetic accident millions of years ago left the ancestors of human beings and a handful of animals—including the guinea pig—unable to produce this vitamin in their bodies. If true, it means people have hobbled from one generation to the next totally dependent on meager dietary sources of vitamin C.

In animals—and in people—vitamin C maintains homeostasis, the term biologists use to describe staying on an "even keel" when faced with stress, infections, heart disease, cancer and other conditions. Vitamin C is essential for a smooth-running immune system, and is also an antioxidant.

New methods of preparing this vitamin have added to its effectiveness and "tamed" it for those who have been put off by its acidity. This new family of mineral ascorbates is called Ester-C, a trademark for a product made by the Inter-Cal Corporation of Prescott, Arizona (see Resources). Ester-C can be found in hundreds of products sold by dozens of distributors. It is non-acidic, so the harshness that might upset your stomach is gone. The unique manufacturing process creates a patented vitamin C complex consisting of ascorbate and C metabolites. These metabolites, naturally present in Ester-C, are the same ones that your body makes at much smaller concentrations. They enhance cellular absorption and utilization of the ascorbate in Ester-C supplements. Inter-Cal is actively investigating new therapeutic uses for this new form of vitamin C, and they are getting exciting results.

Dr. Anthony Verlangieri of the Department of Pharmacology at the University of Mississippi, and Dr. Seth Rose of the Department of Chemistry at Arizona State University, have been the trailblazers in identifying the C metabolites and investigating their role as cellular "door-openers" that allow ascorbate to build intracellular levels not possible with ordinary supplements.

By now, it's well accepted that stressful situations and illness can tax our immune systems to the limit. One of the reasons for this is the rapid depletion of ascorbate from our cells in response to stress and infection. So it makes sense to combat this threat by taking ascorbate supplements like Ester-C that have a good chance of getting into the critical cells, such as the white blood cells that are the first-line defense against bacterial and viral attack.

Research conducted by the Life Management Group of San Diego has provided new evidence that Ester-C is a more effective way of building intracellular levels of ascorbate. Their study used male subjects receiving a one-gram dose of vitamin C in the form of Ester-C calcium ascorbate or ordinary ascorbic acid. They found that, after 24 hours, Ester-C had delivered and maintained significantly higher amounts of ascorbate to the white blood cells. These are the cells that really count, and they need ascorbate to maintain their essential functions in stress and infection.

Scientists often use animal models to answer questions about vitamin C when it's not possible to conduct clinical trials. For example, Dr. Verlangieri showed that Ester-C ascorbate was better than ordinary ascorbic acid at preventing scurvy in a type of laboratory rat that has a requirement for this vitamin. We have known for a long time that humans cannot manufacture their own ascorbate and require it in their diets. Many investigators are now discovering that even some animals may benefit from additional ascorbate, even though they can survive without it in their diets and don't get scurvy the way people do. Studies with dogs and horses with various musculoskeletal disorders—from lameness to hip dysplasia to joint inflammation—are showing that large doses of Ester-C ascorbate can relieve pain and restore mobility in these animals after several weeks.

Dr. L. Phillips Brown, a Massachusetts veterinarian, has compared Ester-C calcium ascorbate to ordinary ascorbic acid in a large population of old, lame dogs in the Best Friends Animal Sanctuary in Kanaab, Utah. He fed different doses of ascorbate supplements to the dogs several times a day and then scored the degree of improvement in pain relief, lameness, and mobility. The results were remarkable. Not only did nearly 80 percent of the dogs improve clinically, but Ester-C ascorbate was significantly more effective than ordinary ascorbic acid. Similar results had been obtained several years earlier by Dr. Geir Berge in Norway. Dr. N. Lee Newman, a Virginia large-animal veterinarian, is beginning to show very similar results with Ester-C supplementation for horses with degenerative joint diseases such as ringbone and hock spavin.

It's tempting to dismiss these results by saying that animals don't require vitamin C because they make ascorbate in their own tissues. But do they make enough? Can their internal supply keep up with the increased demands of aging and with a degenerating circulatory system? At the very least, these intriguing results suggest—for both humans and animals—that the vitamin C requirement may increase with age. It is beginning to look as though certain joints and connective tissue may not get enough vitamin C unless it is supplied as Ester-C ascorbate.

Ester-C can also give you a reason to smile! Researchers have learned that Ester-C ascorbate in the zinc form is just as effective an antiplaque agent as some of the ingredients in your favorite mouthwash. Dr. Steven Silverstein of the School of Dentistry at the University of California in San Francisco has shown that Ester-C zinc ascorbate is very effective at inhibiting the growth of the types of bacteria known to produce dental decay and plaque formation on tooth enamel. In another study, Dr. Silverstein used a high-resolution microscope to produce shockingly explicit photographs of the process of tooth erosion by acid . . . ascorbic acid! Can you imagine the countless numbers of children who have been biting into chewable Vitamin C tablets—and losing their tooth enamel in the process? The good news is that Ester-C ascorbate, which is neither acid or alkaline, doesn't affect enamel in the least. With results like these, you can bet you'll be seeing more Ester-C in oral health products in the near future.

Ester-C mineral ascorbates put the technology of C metabolites at your service to achieve and maintain higher intracellular levels of ascorbate than ordinary vitamin C supplements. Ester-C products are backed up by strong research support and pioneering scientific discovery. If you believe, as I do, that extra vitamin C can enhance your health and well-being, Ester-C mineral ascorbates are the way to get it. I take Ester-C in a formula that includes an aged garlic extract called Kyolic Formula 103.

Great Garlic

Garlic can do more than make food taste good—it can save your life, say the experts. "Garlic is nature's most valuable disease-fighting food!" writes Dr. James Balch, co-author of *Prescription for Cooking & Dietary Wellness*.

Numerous studies showing that garlic—and especially an aged garlic extract called Kyolic—helps prevent several types of cancer, reduces the risk of heart disease, lowers cholesterol, helps prevent Alzheimer's disease, improves memory, boosts the immune system and much more.

These studies, explains Dr. Herbert Pierson, a top nutrition expert, formerly with the National Cancer Institute, "clearly showed garlic's effectiveness in lowering the incidence of cardio-vascular disease and drastically reducing stomach and colon cancer. I was amazed at the number of studies showing how garlic actually can reverse the effects of aging, including memory loss."

Most researchers used an aged garlic extract called Kyolic in their studies because of its potency and purity. Since the development of Kyolic almost four decades ago, aged garlic extract has attracted the attention of some the world's most promising researchers. A wide range of research and clinical studies confirming the superiority of Kyolic have been conducted by various research institutes worldwide. Over 100 studies on aged garlic extract have been presented at various symposiums, including the First World Congress on Garlic in 1990, and published in various scientific journals. Kyolic is also covered by more than a dozen patents and patents pending worldwide.

Here are some exciting findings.

- **Cancer**: In studies "garlic significantly lowered the risk of getting breast and prostate cancer and slowed its progress in subjects who already had the disease," according to Dr. John

Pinto, director of the Nutrition Research Laboratory at Memorial Sloan-Kettering Cancer Center. A Michigan State University study confirmed that garlic can lower the risk of breast cancer. Garlic also helps prevent stomach cancer, several Chinese studies found. And Dr. Vivenne Reeve, a researcher at the University of Sydney in Australia, revealed that she was able to greatly reduce skin cancer in mice by applying aged garlic extract on affected rodents.

- **Heart and Circulatory Disease**: Garlic reduces the risk of heart disease and stroke, according to research by Dr. Robert I-San Lin, who has worked with the U.S. government to help establish nutrition standards. "My research shows that garlic unclogs blocked arteries and prevents cholesterol and other deposits from sticking to the arteries, reducing plaque formation," he said. "Since plaque is the major cause of heart attacks, I think garlic should be mandatory medicine for anyone at risk for heart disease."
- **Alzheimer's Disease and Aging**: "Garlic enhances blood circulation to the brain, which helps prevent senility, Alzheimer's and even Parkinson's disease," said Dr. Lin. A Japanese study showed that garlic can combat age-related memory loss and brain cell deterioration. And a French study found that garlic improves memory and relieves symptoms of depression and fatigue.
- **Immune System**: Garlic contains compounds that boost the activity of white blood cells—the cells that help ward off disease—reveals research by Dr. John Milner, head of the department of nutrition at Pennsylvania State University.

Also, several researchers have even reported that garlic shows promise in killing the AIDS virus.

I have been taking Kyolic aged garlic extract for the past 15 years and know it's one the reasons I'm radiantly healthy and rarely sick. While I use some garlic in my cooking, too much raw garlic is irritating to the digestively system, not to mention its effect on the breath. That's why I take Kyolic. It's the most scientifically researched garlic supplement, rather than a commercial food additive or flavoring. Kyolic is organically grown and aged naturally. During aging, the concentrated active compounds are mellowed and the harsh, irritating, odorous compounds found in raw garlic are converted to dozens of valuable, stable, safe, and odorless compounds, including S-allyl cysteine, that make Kyolic so beneficial. It is the only truly odorless garlic product available.

Kyolic comes in a variety of excellent formulas. (See Resources.) One of my favorites is Kyolic Formula 103 which is a combination of Kyolic aged garlic extract, Calcium, Ester C, and Astragalus. (The herb astragalus is an excellent energizer. It has been used by athletes for building energy reserves, especially in the arms and legs. It is also useful in cold climates for keeping the body warm. And it's a natural interferon support, immune stimulant and overall tonic.)

Fabulous Flavonoids

You should choose a diet containing at least seven servings of fruits and vegetables each day. Dark green leafy or yellow, orange, and red vegetables (such as spinach, squash, carrots and peppers) and some fruits (such as apricots, cantaloupe, mangos, and papayas) are good sources of beta-carotene. Fresh citrus fruits and some vegetables (such as peppers, tomatoes, collard greens, and broccoli) are rich in vitamin C. Cold-pressed vegetable oils, green leafy vegetables, nuts, and wheat germ contain vitamin E.

What we're seeing here is the importance of eating foods with a variety of colors, which will help prevent diseases like cancer, heart disease and other illnesses. Blackberries, blueberries, strawberries, plums, squash, pumpkin, apples, oranges, grapefruit, tomatoes and other fruits and vegetables colored purple, blue, black, red, orange or yellow are nearly all rich sources of carotenoids and flavonoids.

You may have heard of citrus flavonoids including rutin and hesperidin. Biochemical dictionaries say there are 3,000 or more naturally occurring flavonoids, of which only several hundred are colored. However, even colorless flavonoids often contribute to plant coloration by interaction with other flavonoids. As some of the specific effects of individual bioflavonoids are researched and documented, a few of the better known—including quercetin and pycnogenol—have joined rutin on the health food store shelves.

A 1994 report in the prestigious medical journal *Lancet* states that "flavonoids in regularly consumed foods may reduce the risk of death from coronary heart disease in older men." In this study, 805 men, ages 65 to 84 years, were studied over a five-year period for flavonoid intake and incidence of heart attacks. The highest risk of heart attacks was found in those with the lowest flavonoid intake. Conversely, those men who consumed the most flavonoids had the lowest risk of heart attacks. It was also reported that flavonoids also interfere with cancer growth and development.

Eat at the Bottom of the Food Chain

Fruits and vegetables are clearly main ingredients of health, but try to get them free of pesticides and herbicides. These are among the most toxic chemicals known to science, designed to kill living creatures. "Along with other industrial metals and chemicals," writes James Solman in his marvelous book, *The Healing Heart,* "pesticides run off into our lakes, rivers and oceans, polluting both water supplies and marine animals." All of these toxins become more concentrated as they move up the food chain. "From phytoplankton to zooplankton to small fish to larger fish, the metals and chemicals concentrate as they move up. That's why a large fish like tuna has more mercury, for instance, than a smaller fish like cod; tuna is further up the food chain," says Sloman.

Livestock animals also concentrate toxic chemicals in their fat and livers. This toxic concentration as we move up the food chain is confirmed in tests. In a study from 1964 to 1968, for instance, it was found that, compared to the average pesticide residues found in plant foods, dairy foods had about three times as much; meat, fish and poultry had about six times as much.

If you want to lower your ingestion of harmful toxins, eat lower on the food chain. In other words, the closer we come to being vegans (vegetarians who eat no animal products including dairy or eggs), the fewer harmful metals and chemicals we take in. I have been a vegetarian for over two decades and a vegan for a few years—

although I do include honeybee products in my diet. (See Chapter 6 on Bee Products.) A plant-based diet is also a safe, simple way to re-establish a relationship with nature and practice environmental awareness. Eating these foods is eating at the bottom of the food chain. The lower you eat on the food chain the less energy it requires to produce food and the less damage it does to the environment. And it's more economical, too.

Whenever possible, choose organic food. This is a loose term, but generally means fruits and vegetables grown without pesticides or herbicides.

Look at the Labels

I also recommend you read labels when grocery shopping. In its top ten list of the "Best Science of 1994," *Time* Magazine included what it termed "a radical idea" implemented by the U.S. Food and Drug Administration: food labels that actually are useful to consumers. Indeed they are. On packaged foods—cereals boxes, breads, crackers, potato chips, ice cream, just about everything, in fact—manufacturers must now display data on cholesterol, total fat, sugars, sodium and saturated fat. Gone is a lot of the deception behind health claims. "Fat-free" really does mean "fat-free." Gone also are serving sizes so small they wouldn't satisfy a rabbit. Life in the supermarket aisles has definitely gotten easier.

Ironically, those foods that are best for us—the ones naturally lowest in fat, cholesterol and sodium and highest in fiber and other rich nutrients—are the very foods that don't have any labels on them. They're your fresh fruits and vegetables.

A good rule of thumb when reading labels is that if you find it difficult to pronounce one or more ingredients on a label, it's probably best to pass that food by. The label does provide two key pieces of information to help you judge the nutritional attributes of the product: the ingredients list and the nutrition information panel.

Ingredients are listed in descending order by dry weight, so you can get a good idea of their relative proportion. For example, if salt is listed before the vegetables in a package of dehydrated soup mix, the soup contains a lot of salt and very few vegetables. Similarly, if sugar (sucrose) is listed as the first ingredient, or sugar appears in several other forms (corn syrup, fructose, molasses), then a large portion of the product's calories comes from sugar. There's no shortage of "fat-free" products on the shelves, but it appears, in an effort to retain flavor while removing fat, manufacturers have poured on the salt—sometimes quadruple the sodium of the original higher fat product—and have added sugars. Optimally, the total number of milligrams of sodium should not exceed the total number of calories. Simple sugars pump glucose into your bloodstream at breakneck speed, driving up insulin levels, which then trap fat in your fat cells, forcing the body to burn less fat. That's right, the very product—a "fat-free" food—that's supposed to help you get rid of fat tissue is actually promoting fat storage.

The nutrition information panel provides details about the nutrients in the food. The number of calories, the grams of carbohydrates, protein and fat, and the milligrams of sodium per serving size are at the top of the list. In foods where a large proportion of the calories comes from fat, the grams of unsaturated and saturated fat and the milligrams of cholesterol may also be provided. But it's easy to be misled. For example, there is a lot of confusion about two percent low-fat milk. Although people assume that the "two percent" means the milk is 98 percent fat-free, this is not so. The percentages are based on weight, not total calories. An eight-ounce glass of "low-fat" two percent milk has 120 calories and 4.7 gm of fat with 35 percent of the calories coming from fat. Skim milk, on the other hand, has only 85 calories and 0.4 gm of fat with a mere 4 percent of the calories coming from fat. Although I don't recommend eating dairy products, if you choose to, skip the two percent and use skim milk.

The new food labels don't tell you the percentage of calories from fat, but it's now easier to figure out. Just go to the nutrition panel and find the calories from fat. Divide that number by the total calories—ending up with the percentage of calories from fat. If division trips you up, go by grams, using this easy rule: if a product has 1.5 fat grams or less per 100 calories, its fat content is within healthy guidelines; the fat, per serving, is 15 percent or less of total calories.

There's a catch. Though the nutrition panel lists the amount of cholesterol and saturated fat for each serving, it does not tally up under either of those categories the amount of trans-fatty acids in the food—those fatty acids which do not contain saturated fats, per se, but can act like saturated fats in your body, driving up blood cholesterol levels. Trans-fatty acids pop up all over the place—in breads, chips, crackers, cookies, microwave popcorn, you name it. Manufacturers like them because they give margarines and other foods a creamy consistency, and they prolong shelf life. On your ingredient list, they're known as hydrogenated or partially-hydrogenated fats. If you see the word 'hydrogenated' on an ingredient list, don't even bother reading further. Just put it back. It's a product that can raise cholesterol levels and clog arteries.

Under "sugars," the nutrition panel will give you a fairly good sense of the number of sugar grams you're eating. It gets a little tricky, though, because that number includes both added and natural sugars. Your best bet is to stick with the ingredient list. If on the list you're seeing natural sugars, like raisins, date sugar, figs and other fruits, that's good. Your insulin levels won't shoot up nearly as high as with added sugars. However, if the ingredient list sports a lot of "ose" words—like sucrose, glucose, fructose—or if there are other added sugars, like corn syrup, sorghum, honey and mannitol, it's prudent to limit your intake to less than 1.5 grams for every 100 calories. If you're eating 2,000 calories a day, then your "budget" is around 30 grams of added sugar.

The nutrition information panel is especially important if you are interested in controlling calories by trimming the fat content of your diet or in limiting the amount of sodium you consume. However, when making product comparisons, bear in mind that serving sizes are specified by the manufacturer and may vary substantially between similar products.

I also suggest that you do some housecleaning in your kitchen cupboards and refrigerator. This is one of the things I do in my counseling with individuals and families. I actually go to their homes and lend guidance on what to throw out or keep—with the goal of optimum health.

There are some appliances which make being healthy a little bit easier, such as a juicer, blender, stainless steel vegetable steamer and a salad spinner. These are four items that are very important in my kitchen. They help me prepare the kinds of foods that I want to eat, and they compliment the look of my kitchen—cleaner and healthier, reflecting my feelings about myself.

In Victoria Moran's wonderful book, *The Love-Powered Diet*, she says, "Start with small things. Delight in your dishes or your herb plants or the needle work saying on the wall. You'll soon delight as well in how your eating has changed. It's all connected. . . . When you're eating the purest, most healthful foods available to you, you feel good about your body, your thinking is more lucid and your outlook more positive."

Healthful behaviors are more likely to increase if they are easy and convenient. Have healthy foods easily available. When I come home from being out all day and am tired and hungry, there is a greater possibility that I will include a raw vegetable salad with my evening meal, or as my evening meal, if I washed the vegetables and perhaps partially prepared or trimmed them earlier. Sometimes it's harder to stay on track when you have to start from scratch. Do you know what I mean?

Keep in mind, too, that the body craves concentrated foods when hungry. Raw unheated nuts, avocado, whole grains, dried fruit, tofu, etc. are healthy concentrated foods which can be included in lunches instead of taking only fruit or vegetables. If you get hungry during recreational situations which overlap meal times, you may be tempted to eat whatever is handy. I usually bring some fresh fruit to the movie theater (although sometimes I need to conceal it upon arrival!). I've been known to take in vegetarian sandwiches, bottled water, and even home-made fresh juices. I like to observe the motto of the Boy Scouts of America: Be Prepared. Think ahead. "Failing to plan is planning to fail," said Ben Franklin.

Enjoy your food. But remember, food is fuel. Eat to live. Don't live to eat. There is more to life than food. Honor the divine temple that you are and support your self-esteem by selecting foods that support your body and promote optimum health.

THREE

Healthy Weight
Creating a Fit, Lean Body

T*he body is, ultimately, a reflection, a reflection of what is going on inside: emotionally, intellectually, and spiritually.*
                                        —**Victoria Moran**

You've seen the headlines on supermarket tabloids. "Use your zodiac sign to pick the perfect diet," or "Lose 10 pounds in one week on a dessert diet!" Americans are preoccupied with their waistlines and fat. We spend more than 30 billion dollars a year on diet foods, diet programs, diet pills, and other "guaranteed" weight-loss regimens and products. Yet we're getting fatter all the time, according to the National Center of Health Statistics.

Between 1988 and 1991, researchers at the Center measured height and weight in a nationally representative sample of 8,260 adults. One out of three was overweight. This is the highest proportion ever reported. In all, 58 million people weigh at least 20 percent more than the ideal weight for their age, height and sex. And we're getting fat fast. From 1960 to as recently as 1980, only one in four adults met the same criteria for overweight.

While millions of people starve to death in many parts of the world, the United States has the dubious honor of being the fattest country on the globe. The unhealthy numbers show no signs of lightening up. Experts call obesity an epidemic—one that spawns major health problems. Heart disease, endometrial cancer (uterine) and possibly breast cancer, high cholesterol, high blood pressure, immune dysfunction, osteoarthritis, stroke, gout, gallstones, and diabetes are all associated with overweight. Put in a more positive way, losing even a little weight may significantly improve your health and well being. So even if you're only interested in losing ten or twenty pounds to look better, you'll also benefit in many other ways.

Your body has an unlimited capacity for storing fat. Fortunately, it also has ample capacity to use and reduce it. Losing excess fat reduces crowding of your organs and the strain on your lower back, hips and knees. It also boosts your mood, self-esteem and energy levels, helps you sleep better (being overweight is often associated with sleep disorders such as sleep apnea—temporary cessation of breathing), and improves your appearance and attractiveness.

Eating disorders such as anorexia and bulimia are on the rise, and women's magazines are not helping when they continue to use models who are embracing the waif look. Take Barbie, for example, a doll that's part of most little girls' upbringing. This model of good looks and perfect body is giving the wrong message about what a healthy woman's body should look like. Barbie's bodyfat, were she an actual person, would be so low that she probably wouldn't even be able to menstruate. As little girls swarm to Barbie and teens try to emulate her, she has one accessory missing—food.

So how do you know what's an ideal weight for you?

Until recently, we have usually referred to height and weight tables provided by Metropolitan Life Insurance Company (MetLife). Yet, according to Dr. William P. Castelli, medical director of the famed Framingham Heart Study, these MetLife tables, which were revised in 1983 to allow for more weight, have become too lenient. In fact, the American Heart Association has urged people to ignore those guidelines. According to the current MetLife tables, for example, 155 pounds is within the desirable weight range for a 5'5" woman. That may be fine for a female bodybuilder with lots of lean muscle tissue, but it's too high for a normal non-bodybuilder female. These MetLife tables are based on death rates and vital statistics from millions of insurance holders in the United States. They don't account for the fact that many thin people with high death rates are cigarette smokers or otherwise ill. If those people had been eliminated from the current tabulations, says Dr. Castelli, the desirable weights would be lower. Dr. Castelli and other experts are exploring better ways to evaluate optimal body weight based on the latest research on weight-related health risks.

What Your Shape Says About Health Risks

Two approaches, when used together, are emerging as the new "gold standard" for weight: *Body Mass Index* and *Waist/Hip Ratio*.

Body Mass Index (BMI) is a ratio of height to weight. It's determined by a mathematical formula: First divide your weight (in pounds) by your height (in inches) squared, then multiply the resulting number by 705. You should get a BMI that's somewhere between 19 and 30. For example, let's say you weigh 140 pounds and you are 5'8" tall. You would first figure out your height (68") squared which is 4624. Then take your weight (140) and divide it by 4624 which gives you .030. Multiply this number by 705 and you get 21. (See figure 1.)

Numerous studies have already been conducted to validate the efficacy of the BMI and weight-related health risks. The conclusion is that 21 to 22 is the optimal body mass index because there are no weight-related health risks at this level.

One large-scale study indicates that a BMI below 22 is ideal for preventing heart disease in women. This Nurses' Health Study, co-directed by Dr. JoAnn E. Manson and conducted at Brigham and Women's Hospital and Harvard Hospital in Boston followed 115,886 initially healthy American women ages 30 to 55 for eight years. During that time, 605 of the women experienced coronary-artery disease, of whom 83 died. There was no elevated risk of heart disease among women whose BMIs were under 21; the risk was 30 percent higher than that of the lean group for women whose BMI was between 21 and 25, 80 percent higher for a BMI 25 to 29, and 230 percent higher than the lean group for those with a BMI greater than 29. The researchers concluded that "obesity is a strong risk factor for coronary heart disease in middle-age women." They reported in *New England Journal of Medicine* (March 1990) that

CALCULATING BODY MASS INDEX (BMI)

HEIGHT	BODY WEIGHT IN POUNDS											
4' 10"	91	96	100	105	110	115	119	124	129	134	138	143
4' 11"	94	99	104	109	114	119	124	128	133	138	143	148
5' 0"	97	102	107	112	118	123	128	133	138	143	148	153
5' 1"	100	106	111	116	122	127	132	137	143	148	153	158
5' 2"	104	109	115	120	126	131	136	142	147	153	158	164
5' 3"	107	113	118	124	130	135	141	146	152	158	163	169
5' 4"	110	116	122	128	134	140	145	151	157	163	169	174
5' 5"	114	120	126	132	138	144	150	156	162	168	174	180
5' 6"	118	124	130	136	142	148	155	161	167	173	179	186
5' 7"	121	127	134	140	146	153	159	166	172	178	185	191
5' 8"	125	131	138	144	151	158	164	171	177	184	190	197
5' 9"	128	135	142	149	155	162	169	176	182	189	196	203
5' 10"	132	139	146	153	160	167	174	181	188	195	202	207
5' 11"	136	143	150	157	165	172	179	186	193	200	208	215
6' 0"	140	147	154	162	169	177	184	191	199	206	213	221
BMI	19	20	21	22	23	24	25	26	27	28	29	30

FIG. 1 To find your BMI, locate your height in the left column. (If you've lost inches over the years, use your peak adult height.) Move across the chart (to the right) until you hit your approximate weight, then follow that column down to the corresponding BMI number at the bottom of the chart.

"even mild-to-moderate overweight is associated with a substantial elevation in coronary risk."

There's no consensus yet among the experts on how much is too much. Some insist that although a BMI between 23 and 25 isn't ideal, the excess risk for cancer and other weight-related diseases seems to be small. Approximately around a BMI of 26, these health risks appear to rise, although it's not quite clear to scientists where to draw the line. Jean Pierre Despres, Ph.D., associate director of the Lipid Research Center at Laval University in St. Foy, Quebec, says that between 25 and 27 is a gray zone. "A lot of people in this range are perfectly healthy, but others have a substantially higher risk of developing diabetes and premature coronary disease." Most scientists do agree that a BMI over 27 increases risk for many people. But their risk also depends on other factors, including their waist/hip measurement, notes Dr. Despres.

Although less common than overweight in the United States, excessive thinness can also be a problem. It is linked with osteoporosis and other health problems, even early death, especially if weight loss is sudden. The experts feel that someone with a BMI under 19 should be evaluated. "That doesn't mean everyone low is going to be unhealthy, but it's worth taking a closer look," says James O. Hill, Ph.D., associate director of the Center for Human Nutrition at the University of Colorado Health Sciences Center in Denver.

In addition to knowing your BMI number, it's equally important to be aware of your Waist/Hip Ratio (WHR). You get this number by measuring your waist (at the midpoint between your bottom rib and hip bone) and your hips (at their widest point). Then divide the waist measurement by the hip measurement. For example, if your waist is 29' and your hips measure 38', then your WHR is 0.76.

Why is this ratio important? In the last few years, researchers have determined that the fat most associated with health risks is on the upper body—the abdomen and above, rather than the thighs and hips. (This pattern of upper-body fat is often called "central obesity.") "Central obesity is turning out to be the most lethal risk factor associated with excess body weight," says Dr. Castelli. That's because upper-body fat is strongly correlated with visceral fat, which is fat that's packed around our internal organs.

The WHR, though not perfect (it isn't very reliable for women who are very thin, very overweight or for bodybuilders) can, in most cases, prove very predictive of cardiovascular disease risk, especially in women. Researchers at the University of Miami School of Medicine and the University of Minnesota School of Public Health examined data on 32,898 healthy women ages 55 to 69. As reported in the *Annals of Epidemiology,* January 1993, there were nearly three times as many heart-disease deaths in a four-year period among women with the greatest waist/hip ratio (0.86 and over) than those under .80. A high waist-to-hip ratio has also been associated with diabetes, hypertension, stroke, breast and endometrial (uterine) cancers and high cholesterol.

If the ideal BMI is around 21 or 22, let's see what the experts say about the ideal WHR. Most target 0.80 as desirable. If you're a woman, a number greater than 0.85 indicates higher health risks. If you're a man, health risks are related to a ratio greater than 1.0. Dr. Castelli believes that the WHR measurement is even more important than BMI in predicting risk. "If someone has a healthy BMI but a high WHR, it is important to try to bring that WHR down," he explains. "Someone with a higher BMI but a low WHR might not be quite as bad off."

There's another point to consider. Are you overweight or overfat? Weight tables can classify you as overweight when you actually have average or below average bodyfat. Athletes are often overweight because of a large frame or muscle development, but they aren't overfat.

Obesity means an excess accumulation of bodyfat. Usually, obesity and overweight are related. If you're 25 pounds or more overweight by most weight charts, you're probably overfat. At this point, the health risks of obesity surface. When you are 25 pounds overweight, your heart must pump blood through nearly 5,000 extra miles of blood vessels.

An easy way to judge whether you're overfat is by looking in a mirror. If, despite good BMI and WHR numbers, you look flabby, you probably are. You'd do well to measure your body fat and to embark on an exercise regimen that burns fat and tones muscles.

Exact standards don't exist for how much body fat a person can carry without increasing risk. I suggest aiming for body fat of 18 to 28 percent of total weight for women as optimal, slightly higher than for men who optimally have body fat of 12 to 22 percent.

There are several ways to determine your percentage of body fat. You can get calipers that pinch skin folds in various places on the body (which is what I usually use). You can use a bioelectric impedance test (running a mild current through the body to measure resistance) or do underwater weighing. Unfortunately, the latter two methods are not widely available outside health clubs or specialists' offices and are not always reliable. All methods only give you a ballpark figure. And the older and fatter you are, the less reliable the measurement may be. Whatever method you pick, stick with the same one over a year or so. I usually check my percentage of body fat quarterly.

Obesity in infancy and childhood can lead to a life battling the bulge. During the first few years of life, you form new fat cells rapidly. As the rate of fat storage increases, so does the number of fat cells. In obese children, the number of fat cells is often three times that in normal-weight children. As a result, overfeeding children, especially in infancy, can lead to a lifetime of obesity. After adolescence the number of fat cells remains almost constant throughout the rest of life.

Although the extra pounds and less than ideal BMI and WHR numbers could be explained by exercise-induced muscle (which, inch for inch, weighs more than fat), unless you're an avid fitness enthusiast or athlete, it's not likely. "The people in this country are still geared toward overeating," says Margaret McDowell, R.D., at the National Center for Health Statistics. If you don't want your eating habits to get the best of you, consider raising your basal metabolic rate.

Metabolism and Ways to Increase It

Your *basal metabolic rate* is the rate at which your body utilizes energy. Put another way, it has to do with how efficiently your body burns calories. As you may recall from your physiology classes, calories are the measuring unit of heat energy. When your metabolism is higher, you burn more fat and have an easier time losing weight (fat) or maintaining your ideal body weight.

Statistics reveal that most people are not happy with their weight or the shape of their body. Half of the women and a quarter of the men in this country are currently trying to lose weight and reshape their bodies. The sad thing is that a majority of these people are going about it in the wrong way—like swimming upstream. Most people try to lose weight by dieting, which usually involves eating certain foods and cutting back on calories. *Diets don't work!*

Statistics also reveal that two out of three people who go on a diet will regain their weight in one year or less; 97 percent will regain the weight in five years. To make matters worse, a majority of dieters who lose weight will gain back even more fat than they had before they started the diet. They have all violated an important rule in creating and maintaining a healthy, fast metabolism: they lost lean body mass, or muscle.

Lack of exercise is a major reason for the rise of obesity in the United States. Between our desk jobs and our automobiles, we don't move our bodies enough to ward off the gain in fat that naturally tends to come with aging. The problem is, many people do not realize that they need to include deliberate exercise in their daily routine.

In my workshops around the country, people tell me they get plenty of exercise doing household chores or walking around at work. I emphatically tell them that it's not enough! You need *intentional* exercise, like fitness walking and lifting weights or cycling, to call yourself anything but sedentary.

You see, most adults lose about one percent of their muscle every year after about age 40. At the same time, many people gain about a pound of fat a year. But the slide to fat really doesn't have to happen if you participate in appropriate physical activity programs that include both some aerobic and some strength-training exercise, and if you select the proper foods.

So let's go over 15 ways for increasing your metabolism, selecting the right exercises and foods, and making healthy choices for creating a fit, lean body.

15 Steps to a Fit, Lean Body

1. Muscle burns fat. Decreased activity leads to muscle loss. Why is lean muscle tissue so important? More muscle means a faster metabolism because muscle uses more energy than fat. That is because muscle is a highly metabolic tissue; it burns five times as many calories as most other body tissues, pound for pound. In other words, muscle requires more oxygen and more calories to sustain itself than does body fat. When you have more muscle on your body, you burn more calories than someone who doesn't, even when you're both sitting still. So it's easy to understand how people who build muscle have an easier time maintaining a healthy weight. They're simply more efficient calorie burners.

Why does it seem that men can eat more of everything than women without gaining weight? One explanation is that men have more muscle and less fat than women. Because men have more muscle, they burn ten to 20 percent more calories than women, at rest.

The addition of ten pounds of muscle to your body will burn 600 calories per day. You would have to run six miles a day, seven days a week to burn the same number of calories. Ten extra pounds of muscle can burn a pound of fat in one week; that's 52 pounds of fat a year. If you increase muscle mass, you increase the number of calories your body is using every moment of the day, not just during exercise, but also at work, play, and even when sleeping.

The best way to increase lean muscle mass is through resistance training which means weight lifting or resistance machines— barbells, dumbbells or machines, cables, or even "free-hand" movements such as push-ups and sit-ups. All it takes to add ten pounds of muscle is a regular weight training program involving only 30 minutes, three times a week for about six months. Isn't that fantastic? And the wonderful thing about increasing your metabolism through increasing your muscle mass is that you don't have to restrict your calorie intake.

2. Aerobic exercise can increase or decrease metabolism. While the best exercise for permanent fat loss is resistance training (lifting weights) because it increases muscle which burns more calories, low intensity aerobic exercise such as walking is also an excellent way to burn fat efficiently. Cutting 250 calories from your daily diet can help you lose half a pound a week (3,500 calories = 1 pound of fat). But add a 30-minute brisk walk four days a week, and you can double your rate of weight loss. Aerobic exercise increases your metabolic rate for hours after exercising. However, according to Dr. Dean Ornish in his book *Eat More, Weigh Less*, intense exercise (beyond your target heart rate), for an extended period of time, as opposed to short intervals, may actually decrease your metabolism in the long run because you burn valuable muscle tissue.

In a study conducted at the Cooper Aerobic Center, Dr. John Duncan took 102 sedentary women and divided them into three groups. Each group walked three miles, five days a week for six months. The first group walked five mph, the second group four mph, and the third group three mph. He found that the slowest walking group lost the most weight. Running, or any aerobic exercise that raises heart rate above 80 percent of maximum (220 minus your age times 0.8) will cause you to burn more muscle and less fat. An exercise heart rate kept closer to 60 percent of maximum (220 minus your age x 0.6) or 108 beats per minute for a 40 year old person, will burn mostly fat. This is why walking is superior to running as a fat burning exercise. Walking is one of the most underrated of exercises. The risk of injury is lower than for many other exercises, it's inexpensive, and you can do it just about anywhere. All you need is a good pair of walking shoes.

Other good aerobic/endurance activities include hiking, jogging, skating (ice, roller or in-line), cross country skiing, swimming, aquarobics (aerobic exercise in water), bicycling, rowing and stair climbing.

For healthy adults, the American College of Sports Medicine recommends 15 to 60 minutes of aerobic exercise three to five times a week. The intensity or level of effort will depend on the goals and condition of the person exercising. Simply walking at a moderate pace (two and a half to three miles per hour) for 30 minutes or more on a regular basis can do wonders to improve body composition and appearance, cardiovascular risk factors, mood, self-esteem, sleep quality and perceived energy level. And that's just for starters.

3. Break up your exercise. The news from the American College of Sports Medicine and the U.S. Center for Disease Control and Prevention is that exercise need not necessarily occur in one continuous bout (unless you have extra weight to lose, which might make exercising longer more effective). The daily training can be broken up—with equivalent health benefits—into segments. For example, in lieu of spending 45 minutes doing aerobics at the gym in either a class or on the aerobic equipment, you can take a ten-minute walk in the morning, walk up and down stairs during the day instead of taking the elevator, take a ten-minute walk during your lunch hour and finish up with a relaxing 20-minute walk after dinner. Even house and yard work, such as sweeping, mopping, gardening, mowing the grass and shoveling snow, count toward your daily total.

4. Intense exercise helps burn fat. Take the hills on tomorrow's walk. They could give you greater fat-burning power than you got on the level today. A report suggests that a few bouts of high-intensity exercise mixed with low-intensity exercise (that might be a few short hills and some easy walking in-between) may be strikingly more effective in burning fat than one long lower-intensity bout, even if the long bout burns more calories.

Case in point: Seventeen exercisers on stationary bikes followed a moderate-exercise training program (30 to 45 minutes, four to five times per week for 20 weeks). All burned about 300 to 400 calories per session. Ten other exercisers did only about one-third as many bouts of 30-minute bike riding over 15 weeks. They filled the other sessions with short bursts of high-intensity cycling—they went almost as quickly as they could for 30 to 90 seconds and repeated these bursts several times per exercise session. These folks used only about 225 to 250 calories per session, but they lost more fat (according to skin-fold measurements) than did the moderate exercisers (who technically burned more calories). When expressed as calories expended during exercise, their fat loss was *nine times* greater than that in subjects performing lower intensity exercise. Muscle biopsies confirmed that the important step of fat oxidation had occurred in the cells of the high-intensity exercisers to a greater degree than in the low-intensity exercisers, as reported in the journal *Metabolism*, July 1994.

It seems to be a paradox that less exercise time could result in more fat burning. Standard thinking says that high-intensity exercise burns the available carbohydrates as the fuel source before it digs into fat. Researchers think that what happens here may have to do with two things believed to happen *between* and *after* exercise. First, intermittent high-intensity exercise may encourage a higher rate of fuel burning during the recovery periods and after exer-cise—and that fuel may come from fat. And second, high-intensity exercise may have an anorectic effect—that is, you may feel more satisfied with fewer calories (and few fat calories) in what you eat for a while after your workout.

The high-intensity exercise levels in this study were equivalent to sprinting. That level of effort isn't appropriate for everyone, says study leader Angelo Tremblay, Ph.D., professor of physiology and nutrition at Laval University, Quebec. "Something comparable might be vigorous circuit training. Or it could be reasonable—if you are healthy and accustomed to performing vigorous exer-cises—to briefly increase walking to a level where speaking is not possible. You can do that for 60 or 90 seconds, three to five times during a walk." Later, he says, you can increase the number of high intensity bouts. Of course, even if this is confirmed in other studies, it's not an excuse to cut your exercise time. Even trained athletes can't sustain day-in/day-out workouts at super-high intensities.

Endurance exercise may have benefits we're just beginning to tap. Another study, for instance, found that 35 to 45 minutes of endurance exercise three times a week reduced insulin levels in the blood of 70- to 79-year-old men and women.

So pump up the intensity if your doctor says you can. Just find a way to fit that extra vigor into your regular workout program. My favorite way is hiking. I often hike in my local Santa Monica Mountains where I experience frequent bouts of high intensity when hiking up the hills interspersed with more level or declining grades.

5. Grazing decreases fat storage. Liquid meals, diet pills and special combinations of foods aren't your answer to increasing metabolism, weight control or better health. Instead, learn how to eat.

Results of four national surveys show that most people try to lose weight by eating 1,000 to 1,500 calories a day. However, cutting calories to under 1,200 (if you're a woman) or 1,400 (if you're a man) doesn't provide enough food to be satisfying in the long term. Eating fewer than 1,200 calories makes it difficult to get

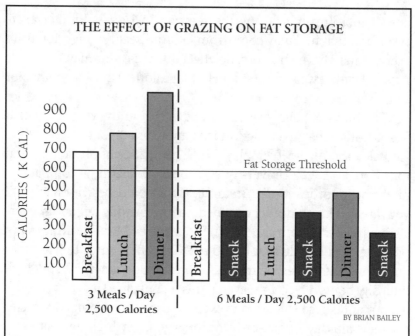

FIG. 2 This graph illustrates how three meals can result in 700 calories being stored as fat. The same calorie intake spread over six meals produces no fat storage.

adequate amounts of certain nutrients, such as folic acid, magnesium and zinc. It also promotes temporary loss of fluids rather than permanent loss of fat.

To increase your metabolism, eat several small healthy meals a day as opposed to two or three larger meals. (See figure 2.) This keeps your metabolism stoked. The typical dieter will often skip meals and, as research points out, the worst meal to skip, if you want to increase your metabolism, is breakfast. This temporary fasting state sends a signal to the body that food is scarce. As a result, the stress hormones (including cortisol) increase and the body begins "lightening the load" and shedding its muscle tissue. Decreasing muscle tissue, which is metabolically active, decreases the body's need for food. By the next feeding, the pancreas is sensitized and will sharply increase blood insulin levels which is the body's signal to make fat.

The secret to keeping your metabolism from slowing is to make sure that you graze throughout the day and that your diet contains at least 10 calories per pound of your ideal body weight. If you are aiming for a weight of 150 pounds, your daily menu should contain at least 1,500 calories. If you have less food than this, you run the risk of slowing down your metabolism. People on restrictive diets and limited calories usually get tired of feeling deprived and hungry. Grazing throughout the day eliminates feeling deprived.

Have you ever wondered how the Sumo wrestlers get so big? They fast and then gorge themselves with food.

6. Choose the right foods that burn more fat. If you change *what* you eat, you don't have to be as much concerned with how *much* you eat. By doing this, you can eat whenever you're hungry until you feel full. You'll lose weight without hunger or deprivation and you won't need to count calories. You need information, not willpower.

The best foods are complex carbohydrates. Low in fat, fast-burning, and rich in vitamins and minerals, they are also high in bulk, which means you can feel full on fewer calories. These foods are whole-grain cereals and grains including brown rice, whole grain breads, legumes, vegetables, fruits and nuts (sparingly). Fruits should be eaten for breakfast or between meals. When you eat fruit with or after meals, the fructose is likely to be converted to fat by the liver.

Whole, natural foods usually have a low glycemic index. A low glycemic index means that blood sugar is not rapidly elevated after a meal. High glycemic index foods, such as sugary foods, put your blood sugar on a rollercoaster. When blood sugar rises too rapidly, insulin is secreted in an overabundance. This excess insulin stimulates fat production and storage. The superfluous insulin will cause too much sugar to be stored, resulting in low blood sugar. Low blood sugar, in turn, will then cause stress hormone release, depression, fatigue and hunger.

The high fiber in this recommended plant-based diet will actually slow digestion and absorption for a more even blood sugar level. Fiber will also bind with some fat and prevent its absorption. High fiber foods are beneficial for speeding up bowel transit time, too. This will take some stress off the liver as less toxins will form.

The body can then more efficiently metabolize fats. (Refer to section on fiber in Chapter 2 for more information.)

Research reported by Jeffrey Bland, Ph.D., in the January 1995 issue of *Let's Live* magazine indicates there may be a significant connection between toxicity in the body and weight problems. Toxicity in the body causes retention of fluids, called edema. The short term solution to toxicity is to drink more water. In other words, dilution is the solution to internal pollution. When toxins are eliminated, the body no longer needs to retain water, and a significant loss of fluid occurs. Water retention alters the body's energy-production systems and affects metabolism, according to Bland. The long term solution is to eat wholesome foods. A plant based diet doesn't create the toxic overload in your body that unhealthy foods do.

Eating healthy foods with a plethora of nutrients increases your mitochondrial bioenergetics (energy production which helps increase metabolism). The nutritional support necessary for promoting this increase in energy production includes adequate levels of B vitamins, trace minerals (for example, copper, iron, and chromium) and nutrients necessary for supporting proper detoxification—including molybdenum, selenium, manganese, zinc, and the antioxidants vitamin E, C, and bioflavonoids, along with pantothenic acid, biotin and folic acid. These nutrients, together with a well-designed nutrition program as presented in this book can lead to improved mitochrondrial bioenergetics, which helps you reset your body weight to a lower set point by improving your body's heat-producing properties.

Investigators at the Department of Community Health at the University of Oregon recently published a paper in which they report on the use of a specific, controlled weight-loss program in moderately overweight women. In this study, reported in the *Journal of the American College of Nutrition, 1994,* 18 sedentary, moderately overweight women followed a seven-week program consisting of a diet of whole foods containing 1,000 to 1,100 calories per day and a specific vitamin and mineral-fortified meal supplement drink, along with a progressive walking program. Mitochondrial energy production was assessed in these women before, during and after the weight-loss program. The weight loss was principally body fat, not muscle. In fact, some women actually gained muscle as they lost fat, causing their bodies to be much leaner at the conclusion of the program.

The bottom line: eat a wholesome diet with lots of nutrients, drink plenty of water between meals, and exercise regularly.

7. **Fat makes you fat.** Overweight people tend to eat a higher fat diet than people of normal weight. Fatty foods slow metabolism. Your body converts dietary fat into body fat very easily. Fats not only have twice the calories, gram for gram, as carbohydrates and proteins (nine compared to four), they also burn only two percent of their calories to be stored as fat. Protein and carbohydrates, on the other hand, will burn about 25 percent of their calories to be stored as fat. In other words, it is considerably more difficult to convert protein and carbohydrates into body fat; your body actually burns calories doing so. Thus, even when calories are the same, a person eating a high fat diet tends to store more excess calories as body fat than someone eating a lower fat diet. Consequently, the closer you can adhere to a low-fat diet, the less fat will remain on you. So, for example, if you eat 3,000 calories a day and decrease the percentage of fat from 40 percent to 20 percent, you can lose one pound of fat in about three weeks—while at the same time eating 20 percent more food from carbohydrates and protein. The bottom line: eating fat makes you fat.

You can also fight fat with fat. Sounds paradoxical, doesn't it? Despite what I just said, not all fats make you fat. As I explain in greater detail in Chapter 4, omega-3 fatty acids can actually increase your metabolic rate. They also rid the body of excess fluids and can increase your energy level. The best source of omega-3 (LNA) fatty acids is organic flax seed oil available in the refrigerator section of health foods stores; other sources include flax seeds and fish. Also explained in that chapter, omega-6 (LA) fatty acids (especially gamma linolenic acid or GLA) are also essential to health and a healthy metabolism but are less likely to be deficient in a healthy diet. Good sources of GLA and omega-6 fatty acids are borage seed oil, black current oil and primrose oil.

8. Alcohol can make you fat. For those of you who drink alcohol, listen up. One of the greatest ways to sabotage your fat loss program is through alcohol consumption. Aside from having seven calories per gram, alcohol shifts metabolism in favor of fat deposition, burdens the liver and stimulates your appetite.

9. Water washes away fat. Water is very important in helping to maintain a healthy metabolic rate. At least two quarts a day, between meals, is essential—more if you're physically very active. In fact, water may be the most important catalyst to increase fat burning. Simply drinking 1 gallon of water throughout the day, cooled (yes, it needs to be cooled) to 40 degrees F, will burn 300 calories, the equivalent of running three miles. And, water suppresses your appetite naturally.

High water intake reduces fat deposits by taking a load off the liver. The liver's main functions are detoxification and regulation of metabolism. The kidneys can get rid of toxins and spare the liver if they have sufficient water. This allows the liver to metabolize more fat. Adequate water will also decrease bloating and edema caused by fluid accumulation. Water does this by flushing out sodium and toxins. A high water intake also helps relieve constipation by keeping your stools soft.

10. Cellulite can be a thing of the past. Millions of people, especially women, have cellulite. In fact, about 90 percent of all women over the age of 18 are plagued with this problem. While these may seem like hopeless odds, there is help.

Cellulite is actually a combination of fat, water and wastes. It frequently appears on otherwise thin women. While fat is typically a generalized condition, cellulite settles predominantly on the hips, buttocks, thighs and knees. Sometimes it even surfaces on the calves, ankles, abdomen, arms and upper back. It most often forms in areas with poor circulation. When circulation becomes sluggish, wastes can accumulate in the connective tissues that surround the fat cells just beneath the skin. Cellular exchange slows down or stops and metabolism becomes sluggish. When cells don't receive adequate nourishment, individual cells can't function properly. Wastes continue to build up until the tissue becomes hard and lumpy beneath the surface and rippled on the surface. Cellulite takes on the characteristic appearance that has aptly earned it the nicknames "cottage cheese" and "orange peel" skin.

Cellulite is the result of a combination of factors. Lifestyle plays a primary role in its formation. Habits and lifestyle patterns such as stress, poor posture, improper diet, lack of exercise, poor elimination and sluggish circulation contribute to cellulite according to Roberta Wilson, author of *The Cellulite Control Guide*. A sound cellulite control program incorporates exercise—aerobics, weight training and stretching, daily skin brushing (to increase circulation), deep breathing, regular massages, and proper nutrition.

Good dietary guidelines for controlling cellulite including the following:

- Eat plenty of fresh vegetables and fruits and a variety of whole grains.
- Increase water intake to at least 80 ounces a day—more if you're physically very active.
- Eliminate salt.
- Avoid sugar, caffeine, alcohol and saturated fats.
- Eat more complex carbohydrates; they provide energy and fiber necessary for proper elimination.
- Eliminate red meat. Gradually phase out other animal products and byproducts.
- Avoid preservatives, pesticides and food additives such as food coloring and flavor.
- Make at least 50 percent of your diet living foods (not cooked).

What I'm suggesting here is what I've described in detail in Chapter 2 on nutrition.

11. Do fat burning supplements work? Despite the latest wave of research into new and better ways to fight fat, I believe that the most efficient fat busters are the same old standbys: exercise and proper nutrition. There's one exception, however, and that's the mineral chromium. Here's what makes taking chromium supplements especially appealing. Most of us don't get enough of this trace mineral in our diet anyway, according to researchers at the U.S. Department of Agriculture. Although chromium is available in such foods as broccoli and brewer's yeast, about nine out of ten Americans consume it at levels well below the 50 to 200 microgram level recommended by the National Academy of Sciences, says Richard Anderson, a USDA researcher and a leading authority on chromium.

Chromium doesn't zap fat directly. Rather, it enhances the efficiency of insulin, the hormone responsible for regulating blood sugar. By helping insulin work more effectively, scientists theorize, chromium may play an indirect role in metabolizing fat and turning off hunger signals in the brain's appetite-control center. Some research also suggests chromium aids in building the body's most efficient fat-burning tissue, lean muscle, which burns fat even while the body is at rest. (As mentioned above, this is why women who add weight training to a program of aerobic exercise will lose fat faster than those who don't. It's also why trying to lose weight only by dieting is an effort doomed from the start. Exercise raises metabolism and makes the body burn fat for energy; dieting lowers metabolism to compensate for the lack of food and forces the body to use muscle for fuel.)

The chromium rush began after a study in which former USDA researcher Gary Evans gave one group of football players at Minnesota's Bemidji State University a daily dose of 200 micrograms of chromium picolinate during six weeks of training; the other group received a placebo. Those taking chromium gained 42 percent more muscle mass and dropped more than three times as much body fat as the control group. Similarly encouraging results occurred in a University of Texas Health Science Center study of overweight adults who didn't diet or work out regularly but still lost weight while taking chromium supplements. In research at Louisiana State University, a group of pigs that ate chromium picolinate (and that likewise avoided dieting and exercise) wound up with more lean meat with less fat than pigs that didn't. Other studies found that chromium helps rats live longer and in humans reduces cholesterol and helps type II diabetes. In terms of losing fat and gaining lean muscle tissue in humans, all the studies indicate that those who get the biggest payoff from chromium are the ones who get regular exercise and avoid eating too much fat.

I take an excellent chromium supplement called Kyo-Chrome made by the highly respected company, Wakunaga of America. (See Resources) This is a blend of odorless Kyolic brand aged garlic extract with chromium picolinate and niacin. It's available in health food stores.

12. Good habits make the difference. Here are some things to keep in mind to help assure success in your program.

Start Strong. People who eat a healthy breakfast generally feel less hungry throughout the day. This also stokes your metabolism.

Curb Your Appetite. Drink a glass of water about fifteen minutes before a meal.

Eat What You Like. Nothing makes a food program more difficult than having to eat foods that you don't like. Make wise choices from the foods you like.

Slow Down. Eat slowly enough to give your body time to release the enzymes that tell your brain when you've had all you need.

Don't Give Up. Falling off your health program once or twice does not mean the effort is hopeless. Simply acknowledge that you over-ate, and get back on the plan.

Reward Yourself. Treat yourself with a massage, a movie, a piece of clothing, a delicious meal at your favorite restaurant, or whatever, for each week that you maintain your health program, achieve goals or maintain weight.

13. Self motivation is the key to success. To stay motivated, make a commitment, get your priorities straight, and set realistic goals.

Make a commitment and follow through on what you say you're going to do. Lose weight because you want to, not to please someone else. You must be internally motivated to lose weight and create a fit, lean body—it's what you want to do.

Be realistic. Don't set yourself up for failure by trying to improve your lifestyle if you're distracted by other major problems. It takes a lot of mental and physical energy to change habits. If you're having marital or financial problems or if you're unhappy with other major aspects of your life, you may be less likely to follow through on your good intentions. Timing is critical. I'm not saying to abandon your health program if you're under stress. Just modify it and start with easy-to-achieve goals like drinking more water, eating more fruit or simply walking daily.

What are your fitness goals? Write them out, both short and long term. Don't set a weight goal that conforms to unrealistic social ideals for thinness. Instead, try achieving a comfortable weight you maintained easily as a young adult. If you've always been over-weight, the weight at which levels of triglycerides, blood sugar, blood pressure and energy improve may be a realistic goal.

Accept that healthful weight loss is slow and steady. Aim to lose no more than one pound a week if you're a woman, two pounds a week if you're a man. (Men's naturally higher metabolic rate makes it easier to lose weight faster.)

In addition to longer goals, set weekly or monthly goals that allow you to check off successes.

14. Moderate doses of sunlight increase metabolism. The sun has been getting a lot of bad press lately. Actually, sunlight in moderation is very good for the body in a variety of ways. It increases your metabolism, as documented in the excellent book, *Sunlight,* by Dr. Zane Kime. Dr. Kime states, "There is conclusive evidence that exposure to sunlight produces a metabolic effect in the body very similar to that produced by physical training, and is definitely followed by a measured improvement in physical fit-ness." He also explains in this book how a vegan diet (vegetarian with no dairy) will greatly decrease the risk of skin cancer.

15. Nourish your spirit. To be healthy, to improve your metabolism, to make healthy food and exercise choices, you must first nourish your spirit. The real epidemic in our culture is spiritual heart disease—feelings of loneliness, isolation and alienation that pervade our culture. Many people who suffer from spiritual malaise use food (or stimulants such as drugs, caffeine, alcohol, sex or overwork) to numb the pain and get through the day.

Stretching, deep breathing and meditation will relax your mind and you will experience a greater sense of peace and well-being. Then you'll be able to make eating and exercise decisions—and other lifestyle choices—that are life enhancing rather than self-destructive.

Dieting alone doesn't work. Dieting combined with regular aerobic exercise is better, but it won't replace the muscle tissue that's lost in aging. But when you combine strength training, aerobic exercise, sensible eating and nourishment for your spirit, you've got an unbeatable combination for reaching and maintaining your ideal weight, improving your metabolism, creating a fit, lean body, and celebrating life.

FOUR

Fats & Oils
Telling the Killers from the Healers

C*ertain types of fats called essential fatty acids (EFAs) are critical to good nutrition because humans cannot make them. Failure to eat enough EFAs is a cause of hardening of the arteries, abnormal clot formation, coronary heart disease, high cholesterol, and high blood pressure. —**Edward N. Siguel, M.D.***

You have probably heard or read that fats are literally killing us. Actually only certain types of fats injure us, while another entire set of fats keep us healthy and vital. The facts are in: Some fats are deadly and others are life savers! The high incidence of heart disease, cancer and numerous other degenerative diseases is not caused by the amount but rather the type of fat we consume, and the profound deficiency of "healing fats" or essential fatty acids (EFAs) in the average diet.

Degenerative diseases that involve fat metabolism have rapidly increased since the turn of the century. During the early 1900s, only one in seven people died of degenerative cardiovascular disease. Today almost half of Americans will die from arterial, vascular, and coronary heart disease. In 1900, only one in 30 people died of cancer. Today nearly one in four die from a variety of cancers.

We can help reverse these disease processes by making prudent food choices, up to a point. However, there comes a time when vital organs are so severely depleted and damaged nutritionally that they cannot recover. In other words, reversal of degeneration is no longer possible and death ensues. This process is caused by extreme free radical pathology, proliferation of metastasized cells and cell toxemia from a lifetime absorption of environmental pollutants in food, air and water. When this state is reached, the final stages of cellular death occur.

It takes 30 years to "feed" a heart attack or cancer; so now is the time to make some positive changes in your eating habits. You may decide to avoid the deadly or toxic fats, or add the "healing" EFA (or essential fatty acid) fats to your diet. It truly becomes a choice of healthy mind over diseased matter. A healthy life starts with a "healthy" attitude.

Even genetic diseases, that affect one in 200 Americans, may be incurable but can still be mitigated and even improved with proper nutrition. Even depression and mental health can be greatly improved with intelligent eating, taking into account age and genetic frailties.

Low-Fat Diets Will Not Save Us

The U.S. Department of Agriculture and Health Department recommends that all Americans over the age of two should decrease their fat intake to below 30 percent of daily caloric intake, and saturated fat intake to below 10 percent of total calories. Although this gesture is laudatory for most "typical" Americans who consume the Standard American Diet (SAD), following that recommendation will not save you from degenerative diseases. At best it will only moderately retard their onset. At worst, contemporary lipid (fat) research reveals that a low-fat diet may actually *speed* the degenerative process. This is because many low-fat diets are low in health-promoting EFA fats as well as being high in damaging saturated and trans-fats.

The subject of dietary fats and oils is a bit complicated and the terminology may be new to you. Nevertheless, I urge you to stick with it because understanding this chapter is truly a main ingredient of health and happiness.

In order to understand the difference between good and bad fats we need to know the composition of fats. The scientific name for fats and oils is lipids. Lipids are made of carbon, hydrogen and oxygen molecules. Both plants and animals produce fats. The exquisite biochemical architecture of fats (and how they function in our bodies) is determined in large part by their molecular structure. This structure can be described as a "caterpillar shape." The molecules look like a series of integrated globes. The lipid molecules are broken down into degrees of chemical reactivity based on the number of chemical bonds.

Fats may be *saturated* or *unsaturated*, according to the frequency of the bonds or "kinks" in the molecules' shapes. The bonds or "kinks" in the molecule also define its stability or reactivity with other molecular substances around it. The greater the number of bonds, the greater the fragility of the lipid. *Unrefined polyunsaturated oils* like flax seed, hemp seed or soybean oil, contain several "kinks" in the polyunsaturated fatty acids. They are made up of long chain fatty acids (in the chemist's shorthand they are called C:18:2 or C:18:3 fatty acids which typically means 18 carbon lengths long, with either two or three bonds in the fatty acid chain).

The inherent fragility of the bond makes them chemically very reactive—acting as an oxygen magnet in the body at the cellular level. The ability for this highly reactive bond to absorb free single oxygen molecules into the permeable cells of the body is what gives these oils their dramatic energy producing properties prized by athletes and sought by people healing from heart disease and cancer. This unique chemical property of essential fatty acids is behind the anti-carcinogenic prowess of unrefined polyunsaturated oils. As explained by Udo Erasmus in *Fats That Heal, Fats That Kill,* cancerous cells hate oxygen and typically behave anaerobically. Increasing our consumption of unrefined super polyunsaturated fats makes us more cancer resistant, more energetic and makes our heart muscle, veins, arteries and skin more supple.

Saturated fats are short and straight (C:4:0), without any "kinks" so they are able to stack densely together. They are relatively non-reactive and remain solid at room temperature, unlike all other classes of natural fats. Saturated fats are most typically found in animal products. For example, lard and butter are almost completely saturated animal fats; coconut and palm oil, on the other hand, are saturated vegetable fats. Saturated fats are also much more stable than unsaturated or super-unsaturated fats and go rancid less easily because of the short carbon chain length. This is why the mass-market food industry prefers to use saturated fats over less stable polyunsaturated fats. The shelf life of foods with saturated fats is much longer—but they are far less healthy.

Unsaturated fats have bonds or "kinks" everywhere there is a double bond. (See Figure 3.) This unsaturated spot or "kink" keeps the individual fatty acid chains or "caterpillars" from stacking and compressing neatly together. This property explains why unsaturated oils are liquid at room temperature. Unsaturated fats can be *monounsaturated* (for example, olive oil) which means it has one double bond or kink in its molecular structure; *polyunsaturated* (for example, corn or safflower oil) which means it usually has two double bonds or kinks; and *superunsaturated* (for example, flax seed and fish oils) which have three or more double bonds or kinks. The superunsaturated oils are "firecracker" reactive in the presence of atmospheric oxygen, whereas a single bond oil like coconut oil is "molasses slow" in the presence of atmospheric oxygen. That is why coconut oil has ten to 20 times as long a natural shelf life as flax seed oil—and why flax seed oil needs to be refrigerated while coconut oil stores well at room temperature or higher.

Whether a fat is health promoting or disease producing is dramatically affected by how it is processed, stored, and used in the diet.

Hydrogenation, Margarine, and Deadly Trans-fats

Have you noticed that the mass market food industry has recently decreased the amount of animal fat in their products to make their products seem more healthy? Don't let that fool you. They have simply replaced them with something even more deadly—*hydrogenated* (or partially hydrogenated) vegetable oils.

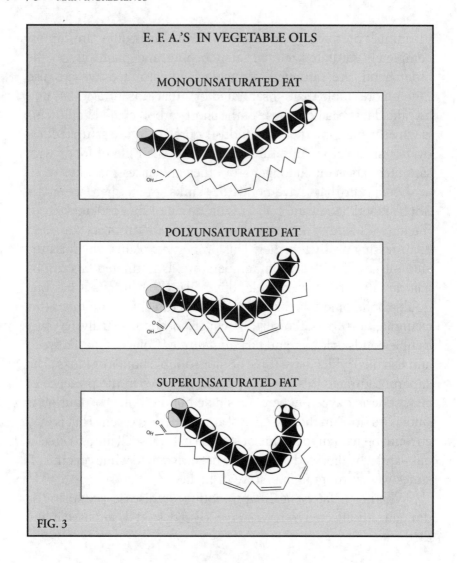

FIG. 3

Hydrogenated fats are highly processed industrial oils made by fusing hydrogen atoms into the fats' molecular structure, thereby disrupting the natural double or triple bonds that shape the molecule. This results in a highly uniform, totally dead (and deadly) food!

Fats from oilseed plant sources are naturally shaped in what is called a cis-isomer molecular structure, which means that it is shaped like a horse-shoe—curved with a steep rounded angle at the midpoint. This gives the molecule a springy quality and is what makes the cells more flexible, because the fatty acids in the cis-isomer configuration are very supple. This structure creates a fluid bend and makes this oil more biologically appropriate for human consumption. By heating natural fatty acids at temperatures of 500 degrees F. in large industrial vats for prolonged periods, and the addition of nickel powder catalysts to stimulate the chemical polymerization or plasticizing of the fatty acids with bubbling hydrogen gas, a 180 degree twist occurs in the molecules' shape, and injures the natural bond of the fat drastically. It dramatically changes its formerly beneficial biochemical properties. The synthetic or man-made version is called a trans-isomer, and consequently this "hardened oil" is called a *trans-fat*. It lacks the fluid kinks, which changes its physical properties from a liquid to a solid.

Trans-fats disrupt the body's metabolism, in part, *by altering the permeability of many cells in our body*. This syndrome is called "leaky gut" and is indicative of many auto-immune disorders. Being unnaturally made solid, trans-fats harden like lard when a cell membrane absorbs too many, causing the cell's permeability and biochemical structure to change. Altered permeability of their cells allows many viruses, toxins and parasites to invade more easily and prevents metabolic removal from the cell.

Dietary scientists have known this critical fact for 20 years yet haven't been overly concerned because they assume that the Standard American Diet (SAD) contains only three to four percent of calories as trans-fats. According to Dr. Mary Enig, a respected trans-fat biochemist at the University of Maryland, the actual amount may be four times higher. Animal studies have shown gross cell abnormalities with just a little over four percent of calories from trans-fat sources.

Human studies have shown increased elevations in the "bad" LDL cholesterol in only three weeks of eating a diet high in trans-fats. The amount of trans-fats in most Americans' diets is rising rapidly due to greater reliance on industrially processed food.

Reducing or eliminating trans-fats from the diet will increase the likelihood that the cell's fluid membranes will be able to transport and metabolize excess sugars, fats and toxins. Regular "cellular housekeeping" helps to keep our blood clean and prevents arterial degeneration and atherosclerosis.

Three recent studies clearly show the deadly effects of trans-fats. More than 85,000 female nurses were studied for eight years by researchers at the prestigious Harvard Medical School in Massachusetts. They tracked the correlation between trans-fat intake and heart disease. The women with the highest trans-fat intake had a 50 percent higher rate of heart attacks and coronary artery disease than those with more balanced diets.

A second study on fats and health was conducted at the Agricultural University in the Netherlands. Three groups of men and women with normal cholesterol were studied. Their diets were identical except for the type of fat consumed; the fats being tracked were saturated, trans-fat and polyunsaturated fats. After three weeks the saturated and trans-fat groups had elevated cholesterol levels. Their LDL cholesterol (the bad, artery clogging kind) rose while the 'good' HDL cholesterol levels fell. Trans-fats increased cholesterol to the same degree as saturated fats. This adverse effect didn't occur in the polyunsaturated group.

A third study conducted in Germany demonstrated the ill affects of saturated and trans-fats on premature infants. Results: the higher the level of trans-fats in the newborn's blood, the lower the birth weight and opportunity of survival.

As mentioned above, trans-fats—like partially hydrogenated soybean, safflower or even coconut oils—are generally solid at room temperature and melt to some degree at body temperature, while natural cis-fats—like unrefined, non-hydrogenated flax seed, safflower, sunflower and canola oils—remain liquid at room temperature and also at body temperature. Trans-fats, when consumed, remain sticky and are likely to clog our arteries. Our blood platelets and other blood cells also become sticky because the trans-fats become incorporated in the blood cell membranes.

Trans-fats also interfere with prostaglandin production (hormone-like regulators in the blood) because they tend to thicken the blood, causing added pressure on the cardiovascular system while at the same time weakening the very arterial walls that carry our blood supply. This weakness is caused by the lower quality of a trans-fat absorbed in the cells throughout the body which are stiffer, making the arterial walls more prone to plaque and easier to damage through thrombosis.

Trans-fat intake promotes ulcers, hypertension and many immune system dysfunctions. Trans-fats exacerbate already low essential fatty acid (EFA) levels, because they compete with the EFAs for absorption by the cells. They do this by clogging up the enzyme reactions that transform EFAs into highly unsaturated fatty acid derivatives. These highly unsaturated fatty acids are necessary for normal function of the brain, sense organs, testes and adrenals. *The detrimental effects of trans-fats include:*

- decreased testosterone production and increased abnormal sperm formation (as demonstrated in animals)
- complications during pregnancy
- correlation to low birth weight babies
- decreased quality of breast milk
- promotion of diabetes
- taxation of the liver's ability to process toxins and stress on the gallbladder
- alteration of the size, number and composition of human fat cells
- alteration of immune functions, promotion of cancer

Malefic Margarine and Other Menu Misadventures

Although trans-fats are usually man-made, some trans-fats do occur naturally in animal products, up to about 12 percent. Butter contains from two percent to 12 percent trans-fat—not a plus for sure, but the trans-fat in butter seems to be in a form that the body can break down and excrete. Margarine, on the other hand, is made from oils that were fluid at room temperature (such as oils like canola, corn, cottonseed, soybean and safflower) but which have been "traumatized" as described above in order to make them solid.

Depending on its type, margarine contains as much as 50 percent trans-fat. When you use margarine, the hardened fat is virtually pure saturated fat with a remnant percentage of trans-fat. In combination, these synthetic molecules are a deadly mixture over a dietary life span.

The detrimental effects of margarine are so well documented that the Dutch government banned the sale of margarines containing trans-fats. The head of Harvard School of Medicine, Dr. Walter Willet, says that over 30,000 American lives are needlessly lost each year to heart disease due to the harmful effects of margarine.

Both butter and margarine should be eliminated from your diet. I recommend, instead, a canola-oil product called Spectrum Spread. It has a similar taste to butter, stays solid enough to be spreadable, but is fluid in the body. Its has no trans-fats (it is not hydrogenated), is low in saturated fat (it's made from expeller-pressed canola oil), is low in sodium, and is made from a chemical-free canola oil.

The main sources of synthetic trans-fats are from margarine, shortening, processed animal products and any partially hydrogenated high-heat, cooked fats and oils like deep fried foods. (See Figure 4.) Most supermarket breads, cookies, crackers, chips and packaged foods are loaded with partially hydrogenated oils, a primary source of trans-fats. Trans-fat content does not appear on food labels because trans-fats are not officially classed by the FDA as saturated fat, so label reading becomes more difficult for health-minded consumers. Just remember to avoid all products with hydrogenated and partially hydrogenated oils as an ingredient.

We now know the detrimental effects of trans-fats on our cardiovascular system, immune system, reproductive system hormonal systems, metabolism, liver function and cell membranes. So why would we ever consume any margarines, shortenings, partially hydrogenated oil or any refined oils that are so obviously bad? (By the way, over 80 percent of the margarine companies are owned by tobacco companies, as reported by the Center for Science in the Public Interest in their *Survey of Margarine & Hard Yellow Fats, 1993.*)

TRANS- AND SATURATED FATS IN FOODS

TRANS-FAT	PRODUCT TYPE	SATURATED FAT
0%	Spectrum Spread	4.8%
51%	Corn Oil Margarine	13%
47%	Soybean Margarine	11%
42%	Safflower Margarine	6.4%
30.6%	"40% Reduced-Fat" Corn Oil Margarine	7.8%
6-25%	Partially Hydrogenated Soy Bean Salad Oil	14%
9%*	Lard	40.2%
0%*	Palm Oil—Refined	51%
9%*	Beef Tallow	36.9%
2-11%	Butter	60.2%
0%	Coconut Oil—Refined	92%

FIG. 4   * = Estimates

Fortunately, trans-fats are not found in the plant world: they do not occur in fruits, vegetables, nuts or seeds.

Average Trans-fat Composition of Foods

(Number in Parentheses Shows the Range)

Margarines	
Stick	31% (10 to 48%)
Tub	17% (5 to 44%)
Low Fat	(up to 18%)
Butter (Milk Fat)	15%
Vegetable Shortening	20% (up to 37%)
Salad Oils	(0 to 14%)
French Fries	(up to 37%)
Candy Bars	(up to 39%)
Bakery Products	(up to 34%)

The Free Radical Threat

While trans-fats are definitely injurious to our well-being, healthy oils can also be turned into toxic substances called *free radicals* by damage from air, heat, and light (see Chapter 5 on Flax Seed). Many of the oils available in stores are damaged by processing. Unfortunately, the potentially healthiest oils—unrefined cold pressed organic oils—are particularly susceptible to damage because these are the most biologically active. The more polyunsaturated the fat, the more likely it is to form free radicals if not properly protected.

Free radicals are unstable oxygen molecules that can disrupt cellular functioning, encourage tumor formation and accelerate the aging process. Free radicals have also been implicated in damage to arterial walls. Damage to arterial walls is probably the first step in arteriosclerosis and atheroma formation (a condition characterized by the deposit of fat in the inner linings of the arterial walls). The free radical causes an injury to the arterial wall cells and a cholesterol-laden plaque forms, acting like a bandage over the injury. Free radicals oxidize cholesterol and triglycerides to a more deadly artery clogging form. The combination tends to form stiff, hard arteries with reduced blood flow, exacerbating hypertension and other coronary related diseases. If this happens often enough, arteries will restrict blood flow and close off, causing strokes, heart attacks and vascular disease.

The body can slowly repair and unclog these vessels if chronic damage by free radicals is stopped or slowed down. Fortunately, free radicals can be neutralized by free radical scavengers (antioxidants) such as vitamin E, beta-carotene, vitamin C, selenium and hundreds of other antioxidants found in unrefined oils (especially low temperature, expeller-pressed wheat germ oil), fresh vegetables, fruits, whole grains, legumes and raw nuts and seeds.

Animal products are high in free radicals and almost totally deficient in antioxidants as the higher ordered species tend to suffer from the same biological stresses that humans do.

Health-Promoting Oils: Essential Fatty Acids

There are just two essential fatty acids: linoleic acid (LA) and alpha-linolenic acid (LNA). LA is also called omega-6 and LNA is also called omega-3. Consuming both in balance in our diets is very important to maintain long term health. It is estimated that about 60 percent of the population gets too much LA while 95 percent gets too little LNA. I discuss essential fatty acids in greater detail in Chapter 5 on Flax Seed.

LA is found in high proportions in vegetable oils like safflower oil (75 percent LA) and sunflower oil (65 percent LA). Consuming large amounts of refined polyunsaturated oils rich in processed LA fatty acids has been linked to increases in some types of cancer. Excess refined LA consumption without the proper balancing ratio of LNA oils tends to suppress immune function. So getting more of the LNAs and less of the LAs is the best plan for better health and longevity.

Most American diets are sadly deficient in LNA. LNA tends to be processed out of most fresh food. It is found in very high proportions in flax seed oil, which is by far the richest source found in nature. Flax seed oil is about 50 to 55 percent LNA, about five to ten times higher than most other available nut or seed oils. (See Chapter 5 on Flax Seed.) Other significant sources of LNA include canola oil at ten percent, soybean oil at five to seven percent, and walnut oil at three to 11 percent. Most other common oils have trace amounts or none. Many dark green leafy vegetables have a micro percentage of LNA but not enough for good health.

Gamma-linoleic acid (GLA) is another important super unsaturated fatty acid identical to LNA except for the position of one of its double bonds. Because of their similar molecular structure their health benefits are similar, although GLA is faster acting than LNA in alleviating some conditions like premenstrual syndrome (PMS) in females. GLA is a great supplement for a stressed body or anyone over 40. Our bodies don't always make enough GLA. People with liver problems, inflammatory diseases and PMS will experience tremendous benefits from GLA included with a sound nutritional program.

Dr. Zane Kime claims that skin cancer is promoted by a poor diet, particularly one high in refined oils and animal products. Recent research has tied skin cancer to a diet too high in refined LA fatty acids and substantially deficient in LNA fatty acids.

Another physician, Dr. Edward N. Siguel, author of *Essential Fatty Acids in Health and Disease,* states that cardiovascular disease and cancer can be prevented in many cases by controlling the balance of EFAs in our diet. Siguel claims that EFA deficiency is the genesis of heart attacks. Siguel also states that progressive EFA deficiency is the main contributing factor in heart failure in those who, over a 25 or more year span, chose diets too high in trans-fat and saturated fat at the expense of the LNAs and LAs.

Flax Seed Oil

One of the best nutritional oils for reversing the degenerative process is flax seed oil. I consider flax seed oil to be so sensational that I have given it a chapter of its own.

Wheat Germ Oil

I use wheat germ oil (Spectrum Naturals—see Resources) for its great taste and beneficial nutrients. It contains 50 percent LA and is one of the richest sources of vitamin E, octacosanol, and beta-sitosterin. Octacosanol is a 28-carbon fatty alcohol that is a potent source of immediate energy prized by competitive athletes. It also protects heart function and may help in nerve regeneration. Beta-sitosterin is a natural sterin which, like phytosterol, assists in the self-digestion of fats.

Because of its highly reactive nature, LA can form free radicals. Therefore vitamin E is needed to protect us from this damaging process. The vitamin E in wheat germ oil is a group of natural mixed tocopherols that are comprised of d-alpha, beta and gamma types, and not just d-alpha like most synthetically manufactured vitamin E. Beta and gamma tocopherols are also free radical scavengers that work in harmony with the fatty acids to regulate enzyme functions associated with free radical control.

Borage, Black Currant and Evening Primrose Oils

These oils are the primary sources of GLA which, as mentioned above, is a close cousin of the important LNA. These oils usually come in capsules and the oils are often contaminated with solvents used to extract the oil, or with pesticides used in growing the plant. I choose cold-pressed organic oils to avoid these problems. The only reason I prefer borage oil is because it has 24 percent GLA. Black currant contains up to 18 percent and evening primrose contains nine percent.

Our bodies can make GLA from LA if conversion isn't blocked. Conversion of LA to GLA can be blocked by eating any of the unhealthy fats or refined vegetable oils previously mentioned. Dietary deficiencies, high sugar consumption, viral infections, diabetes and just plain aging can also block conversion. Consuming GLA will bypass this blockage but that is not a reason to continue with an unhealthy diet. About 20 percent of the population is missing the enzyme conversion synthesis to make GLA from LNA. So if you are getting little improvement from LNA, you will need to increase your intake of borage oil.

Olive Oil

In 1958, Dr. Ancel Keys headed an international team of scientists that set out to discover the causes of heart disease. The evidence at the time seemed to implicate fat as the major cause. Keys and his wife traveled through Europe and Africa measuring cholesterol levels. Their most significant finding was that affluent people, who ate more meat and dairy products, were more likely to have high cholesterol and suffer heart attacks than poor people.

Another piece of supportive evidence was that, during World War II, heart disease plummeted in countries with shortages of meat and dairy products. In Holland, Belgium, Denmark and

Luxembourg, civilian populations were denied their normal intake of dairy foods. Diets were largely vegetarian and grain-based during this time, with caloric levels reduced to 25 to 60 percent of previous levels. Although trauma rates were exponential due to the war casualties, cancer and heart disease rates plummeted (*Morbidity & Mortality*, 1966).

Starting in the late 1950s, Keys and his research team studied 12,000 healthy middle aged men from seven countries for 20 years. They discovered that the highest incidence of heart disease (28 percent) was in Finland. The Finns ate 24 percent of their calories from saturated fat (mostly dairy products).

The lowest rate of heart disease, however, didn't go to the Japanese who had the lowest fat intake, but to the men living on the island of Crete. The Japanese had only nine percent of their calories from fat and only three percent from saturated fat. The Japanese heart disease rate was low (five percent), yet not nearly as low as that of the 655 men studied from the Greek isle of Crete. After ten years, only two percent of the Cretan men developed heart disease and none of them died. Amazingly, the men from Crete had consumed about as much total fat as the Finns. Their saturated fat intake was eight percent—almost twice that of the Japanese. However, the Cretan diet was low in meat and dairy products; it consisted of beans, fresh fruits and vegetables, with over half of the calories coming from whole grain bread and olive oil. The key differential here is the high consumption of chlorophyll-rich olive oil, which is high in monounsaturated fatty acids.

Another health benefit of olive oil is superior blood sugar control. Four independent medical research centers studied 42 non-insulin dependent diabetics. Half of the group ate a diet with the traditional 55 percent of calories from carbohydrates and 30 percent from fat. The other half ate only 40 percent of calories from carbohydrates and a whopping 45 percent from fat, with mono-unsaturated olive oil as the predominant fat. The low-carb, high-mono diet resulted in better diabetic control—lower day-long blood levels of glucose, insulin and triglycerides. These benefits persisted throughout the 14 week study. Cholesterol and blood lipid levels were not increased.

Olive oil seems to protect against heart disease and is associated with low cancer incidence and overall good health.

"Refined" Means Not-So-Fine

Refining an oil takes away its natural flavors and compromises many of the nutrients, such as phospholipid (helps emulsify fat in the body), lecithin (makes oils easier to digest), carotene (anti-cancer compounds), tocopherols (anti-oxidants, free radical scavengers), and EFAs (essential fatty acids which assist in cellular integrity).

Olive oil is high in monounsaturated and polyunsaturated fatty acids that protect our body's cells from mutation, but only if it is marked as either virgin or extra virgin olive oil. "Extra virgin" simply implies that it is the first oil pressed out of the olive, as opposed to later pressings. But because the liquid constituents of olives are typically 25 percent oil and 25 percent water, what forms is a paste. The oil residue must be centrifuged or decanted to release the oil from the water. The oil separation process is called "extra-virgin," simply another marketing gimmick to differentiate an oil. Therefore, virgin or extra-virgin olive oils are the only mass marketed oils that have not been heated above 150° C (302° F). Oils heated higher than this not only lose their nutritional benefits, but they become nutritionally damaging.

Refined oils are heated to much higher temperatures. In the refining process, poisonous solvents (such as hexane, a cousin to gasoline) may be used to extract the oil left behind after pressing. In addition, phosphoric acid (an extremely caustic chemical) may be used to degum the oil—which removes several health-promoting substances such as lecithin, chlorophyll and several trace minerals. The oils may then be bleached and deodorized with other solvent chemicals and heated up to 270° C (518° F) for 30 to 60 minutes. Fully refined olive oil loses over 100 volatile compounds that give olive oil its unique flavor and aroma. It is the lowest grade of olive oil. The final product of all this is a mutated oil stripped of all its healthy components and the nutritional integrity of the EFAs. All refined oils are severely damaged.

Beware of the term "pure" olive oil on the label! "Pure" olive oil is a fully refined solvent-extracted low-grade oil.

I recommend choosing organic oils whenever possible. Oils from Spectrum Naturals, which are available in health food stores, are top quality. Organic oils are pesticide-free and unrefined and make a better overall choice for healthier eating. The bottom line on buying healthy oils is to get organically grown, cold or mechanically pressed oils that are protected from light, air and heat.

Cooking: Go Low & Slow

Cooking is an art, and unfortunately all good art requires time and attention to become a masterpiece. High cooking temperature destroys the healthy properties of biologically intact oils. The more unsaturated the bonds of the oil and the higher the ratio of essential fatty acids (EFAs), the greater the polymerization (or plasticizing) of the oil. Your frying pan when used on the high heat setting becomes a mini-refinery. If you start burning the oil, (i.e., smoking it or having it pop and fizzle with smoke emerging) you have a free-radical factory in your frying pan.

High temperatures create ketones, aldehydes and tri-terpine alcohol—which all break down to products which can become carcinogens. In addition there are deadly dienes, trienes (newly discovered—you'll be hearing more about these in the coming years) and other destructive compounds created, plus dozens of other post-oxidation products which can be just as detrimental as trans-fat. Oils that have underdone thermal conversion at 215° C (410° F) for 15 minutes or more have been implicated in the formation of atherosclerosis when fed to lab animals in research experiments. High heat cooking becomes an unhealthy culinary practice when we abuse a delicate oil.

Our bodies can cope with an occasional dose of a toxic substance like a trans-fat. But over a period of ten, 20, or 30 years these toxic and unnatural substances accumulate and interfere with the normal biological chemistry of our bodies. These corrupted materials create corrupted organs and muscles. Cells lose their DNA reproductive integrity, leading to degenerative disease and rapid aging.

I do not recommend frying not only because of the fat damage but also because it can turn proteins into carcinogens such as acrolein. Frying also destroys much of the nutritional value of all foods. In Udo Erasmus' book *Fats That Heal, Fats That Kill,* he recommends (if you really insist upon frying foods) using naturally occurring saturated fats like those of the least processed tropical oil (coconut). There are new varieties of high-oleic oils (super-canola), hybrids which also take heat quite well.

If you must fry, use these oils in limited amounts. Although refined saturated fats are very unhealthy, they are at the same time much less reactive and form fewer toxic fats when heated at high temperatures. Damage occurs rapidly to unsaturated fats and even more rapidly to essential fatty acids (EFAs) which tolerate heat quite poorly.

Most fast food and other restaurants deep fry foods in hydrogenated vegetable oils that have been kept at high temperatures, often for days.

Instead of frying, I like to take traditional stir-fry vegetables and steam them for a few minutes. I then add flax seed oil that has had garlic pressed into it and allow the vegetables to marinate for about 15 minutes. Another "healthier" way of frying is to stir-fry with small amounts of water, adding a little oil later on. Keeping some water in with the oil keeps the temperature down to 100° C (212° F), which is a non-destructive temperature. Food will retain more nutrients and taste better using this innovative method. For good results, I recommend organic canola or virgin olive oil for this lower temperature method.

The simple technique of boiling food in water doesn't damage even the most sensitive EFA rich oils. Baking, on the other hand, does damage sensitive oils on the outside of baked goods such as the crust of bread. However, the majority of the oil in the center of the loaf does not get destroyed, because the center of a cooked loaf of bread or cake is essentially steamed by the baking action. If you don't use non-stick pans, then use tropical oils (coconut) or try lecithin to prevent sticking. The small amount recommended should not harmfully affect your overall dietary intake.

The more saturated or damaged oils you consume, the more antioxidants you need in your diet to neutralize the production of excess free radicals that are formed by consuming these oils. (See Chapters 2 and 5 on Nutrition and Flax Seed for more information.) If you eat a lot of commercial cookies, crackers, baked goods, candies, or some sweets like chocolate, you need to increase consumption of both EFAs and antioxidants. Antioxidants are especially found in vitamin E oil (from wheat germ), vitamin C, vitamin A, beta-carotene, and selenium.

Hundreds of independent research studies have shown the disease producing effects of animal fats, trans-fats and too much refined LA fatty acids. Research has also demonstrated the disease fighting effects of the unrefined LNA fatty acids.

Fats and oils are a sharp, double-edged sword in your nutritional arsenal: valuable but requiring careful handling. It is well worth your while to understand them. You now have the basic knowledge to improve your health. It is up to you to choose health one tablespoon at a time.

FIVE

Flax Seed
Nature's Miracle Medicine

T he value of flax, one of the wonder grains of the world, will be "newly discovered" by researchers in the next few years. But their work will simply confirm and give better scientific explanations for its curative properties, which have been known since antiquity.
— **Udo Erasmus**

With its rich satin brown hues, smooth and almond shaped, the tiny flax seed is a surprise miracle factory of healing substances. Often referred to as "nutritional gold," flax seed is rapidly becoming a wonder grain of health. It has the potential to heal and prevent cardiovascular disease, cancer, diabetes and many other degenerative conditions, as well as to improve skin and vitality.

Its history is as rich as its medicinal benefits. For more than 7,000 years, flax seed (also known industrially as linseed) has been consumed by humankind. The main foods mentioned in the Bible are flax, wheat, barley, corn, wine and manna—flax being referred to most often. It is one of the oldest known cultivated plants and certainly one of the most useful, for not only is the seed a first class food, but flax fiber makes a first class cloth—linen.

According to archaeological authorities, flax fiber was used by Stone Age people for constructing ropes and fish nets, and the flax seed was used for food. Flax was cultivated in Babylon in 5000 B.C. As early as around 3000 B.C. ancient Egyptians used it to make linen mummy wrappings; the oil was used as a cosmetic and applied to wall paintings for the tombs and temples. Greek and Roman writings dating back to 650 B.C. reveal some of the healing properties attributed to flax. In the fifth century B.C., Hippocrates wrote about using flax to relieve inflamed mucous membranes and for relieving abdominal pains and diarrhea. Flax was also historically used in hot compresses to treat both external and internal ailments. Ancient East Indian scriptures state that a yogi must eat flax daily in order to reach the highest state of contentment and joy. More recently, Mahatma Gandhi observed: "Whenever flax seed becomes a regular food item among the people, there will be better health." In Vedic medicine, flax is considered a "cooling" oil— reducing inflammation.

Until recently, in the West you were more likely to find flax derivatives in your house paint, linoleum floors, and bed linens than on your dinner plate. The English word "linoleum" from the combined words 'linseed' and 'oleum' (meaning "oil-of-the-linseed") illustrates its use as a polymerized vegetable veneer when applied to and cured upon coarse linen fabric or jute cloth. This invention made up the popular linoleum tile material found in many early American kitchens. The word "linen" comes from the Dutch and German root word meaning fiber or stem of the flax plant. As a result when we say linens we really mean cloth made from flax. The world's finest linens still come form Ireland and Belgium where exquisite linen lace is hand shaped.

Today edible flax seed is being rediscovered for its abundant healing properties. Flax seed and its healing oil are being hailed as the latest cure in the fight against cancer and coronary heart disease by plant biochemists and health researchers.

What makes this plant so salutary? Why do I consider the facts on flax worth a chapter of its own? During the last decade research scientists have uncovered components of the flax seed which offer extraordinary nutritional advantages. A real powerhouse, this seed packs a quadruple whammy: (1) a high-dose of LNA (omega-3) fatty acids, a healthy fat which helps lower cholesterol, (2) a proper ratio of LNA to LA (omega-6) fatty acids, (3) fiber, especially cholesterol-lowering soluble fiber, and (4) lignans, a kind of fiber that is looking more and more like a potent blocker of some kinds of cancer. All this and it tastes good, too. It's hard to believe that flax is full of fat and still good for you.

Let's look more closely at flax and its highly regarded nutritional components. Flax is an annual plant with small green leaves and delicate blue flowers. Its Latin name is *Linum usitatissimum*, meaning "the most useful." This miracle grain is truly one of the most nutritionally complete foods ever studied. Flax seed is a top quality food because it contains most of what makes a complete diet. According to Udo Erasmus in his book *Fats That Heal, Fats That Kill*, the components of flax are used to treat many ailments which wouldn't occur if flax seed were a regular part of the diet.

What Flax Seed Offers

Protein: Flax seeds contain high-quality, easily digestible protein with all the amino acids (the building blocks of protein) essential to health. This means that it is a complete protein. These essential amino acids are leucine, isoleucine, lysine, valine, threonine, methionine, phyenylalanine, and tryptophan. Flax seed also contains histidine and arginine which are amino acids essential for infants. When all of the essential amino acids are supplied, our body can manufacture from them the other dozen amino acids required to make proteins. Complete proteins are essential for building muscles, blood, skin, hair, nails and internal organs, including the heart and the brain.

Complex Carbohydrates: Flax seed provides instant calories for energy and assists in digestion and regulation of protein and fat metabolism.

Fiber: Flax seed is an excellent source of both soluble and insoluble fiber and keeps the digestive tract from becoming clogged with mucus. Fiber helps to keep everything moving, maintains healthy intestinal flora and helps to keep the colon clean. It also helps to keep cholesterol and bile acids from being re-absorbed into the body though the intestinal walls. Bile acids are produced when foods progress into the small intestine. The gall bladder secretes bile acids to assist in breaking down fats in the foods. Bile is actually produced in the liver and concentrates in the gall bladder as a dietary fat emulsifier. Bile is rich in enzymes that break apart triglycerides. A healthy person's bile excretion will absorb 95 percent of fat consumed. However, as liver and gallbladder efficiency are taxed from too much fat, wear and tear on these organs takes place. Fiber from flax helps in binding excess fats and allowing their excretion into the large intestine and ultimate expulsion from the body, according to Elson Haas in *Staying Healthy with Nutrition.*

Mucilage: Structurally, mucilage resembles hemicellulose (the most popular source is oat bran), but it is not classed as such due to its unique location in the seed portion of the plant. It is generally found within the inner layer (endosperm) of the plant seeds, where it retains water to prevent the seed from drying. Mucilage is a thick gum found in many plants, especially flax seed (12 to 15 percent of volume), which makes flax seed one of the best natural laxatives available. Like the pectin found in apples, mucilage in flax is important in maintaining bowel regularity. Due to the presence of essential fatty acids in the mucilage, it tends to soothe and protect the delicate stomach and intestinal linings and keeps the contents moving progressively along.

One of the most highly respected natural healers, Bernard Jensen, D.C., reveals that many degenerative diseases start in the colon through the toxic effects of constipation and poor peristaltic action of the colon muscle. When flax seed (oil and ground meal) is taken with fluids, the mucilage assists in alleviating constipation, increasing stool bulk and softness, and speeding up transit time (hastens the movement of stool out of the body). All this helps prevent toxic buildup in our bowel. As a result, the stools smell less foul, breath freshens, and there is less stress on the liver and eliminative organs, including the kidneys and skin. You can chew flax seed, although sometimes the small seeds can get stuck in your teeth. I prefer the oil and ground meal.

Flax mucilage also has the ability to buffer excess acid in sensitive stomachs and helps to stabilize blood glucose due to its absorptive properties. Insulin production is thus more stabilized as the pancreas is not force-cycled through dramatic highs and lows of excess sugars in the diet and the resulting overage/shortage of blood saturated/starved glucose levels between snacks or meals. Sufficient quality fiber from foods such as flax retards the cycles of sugar highs and lows frequently associated with such progressive diseases as hypoglycemia and late-onset adult diabetes, both of which have a defective glucose metabolic factor.

Minerals: Flax seed contains most known major and trace minerals—phosphorous, magnesium, potassium, calcium, sulfur, sodium, chlorine, zinc, iron and adequate trace amounts of manganese, silicon, copper, fluorine, nickel, cobalt, iodine, molybdenum, and chromium.

Vitamins: Flax seed contains fat-soluble vitamins E and carotene, and water-soluble vitamins B1, B2, and C. The tocopherol compounds found in vitamin E act as antioxidants in the body (see Chapters 2 and 4 on Nutrition and Fat for more information), protecting other molecules and cell components from damaging reactions with oxygen. Vitamin E is an antioxidant substance which works as a synergistic ally with vitamin A and vitamin C and as a regulator of cell respiration. Flax is particularly high in minerals and vitamin co-factors.

Lignins and Lignans: Unlike many other plant fibers, flax seed is high in *lignan* and *lignin*. Lignin is an insoluble fiber which our bodies convert to several kinds of *lignans*. Flax seed is the richest known source of lignans, containing 100 as much as the next best source—wheat bran. While all vegetables provide lignin precursors to some degree, flax provides much more, about 800 micrograms per gram, as compared to only eight micrograms per gram in common fiber such as bran. Lignans have only recently attracted the attention of researchers. They have been found to be useful in treating viral, bacterial and fungal infections as well as cancer. In fact, high levels of lignans in the bowel are associated with reduced rates of colon and breast cancer.

The lignans formed from flax are "pseudo-estrogens" that block estrogen receptors in the body. The molecular shape of the lignans are such that they bind with the estrogen receptors in the body, thus "smoothing out" the hormonal and metabolic effect of estrogen release in the body. Over-production of estrogen can stimulate colon and other forms of cancer. Thirty to 50 percent of all malignant colon tumors contain numerous estrogen receptors. It is also significant to note that the rates of colon cancer tend to correlate with those of breast cancer, and that both seem to be high in people with low-fiber diets.

Studies reveal that lignans resemble estrogens and attach to estrogen receptors in the body, but do not have the tumor-stimulating effect of hormonal estrogen. Hormonally induced syndromes, like hot flashes or elevated body temperature, are slightly mitigated by these lignans and lignins. Further, research shows that lignans derived from flax also work to reduce levels of unbound estrogens in the blood, which explains how they can also help prevent breast cancer. Perhaps the presence of lignans, derived from plant fiber, may be one of the main reasons why vegetarians have substantially lower cancer rates than meat eaters.

Essential Fatty Acids (EFAs): EFAs are part of every cell in our bodies, where they play important roles in maintaining the structure of the cells and in producing energy. Our glands need EFAs to carry out the minute secretion of hormones and other biological regulating substances. In our muscles, EFAs help the cells to recover from use and abuse. In addition to fulfilling these basic roles, the EFAs are critical to infants' pre-natal and post-natal development, especially brain development, and for growth spurts throughout childhood.

Our bodies do a remarkable job of creating most of the nutrients we need from the resident cell materials on hand, except in some cases. The nutrients our bodies can't synthesize are called the essential nutrients, and these we must make sure are adequately supplied in our diets. Of the 45 essential nutrients, two are fatty acids: called LNA (alpha-linolenic acid or omega-3) and LA (linoleic acid or omega-6). Besides being an excellent source of the essential LNA fatty acids, flax seed also contains important trace nutrients such as phospholipids, phytosterols, and beta-sitosterin. These naturally occurring compounds assist in the digestion of fats and are just beginning to be recognized for their immune-enhancing properties.

The Modern Diet and LNA Deficiency

In the past 100 years, modern food processing developments have drastically reduced the nutrient value, including the LNA content, of many of the foods we eat. Processing and refining is usually undertaken to stabilize the fragile nutrient substances in foods. To preserve foods from spoilage, fresh foods are sterilized, partially denatured and chemically retarded. Although this extends shelf life, it reduces the life-giving energy in these packaged, bottled, canned or freeze-dried foods. Modern culture has taught us to accept such sub-foods, which are in fact frequently a health detriment over the long run. In his book *The Omega-3 Phenomenon,* Dr. Donald O. Rudin explains that modern food processing and food selection opportunities severely distort the availability of many essential nutrients—especially limiting the LNA essential fatty acids. Whenever high heat and caustic agents are used to sterilize food, the incidence of peculiarly twentieth century diseases such as cancer, heart disease and arthritis skyrockets. Heart disease and many cancers are linked to distortions of dietary fats. Dr. Rudin calls LNA "the nutritional missing link" and attributes its profound absence in most foods to the cause of many degenerative conditions.

For the body to stay healthy, we must have a proper balance of LNA and LA fatty acids in our diets. For example, when your body is homeostatic (balanced in health), you receive pain messages only when you've experienced real injury or when blood clots form at the initial phase of wound healing. Without such homeostatic balance, the LA's (when consumed to excess and in absence of LNAs) can produce pain messages in the brain for no reason or form an unwanted clot spontaneously.

Most Americans who eat highly refined and processed foods, such as regular patrons of fast food restaurants, get excess amounts of refined LA's and insufficient amounts of unrefined LNA fatty acids. The hamburger cooks and fish fryers of fast food restaurants usually cook with highly refined, unstable polyunsaturated oils such as corn, sunflower, safflower, and soy oils. These oils are very highly concentrated with LA fatty acids and deadly trans-fats (see Chapter 4 on fats for more information on trans-fats). Studies have shown trans-fats to be worse than saturated fat. The physiology of fast food consumers remains in a perpetual state of fatty acid imbalance. Consequently, they are more predisposed to degenerative diseases such as heart attacks, cancer, arthritis, stroke, kidney impairment, liver disease, auto-immune disorders and skin disorders.

According to Udo Erasmus, a highly regarded lipid (fat) scientist, North Americans typically consume only about 25 percent of the quantity of LNAs needed for optimal health. He suggests an intake of LNAs equivalent to about two percent of total calories, or about 14 grams per day. *Flax seed is by far the most potent natural source of LNAs.*

Comparison of LNA Sources

Percentage of LNA Fatty Acid by Total Weight of Seeds	
Flax seed	57%
Chia seed	30%
Hemp seed oil	15%
Pumpkin seed	15%
Canola oil	10%
Soy bean oil	8%
Walnut	5%
Fresh leafy vegetables (average serving)	0.009%

Fish oils have been touted for the "heart saving" LNA fatty acids found in the flesh of deep-sea fish such as salmon and mackerel. But what are these animals doing with so much plant-derived essential fatty acids in their fat? They obtain them from the algae and plankton that comprise the foundation of the ocean's food chain. Unfortunately, research shows that along with a concentration of LNA, fish also concentrate in their bodies traces of pesticides, heavy metals and other industrial pollutants such as PCBs. According to Ralph Nader and other respected environmental activists, even our deep-sea waters are now polluted, and the fish store the pollutants in their livers and fatty tissues. Organic flax seed contains no such toxic residues.

The Proven Benefits of LNA

In the last ten years a plethora of scientific studies have been released on flax seed and its oil. At a recent conference held at the Flax Institute of the United States in Fargo, North Dakota, scientists focused attention on flax seed and its role in healing and preventing numerous degenerative diseases. In fact, it was reported that LNA deficiencies contribute to many conditions and may be the ultimate cause of many wide-spread degenerative diseases. At this same conference, a report from Canada's Department of Health and Welfare (comparable to U.S. Food & Drug Administration) dispelled any fears about flax seed's possible toxicity.

Research and clinical experience demonstrate the following benefits from regular consumption of flax seed:

1. Cancers. For over thirty-five years, German lipid researcher Johanna Budwig has been using flax seed oil successfully in cancer therapy. She has more than 1,000 documented cases of successful cancer treatment with flax seed oil as the main treatment. In his New York City clinic, the now-deceased Dr. Max Gerson used fresh flax seed oil as the principal cancer fighting agent. Nobel humanitarian Dr. Albert Schweitzer wrote of Dr. Gerson: "I see in Dr. Max Gerson one of the world's most eminent medical geniuses."

More recent research shows that LNAs kill human cancer cells in tissue culture without harming the normal cells. Breast, lung and prostate cancer cell lines were studied. As mentioned above, research evidence suggests that lignans may fight off chemicals responsible for initiating tumors, and block estrogen receptors which may reduce colon cancer risk. And according to Dr. James Duke of the U. S. Department of Agriculture, flax seed contains 27 identifiable cancer preventive compounds. Additional studies show that LNAs inhibit tumor formation (smaller tumors, less metastasis, longer survival time). The National Cancer Institute is currently researching flax seed for its potential ability to prevent cancer.

2. Heart Disease. Dr. Gerson also treated heart patients with flax, using fresh organic flax seed oil for its cholesterol-lowering ability. LNAs lowered blood cholesterol and triglyceride levels an average of 25 percent, and this treatment lowered the triglyceride levels of some patients as much as 65 percent.

One of the unique features of flax seed oil is that it contains a substance which resembles prostaglandins, which may well be part of its potent therapeutic value. The prostaglandins regulate blood pressure and arterial function, and have an important role in calcium and energy metabolism. No other vegetable oil examined so far matches this property of flax seed oil.

At the Department of Clinical Chemistry in Denmark, Professor H. O. Bang conducted studies on cardiovascular stress in populations with diets high in animal fat. Interestingly, populations like those of the Greenland Eskimos, who consumed diets high in LNAs derived from ocean fish and northern cetaceans (whales & sea mammals), had only three cases of heart trouble among a population of 2,400 people over four years of study. Two of those cases involved people over 78 years old, and the other case was complicated with rheumatic fever.

It's interesting that some studies have suggested that high fat intake is a cancer risk, but Greenland Eskimos have a high total fat intake and relatively low rates of cancer. They also have a very low incidence of ischemic heart disease (the leading cause of death in the industrialized world), attributed to their diet which contains high levels of LNAs. This suggests that the prevention of cancer and heart disease is less related to the quantity of dietary fat and more related to the *quality* of fat.

Further studies showed that when Greenland Eskimos moved to Denmark and adopted the Danish diet, which includes significant saturated fat, they experienced a higher heart attack rate, even though the total caloric fat content of their diet decreased. Although the Eskimo people did not consume flax, they did consume large amounts of LNA fatty acids present in northern species of fish and sea mammals like seals and walrus. Prof. Bang concluded that the relative deficiency of essential fatty acids common in Western diets plays an important part in the causation of atherosclerosis, diabetes, hypertension, and certain forms of malignant diseases.

It was further revealed that Greenland Eskimos of all age groups and both sexes had levels of total cholesterol and 'bad' LDL cholesterol that were significantly lower, and levels of 'good' HDL cholesterol that were higher, than when they lived among Danes. In other words, even though the Eskimo diet is higher in fat, their intake of LNAs was much higher and their blood lipid (fat) levels were healthier.

Similarly, LNAs blood regulating capabilities prevent spontaneous blood clots caused by an excess of LA fatty acids. This has implications for preventing strokes, if used at an early enough stage in a remedial lifestyle change using both exercise and improved diet.

3. Diabetes. Late-onset adult diabetes is suspected to originate partially from a deficiency of LNAs and an excess of saturated and trans-fats in the diet. Although this syndrome can take as long as 30 years to emerge as a full blown disease, reversal of symptoms can occur with positive changes in the diet and proper supplementation of LNAs from flax seed oil. A concurrent lack of vitamins and minerals makes the disease worse. LNAs may also lower the insulin requirement of diabetics.

4. Inflammatory Tissue Conditions. LNA fatty acids decrease inflammatory conditions of all types—a confirmation of ancient Vedic medicine mentioned above that considers flax a "cooling" agent. Inflammatory conditions are the diseases that end in "itis," including bursitis, tendinitis, tonsillitis, gastritis, ileitis, colitis, meningitis, arthritis, phlebitis, prostatitis, nephritis, splenitis, hepatitis, pancreatitis, otitis, etc., as well as lupus. Many of these inflammatory conditions may be eased by use of LNAs.

5. Skin Conditions. Pedigree show animals are fed linseed oil, made from flax seed, to keep their coats glossy. Along the same lines, recent research has shown that skin conditions in humans, such as psoriasis and eczema, have improved dramatically when flax seed and flax seed oil was added to the diet. These skin conditions exacerbate from lack of LNAs in the diet. You will see that your skin gets smoother, softer and velvety from taking flax seed oil *regularly* in your diet. It's also helpful for treating dry skin, dandruff, and sun-sensitive skin.

6. Sexual Disorders. Dr. Budwig has found flax seed oil to be a natural aphrodisiac. The most common physical cause of impotency in men and non-orgasmic response in women is block-age of blood flow in the arteries of the pelvis. Decrease of blood flow prevents full expansion (erection) of the penis and/or the clitoris. Thus ejaculation and/or orgasm cannot occur. The solution is to unblock narrowed arteries in general, and the consumption of flax seed oil will help. Flax seed oil is quickly gaining a reputation as one of the best aphrodisiacs of the 90s.

7. **Calmness Under Stress.** Many people find increased calm-ness to be the most profound effect of using fresh flax seed oil. It brings on a feeling of calmness often within a few hours. This may be partly due to that fact that, under stress, LNA fatty acids appear to slow down the over production of stressing biochemicals like arachidonic acid.

The "fight or flight" stress response is mitigated by the LNAs which compete against the "arachidonic acid cascade" which hap-pens when we are chronically stressed. Arachidonic acid in our blood thickens the blood platelets in anticipation of wounding and bleeding which is an ancient natural defense mechanism. The LNA fatty acids keep these in check.

8. **Water Retention.** The LNA and LA fatty acids in flax seed oil help the kidneys excrete sodium and water. Water retention (edema) accompanies swollen ankles, some forms of obesity, PMS, and all stages of cancer and cardiovascular disease.

9. **Vitality and Athletic Ability.** One of the most noticeable signs of improved health from the use of flax seed oil is progressive and increased vitality and energy. Athletes notice that their fatigued muscles recover from exercise more quickly. LNAs also increase stamina. Flax does have a "cooling" effect on inflammatory condi-tions, but it also generates a healing "heat energy" in the body due to the fact that the fatty acids are burned up for energy production. Its vital energy is enormous and is attributed to the triple bonds in the flax molecules which make them very receptive to other bio-chemicals, speeding up biochemical processes like metabolism. In simple terms, flax increases metabolic rate and the efficiency of cellular energy production. It stimulates respiratory and cellular oxidation, by which energy is produced which we experience as warmth. For athletes, or anyone wishing to reduce fat and create a

fit, lean body, this is great news! As discussed in Chapter 4 on Fats and Oils, flax seed oil is a healthy fat that doesn't make you fat. Adding flax seed to your diet will enhance all life processes, because all our life processes depend on energy production.

10. Other Conditions. LNAs are necessary for visual function (retina), adrenal function (stress), and sperm formation. They often improve symptoms of multiple sclerosis. In fact, when LNA consumption is high, MS is rare. Flax seed oil can also be helpful in cystic fibrosis (LNA helps loosen viscous secretions and relieves breathing difficulties); some cases of sterility and miscarriage; some glandular malfunctions; some behavioral problems (schizophrenia, depression, bipolar disorder); allergies; addictions (to drugs or alcohol); and some deviant behaviors, according to Udo Erasmus, in *Fats That Heal: Fats That Kill.*

When to Expect Benefits from LNA Supplements

From the excellent book by Dr. Donald Rudin and Clara Felix, *The Omega-3 Phenomena*, some remarkable facts are brought forth not only about clinical results from ingesting a significant daily level of LNA, but also the length of time usually required before results are noticed. This landmark book reveals the scientific evidence from Dr. Rudin's research with 44 patients over a period of several years, showing how the critical LNA fatty oils profoundly affect a broad range of contemporary health problems, including those of the heart and arteries, the brain, the emotions and general body functions. The general consensus from clinicians and researchers indicates that about 14 grams of combined LNA fatty acid and LA fatty acid per day is optimum. This equates to 8.5 grams of LNA per 100 pounds of body weight and 4.5 grams of LA per 100 pounds of body weight per day. Ideally this should be consumed in equal portions before each meal. Thus a pre-meal ratio would ideally be about 4.7 grams per 100 pounds. This is about one teaspoon before meals.

The following charts excerpted from Dr. Rudin and Clara Felix's forthcoming book, *The Omega-3 Phenomenon*, were typical periods of time in which human subjects of the pilot study noted beneficial effects of the LNA flax seed supplements. You'll see that a long wait is not always necessary before results are visible.

Time After Taking Oil Supplement	Reaction
2 hours	Mood improved, feeling of calm • Depression relieved
2-7 days	Skin smoother, with less flaking and scaling • Backs of hands and fingers smoother
2-14 days	Fewer hallucinations • Relief for disturbed mental patients • Relief from feelings of anxiety
2-6 weeks	Osteoarthritis relieved, with easier movements and less inflammation and pain • Bursitis and other soft-tissue inflammations reduced • Tinnitus and noises in the ears subside • Dandruff and flaking of the scalp less noticeable • Dry skin alleviated
2-4 months	Rheumatoid pain diminished • "Easy bruising" reduced • Choking spasms subside • Fewer muscular spasms • No nighttime leg cramps • Relief from ocular spasms • Relief from itching and burning sensations • Improved skin color • Reduced sun sensitivity
3-6 months	Diminished food allergies • Healing of chronic infections • Disappearance of rough, bumpy skin on upper arms • Improved alcohol tolerance • Improved cold tolerance • Lessening of fatigue • Overall increased calm and feeling of well-being on a more consistent basis as supplementation is maintained and fully incorporated into the diet.

As you can see from this table, the response time can vary from hours to months. Improvement in some cases can continue for up to one to two years before leveling off. Allergies often require a long time for improvement. Nothing is guaranteed, because each person's makeup is so individual. Persistent emotional or physical problems may improve only after several months, if at all.

Here's another summary of the benefits of LNA supplementation from *The Omega 3 Phenomenon*.

Benefits of the Omega Program

Biochemical Effect	Clinical Result
Normalizes the body's fatty acids	Smoother skin, shiny hair, soft hands • Increased stamina, vitality, agility, and a zest for life
Normalizes and rebalances prostaglandin	Smoother muscle action • Improvement of many other functions
Reduces appetite provocation	Eliminates binging or addictive need for food
Stabilizes insulin and blood sugar levels	Keeps stamina high for long periods
Strengthens the immune system	Avoids or overcomes food allergies • Fights off some diseases more effectively
Increases fiber and aerobic bacteria	Promotes proper function of the digestive tract to avoid gas, constipation, and other disorders
Normalizes blood fats and lowers cholesterol	Stronger cardiovascular system • Clear thinking
Corrects the body's thermogenic-system (ability to burn off calories)	Burns off fat • Increases cold-weather resistance • Increases comfort
Brings enjoyment of total good health	Improved quality of life

The Delicate Flax Seed Oil

Producing an oil from flax seed without damaging or destroying the vital LNA is no simple task. Erasmus summarized the challenge in his book *Fats That Heal, Fats That Kill* this way, "As essential as linoleic (LA) and alpha-linolenic acids (LNA) are to our health, they are also very temperamental and easily destroyed by light, air and heat. For this reason, care must be taken in processing, packaging, and storing oils containing EFAs. In nature, these oils are packaged in seeds in a way that keeps light, air, and heat out. In the seed, oils can sometimes be kept up to several years without spoiling."

He goes on to state that "when the oil is extracted from such seeds, care must be taken to make sure that light, heat, and air are kept out of the oil from before pressing, until the oil is consumed;

but to set such conditions is expensive and such care is not usually taken."

It was the knowledge that extraordinary precautions were necessary to produce an oil rich in LNA fatty acids that inspired the Spectrum Naturals company to develop a revolutionary new oil extraction technology. They call it the SpectraVac process because it presses the oils in an inert gas environment and in a vacuum, eliminating the destructive effects of atmospheric oxygen, high heat and toxic chemicals. Spectrum Naturals uses this process to make Veg Omega-3 Organic Flax Oil and other nutritional supplement oils. This unique oil removal process eliminates the damaging consequences of light, air and heat.

Spectrum Naturals uses in-line refrigeration between the seed press and oil storage and settling vessels (which are also refrigerated). This extra step provides the oil maximum protection from damaging heat. (Some other flax seed brands are refrigerated only at the retail outlet.) Spectrum Naturals also ships the fragile oil by refrigerated truck and requires retailers likewise to keep it under refrigeration. The bottles are opaque black to keep light out. No one can protect as well as Mother Nature, but Spectrum Naturals takes every step they can to try to measure up. I know first-hand about this extraordinary process because I asked for a tour of their SpectraVac process and was very impressed. Spectrum Naturals has done such an excellent job of establishing methods for nutritional oil handling that the Natural Products Quality Assurance Association has used its standards in measuring natural oils manufacturing in the organic and natural foods industry. This Association, headed by Dr. Jeffrey Bland, seeks to educate the consumer on the important issues of natural food safety and health.

Make sure your keep the oil in your refrigerator and use it up within six weeks or it will turn rancid. I keep mine in the freezer as it remains a liquid and lasts longer—up to three months.

I think Udo Erasmus said it best in his critique of fresh flax seed oil in *Fats That Heal, Fats That Kill*: "The fresh oil of the very useful flax seed is the very best oil there is, in every way. It looks good: a rich, deep golden color like fresh liquid sunshine—which by the way, it is. The aroma is a gentle, pleasant, nutty bouquet. It has a variety of flavors. It varies depending on where it is grown to being robust and slightly bitter to light and nutty. Its texture is so light that it is hard to believe that it is oil at all. We usually associate oil with a 'heavy', 'oily' texture. Not so for flax."

I include it in blender drinks (see Chapter 7 on tofu for a recipe), use it as the oil in salad dressings, and sprinkle it on steamed vegetables, potatoes and brown rice.

Fortified Flax Meal

Another beneficial way I get LNAs into my diet is by eating flax seed meal. Keep in mind that if you swallow flax seeds whole, your body will not get the nutrients they contain, because they are protected by a tough seed coat. In fact, after the seeds go through you, you could actually plant them and they would still grow. If you eat them whole, they must be chewed and chewed and chewed. To break the seed coat and make the nutrients available for digestion, you can either grind the flax seeds yourself or get flax seed meal at your health food store.

I use Fortified Flax from the Omega-Life company (see Resources), which is a whole unrefined organic flax seed meal that is fortified and stabilized in a unique grinding process. Zinc, iron, niacin (B3), B6 and B12 are added to the product to keep it fresher and to help in the digestion and assimilation of nutrients. This meal provides all the advantages of flax seed oil and none of the disadvantages like quick rancidity and free radical or trans-fat acid formation. Fortified Flax is sealed in an oxygen-barrier liner so no refrigeration is necessary until opening (although you may refrigerate or freeze it before opening to extend its freshness).

In a study conducted under the care of Milwaukee Wellness Clinic, it was found that in only three weeks of taking two tablespoons daily of Fortified Flax, serum triglycerides levels dropped almost 50 percent in subjects with above normal levels. In her book *Seven Weeks to Sobriety,* founder and director of the Minneapolis Recovery Center, Dr. Joan Matthews Larson, suggests two tablespoons of Fortified Flax and mega-nutrients as part of a daily regime for recovering alcoholics. Dr. Larson has had a 75 percent success rate.

Dr. Herbert Pierson, formerly with the National Cancer Institute, has researched flax and found anti-cancer compounds in it. On an appearance on the "CBS This Morning" television show, he demonstrated the breakfast drink he makes for his family consisting of Fortified Flax, fruit juice and other ingredients. Similarly, Dr. Doris Rapp of Buffalo, New York, suggests Fortified Flax for children with allergies in her book, *Is This Your Child?*

Further research also shows that the use of this type of freshly ground flax seed can also improve digestion, prevent and reverse constipation, stabilize blood glucose levels, improve cardiovascular health, inhibit tumor formation, and bring about other benefits.

Make sure you take this ground flax seed with plenty of fluid, because its mucilage absorbs five times its own weight of water. In addition to taking one tablespoon of Spectrum Naturals Flax Seed Oil, I use from one to three tablespoons of Fortified Flax per day. I mix it in juice or water, blend it (see Chapter 7 on tofu), or sprinkle it on cereal, cooked grains and soup. I also add it to my home-made breads. I prefer, however, to use the oil and meal raw, without heating them.

Nature has provided us with everything we need to be radiantly healthy and free from disease. This is especially true when it comes to this marvelous plant, flax. Our ancestors knew instinctively that flax is nourishing, soothing, and healing. Their intuitive wisdom is now being confirmed by modern scientific analysis.

SIX

Bee Products
Longevity Plus

I believe honeybees have advanced communal living further than any other creature that exists on our globe. Possibly, we owe them our lives. —**Murray Holt**

If a nutritionist were to take all of the research and knowledge now available to develop the perfect all-round dietary supplement, he or she would come up with a combination not far removed from the three lesser-known bee products discussed in this chapter.

A miracle of nature might be one way to describe the honeybee. The honeybee, *Apis mellifera*, is the only insect that produces food eaten by people. No more than three quarters of an inch long, it builds a technically perfect structure, the honeycomb. Apiculturists, who raise bees, harvest bee products and study their relation to human health, have determined that the honeybee has its own language to tell its fellow bees exactly where to find pollen and nectar (the main diet of honeybees).

Scientists estimate that the honeybee has existed for over 50 million years. Impressive? Sure. But even more incredulous is the fact that the bee has undergone no major change for 50 million years—a remarkable record compared to the evolution of most other species over the course of just a few million years.

Honey

Everyone knows that honeybees make honey. Honey has been used as a food and for medicinal purposes from since the beginning of recorded history. Primitive tribal cultures learned to look for "bee trees," trees containing hollows in which wild bees built their honeycombs. This sweet substance was used both as food and medicine in ancient China, Egypt, Babylon and several Middle Eastern nations. Hippocrates, the "father of the healing arts," advised honey for use by his patients. He prescribed honey-water drinks to restore strength in convalescents. This drink is still helpful. Prized for its flavor and quick energy pickup, honey has been a delightful food source from ancient times to modern times by people of all ages.

Several cautions are in order. First, never give honey to babies. Modern research has shown that honey often contains spores of bacteria that can be harmful to babies up to one year old. The bacteria multiply rapidly in the babies' intestines, producing a powerful toxin that causes infant botulism. Authorities say this "caution" applies both to pasteurized and unpasteurized honey.

For adults I add three more cautions. First, use raw honey whenever you can because of its higher food value. Pasteurized honey lacks important enzymes. Second, I believe that cooking with honey changes its chemical composition, and I do not recommend using it in place of sugar in breads, granolas and other products exposed to high heat. Third, honey is a concentrated sweet and should be avoided by people who have an abnormal reaction to glucose.

The vitamins in honey are vitamins K, pro-vitamin A (carotene), folic acid and pyridoxine. Raw, unfiltered honey, which contains some pollen particles, includes vitamins C and B-complex, in addition to others. Minerals in wildflower honey include potassium, iodine, silicon, chromium, manganese, magnesium, zinc, iron, phosphorus and others.

Enzymes in honey are phosphatase, invertase, diastases, inulase, lipase, glucose oxidase and catalase, which breaks down hydrogen peroxide. Enzymes are absent in nearly all processed foods, and yet are among the most valuable of nutrients. Only raw or living foods like honey contain live enzymes.

Primitive tribes in various parts of the world are known to put honey on wounds, boils and slow healing sores to speed up healing. Honey contains some natural germicidal ingredients that help protect against infection.

In his book *Bee Well, Bee Wise,* Bernard Jensen, Ph.D., D.C., states that, "Honey is alkaline-forming and helps counteract the acidity which in many people promotes arthritis, rheumatism and other chronic diseases. Its hormones and nucleic acids support the glandular system, tissue repair and youthfulness."

The antibiotic properties of honey have been verified by several studies, including that of Dr. Jack Tomlinson and Dr. Stanley Williams at San Francisco State University. They published a report in 1985, titled "Antibiotic Properties of Honey." The antibacterial activity was attributed to plant substances gathered by bees in their nectar and pollen collecting work. The strength and efficacy of the antibiotic action varied in honey from place to place.

Raw honey is a superior food, an excellent natural sweetener and is certainly a health-builder.

Did you know that these tiny miracles of nature—the honey-bee—also produce three other products of unique benefit to us all besides honey? They are bee propolis, pollen and royal jelly.

Propolis

Evolution is the result of adaptation to the environment—in other words, survival of the fittest. What can be the reason that the honeybee has kept the same form through such a fantastic number of years? Scientists believe the answer lies in a natural antibiotic produced by the bees called propolis. Propolis is a somewhat gummy substance used by the bees to ensure the cleanliness of the hive, whether the hive is a tree hollow or a manmade home. How else could 50,000 bees crawling over each other live healthily in a small hive?

The famous French scientist, Prof. Remy Chauvin, discovered this remarkable fact. In the mid-60s, he carried out a comprehensive study on bacterial cultures parasitic to insects, and has been studying bee products ever since. He discovered that there was something special about the bee which other insects did not possess—an antibiotic that makes the bee almost entirely immune to attacks of bacteria (they only occasionally get foulbrood due to lack of care by beekeepers) and immune to viruses. The substance is propolis. The discovery was all the more important because propolis is 100 percent effective in killing bacteria.

Propolis is a resinous material gathered by bees from the leaf buds or the bark of poplars, chestnuts and other common trees. When the bees find it, propolis is the juice or sap which the trees themselves secrete to fight infection and disease and to heal cuts. Workers bees collect the various biologic compounds between about 10am and 3pm, when the temperature is greater than 68° F. An important step in the production of bee propolis takes place when the bees add a glandular secretion to the propolis before depositing it in the hive.

Propolis in the hive serves two purposes. First, it seals and tightens the hive when building and repairing. When the resinous propolis solidifies in the cracks and openings of the hive, it reinforces the hive structurally, acts to control the internal environment, and protects against intruders. Second, it protects the bees from bacterial and viral infection. Because the entrance to the hive would be the easiest way for infection to enter the colony, the bees deposit propolis behind the entry way so that all entering bees cross over it. In this way, propolis protects the hive's inhabitants from infections.

Perhaps the following example will shed some light on the remarkable effectiveness of propolis in fighting bacterial and viral infection. If a rodent enters the hive and is stung to death, it will remain in the hive since the bees are not able to remove the intruder. To prevent decay, the bees encase the rodent in propolis and then wrap wax around the entire mass. So embalmed, the body will remain intact without decay or decomposition for five to six years. Thus nature has provided bees with this amazing substance to keep them and their hives free of germs in spite of as many as 50,000 of them being crammed into close quarters in the hive. I've heard it said that bee hives contain less bacteria and are more sterile than hospitals.

In the hive, propolis is generally greenish–brown or chestnut in color. It exudes a pleasant aroma of poplar buds, honey and vanilla. Beekeepers gather it from the hive in the summer by scratching it loose from the frame and comb and rolling it into lumps of up to 200 grams. To preserve it, the propolis is stored in a dark cool place. From 150 to 200 grams of raw propolis can be taken from a bee hive in one season.

Nineteen substances of different chemical structure have been identified in propolis, and there are others that have not yet been identified. It's 50 to 55 percent resin and balsam, 30 percent wax and 8 to 10 percent pollen. Some researchers think the therapeutic properties of propolis come from substances called flavonoids found in the resin. Propolis is also rich in amino acids and is a strong source of trace minerals such as copper, magnesium, silicon, iron, manganese and zinc. It is high in vitamins B, C and E, and beta-carotene.

Researchers around the world are hailing the powers of propolis. It has a wide range of successful therapeutic uses. It is rich in antibiotics and works to raise the body's natural resistance. It stimulates the thymus gland and thus boosts immunity and resistance to infection.

The antibacterial power of propolis surpasses penicillin and other common drugs because bacteria and viruses have been unable to build a tolerance to propolis. In Sarajevo, Yugoslavia, Prof. Izet Osmanagic tested volunteers who were exposed to influenza. He gave 88 students bee propolis; 182 did not receive any. Of those who didn't take propolis, 63 percent became ill. Of those who took propolis, only 7 percent became ill.

Propolis is also a powerful anti-viral that is effective against pneumonia and similar viral infections.

Propolis is very effective in treating stomach and other intestinal ulcers very often caused by stress and poor diet. In Austria, Dr. Franz Klemens Feiks of the Klosterneuberg Hospital tested bee propolis on 300 patients with gastric and duodenal ulcers. He gave half the patients normal medication and the other half bee propolis.

Within three days, 70 percent of the bee propolis group obtained relief. Only 10 percent of the normal medication group got relief in the same time.

Bee propolis speeds the healing of broken bones, and accelerates new cell growth.

It is also part of almost every natural treatment for gum, mouth and throat disorders. This includes its effectiveness in treating sore lips and gums, sore throat, and nasal congestion. Used topically or taken internally, it helps heal skin blemishes and bruises.

Research on propolis and serum blood fats has confirmed its ability to lower high blood pressure, reduce arteriosclerosis and lessen the risks of coronary heart disease.

New research is currently being done on propolis and its healing effects on certain skin cancer and melanoma tumors. Anecdotally, Dr. Mitja Vosnjak, former deputy minister of foreign affairs in Yugoslavia, reported at a medical conference that a friend dying of stomach cancer was advised to take 1/2 teaspoon of propolis three times a day. Within a few weeks, the patient had "no pains, no cramps and no bleeding." After six months he was gaining weight and the cancer seemed to be in remission.

Propolis is available in several medicinal forms including an extract (natural liquid honey paste), powder and chips, capsules, lozenges and tinctures.

Is bee propolis one of America's new answers to good health? Many leading authorities around the world believe it is. One of these authorities has put bee propolis on a pedestal of its own. He is Maurice Hanssen, former Chairman of the National Association of Health in England and author of the book, *The Healing Power of Pollen and Propolis*. In an interview he made quite clear he believes that "bee propolis is perhaps as important as the discovery of penicillin."

Bee Pollen

No ordinary food is good enough for the honeybee. It needs incredible amounts of energy to fly on the average of 15 miles per hour and between as many as 1,200 flowers in one flight from the hive. Besides energizing themselves on nectar, these little honey-bees collect and eat one of the wonder foods of nature—pollen grains from flowers—as they pollinate the flowers at the same time.

Pollen is a food that is basic to all life. It is the male seed of flowers and fertilizes the plant. Without the pollen-carrying honey-bee, many crops and species of plants would fail to be fertilized and would die out. In the process of gathering pollen, bees carry pollen from flower to flower, fertilizing them and assisting in the pollina-tion of fruit orchards, fields of clover and wild flowers. This process is essential to the production of fruit, because certain species of plants are fertilized only by insects. This is why you may have seen rows of white boxes near citrus groves, apple orchards and clover fields. Farmers pay commercial beekeepers a fee for bringing in beehives to fertilize their crops.

After two decades of research on honeybees and their products, it is evident to me that if we did not have pollen, plant life would not exist as it does today. Neither would animal life or human life be possible. As expert apiculturist Murray Holt said in *The World of Bees,* ". . . our whole food structure is based on pollen and pollina-tions. . . ." God sure has a remarkable blueprint to all existence.

This wonder food, pollen, is the main diet of honeybees. They add nectar to it and fly it back to the hive in "pollen baskets" on their back legs. Some of the bee pollen falls to the bottom of the hive and that, no doubt, is how it was discovered by the earliest humans, who must have been amazed at the energy and industry of the honeybee. Historical accounts reveal that bee pollen has been a main food source from the beginning of recorded history.

Bee pollen is mentioned several times in the Bible, was a common health food of the early Romans, and was eaten by athletes in the original ancient Olympic Games in Greece. It is intriguing to me that bee pollen remains one of the only foods left that is still available now just as it was thousands of years ago, and still renders the same remarkable benefits today as it did then.

Bee pollen contains every nutrient needed to help create new living cells: plant, animal and human. Scientists at the Bonny Laboratories of Geneva, Switzerland, discovered that there is total nutrition in bee pollen. They reported that, "generally speaking (there are variations from one type to another) bee pollen contains 35 percent protein of which approximately half is in the form of free amino acids; this is material essential to life, which can be assimilated immediately by the body."

According to scientists from all over the world, pollen may be the most complete food in nature because it is a highly concentrated source of essential nutritional elements. It contains all water-soluble vitamins (it's especially high in B and C), all 22 amino acids, twenty-seven minerals (including calcium, magnesium, zinc, copper and iron), trace elements and different enzymes. Weight for weight, bee pollen contains more protein than meat, fish, eggs and dairy products.

Doctors in some other countries are far more advanced in recognizing the real value of bee products than most physicians here in the United States. They are using bee pollen to treat such problems as colds, ordinary tiredness, fatigue and allergies. Bee pollen also relieves respiratory problems such as bronchitis, sinusitis and the common cold. Equally impressive, pollen helps balance the endocrine system, showing especially beneficial results in menstrual and prostate problems.

Because of its full spectrum blood building and rejuvenative properties, bee pollen is particularly beneficial for the extra nutritional and energy needs of athletes and those recuperating from illness. It is well known to be the supplement of choice by world-class athletes as an energizer and to help give that special edge. In fact, the man *Sports Illustrated* once called the fastest human in the world, Steve Riddick, made bee pollen a regular part of his training program.

Another famous pollen fan is the former heavyweight boxing champion, Mohammed Ali, who used a special secret drink containing bee pollen the night of his match with 25-year-old Leon Spinks. The 36-year-old Ali won the world heavyweight championship for the third time, dancing all around his younger opponent and out-boxing him, seemingly tireless despite his age.

Perhaps the best-known bee pollen fan of our time is former President Ronald Reagan, known to take bee pollen on a daily basis. He loved it and kept an abundance of it on hand at the White

House, which he freely gave away to visitors and friends. He claimed it gave him lots of energy.

There is one other particularly remarkable apparent benefit of pollen. Healthy longevity seems to be a universal desire on the part of human beings, and bee pollen has come to the forefront in demonstrating its propitiousness for long life and robust health. Studies from around the world corroborate this fact. One succinct example comes from the former Soviet Union. Dr. Nicolai Tsitsin, biologist and experimental botanist of the Longevity Institute, sent letters to more than 200 people living in the Soviet Union who claimed to be more than 100 years old. Three questions were asked: their age, how they had earned a living most of their lives, and what had been their principal foods. The responses were remarkable in that, without exception, of the 150 responses returned, all reported that a principal food was bee pollen and a large number of them were beekeepers. The longevity factors in bee pollen apparently gave the beekeepers robust health even at the age of one hundred, according to Dr. Tsitsin.

Honeybees, of course, do their fertilizing work incidentally to their main job of gathering food for the hive. When a worker bee comes to a flower, she crawls down to the stamen and gathers the loose pollen with her jaws and front legs. Her back legs contain pollen "baskets" on the lower parts which the bee packs with the golden grains she has brought from the flower. The hairy combs on the bee's middle legs brush the pollen into the back leg baskets where it is tamped down into a single pellet. The pollen is moistened by nectar before being packed into the bee baskets. Each load of pollen weights about 10 milligrams.

Pollen is collected by pollen traps fastened to commercial bee hives and collection is limited to amounts that will not interfere with survival of the honeybees. The wonderful thing about bees is that they always gather much more pollen and make much more honey than they need for themselves.

There are two kinds of pollen: windblown pollen (already dried up and contaminated by all kinds of dirt) and insect-carried pollen. It is the windblown pollens that cause allergy problems. Ragweed and other pollens carried by the wind make millions of people miserable every year, triggering sneezing, swollen sinus membranes, itching and watery eyes and other symptoms.

Bees' instinct tells them which pollen is freshest with 'alive' nutrients. The kind of pollen carried by bees is a much heavier and somewhat stickier pollen than the wind-borne kind. Honeybee pollen relieves allergy symptoms in some allergy sufferers. (Sometimes unheated raw honey, which is laced with pollen particles, will also desensitize a person to the allergens associated with certain pollens.)

Bee pollen is available in fresh granules, capsules, chewable wafers, and a variety of mixtures with propolis and royal jelly.

Royal Jelly

Among the remarkable bees, unquestionably the most remarkable is the queen bee. Let's take a look at the life of a queen bee. She is fertilized only once, speeding high in the sky, on perhaps the only flight from the hive she will ever take. From that moment on she can lay as many as two thousand eggs a day during the spring and summer seasons. And, as incredulous as this may seem, but irrefutably true, she can lay that many eggs for her lifespan—up to six years! The queen bee is a mother of a quarter million bees and, at a rate of over 2,000 eggs a day, her eggs will total more than twice her own body weight. The average life span of the queen lasts between four to five years, as opposed to the considerably shorter life of workers, who average 5 months or less. Any creature that has that amount of energy and vitality has to be respected.

And what do the queen bees eat? From the earliest stages of egg development and throughout their lives they live on one food: royal jelly. A thick, milky substance secreted from the pharyngeal glands of a special group of young nurse bees between the sixth and twelfth days of their lives, when combined with honey and pollen, produces royal jelly.

In the larva stage, all bees are absolutely identical and feed on royal jelly for the first three days. From the fourth day on, only the special larva selected to become the new queen continues to be fed with royal jelly throughout her entire life. The worker bee larvae, however, are fed on regular honey and pollen. According to this feeding pattern, the fertilized eggs give rise either to sexually immature females, which are the smaller "worker" bees, or to the larger queens. Nutrition is therefore the only distinctive difference between the worker bees and the queen—a fascinating discovery. In other words, although queen honeybees and sterile female worker bees have identical DNA, queens often live 12 times longer. The one difference: queens eat royal jelly. Royal jelly can truly be called a miracle food!

Let's take a closer look at the nutritional breakdown of royal jelly. It is a powerhouse of B vitamins; the minerals calcium, iron, potassium and silicon; enzyme precursors; and eight essential amino acids. In fact, like bee pollen, it contains every nutrient necessary to support life. Tantalizingly, four percent of royal jelly's composition still defies analysis. Perhaps this mystery element makes an important contribution to its impressive performance.

In recent years a startling discovery has been made by scientists. Some samples of royal jelly have been found to contain the male sex hormone testosterone. Now for you men reading this, this is great news indeed! It may provide a more enjoyable love life. But it's also good news for women, too. Both men and women make testosterone, although males produce a greater quantity than females. In females, this hormone is produced in small quantities in the ovaries and adrenal cortex to stimulate the female libido. Not to worry, ladies. It may improve your love life, too. Taking royal jelly will not cause you to grow a beard or hair on your chest!

Dr. H.L. Heyl of France discovered a gonadotropic hormone in royal jelly, similar to that discovered in bee pollen, that would activate the sex glands. This isn't surprising since royal jelly is produced from the pharyngeal glands of "nurse" bees who stuff themselves with pollen and honey to make it. Heyl's studies of female lab rats injected with royal jelly under the skin shows that their ovaries gained weight and their egg-producing activity was increased.

Royal jelly restored potency in a high percentage of 40 sexually dysfunctional men, ages 20 to 52, in a Yugoslavian study. This study, by Dr. Osmanagic, involved men who had been unable to have sex for two or more years. In one month, nearly 58 percent of the men reported improvement in their general and sexual condition. Wives of two participants got pregnant.

There is yet another miracle hidden in royal jelly—a fatty acid called hydroxydecanoic acid. While the name may be hard to pronounce, its benefits to the body are well defined. *One remarkable fact is that it appears nowhere else in nature.* Another is that it's a top-notch bactericidal. In tests carried out as far back as the mid–30s, hydroxydecanoic acid was found to kill the harmful organisms *Escherichia coli* and *Salmonella typhosa.* These studies were confirmed thirty years later when scientists discovered that penicillin was only four times as effective against some organisms as this fatty acid, and that the acid had approximately the same potency as chlorotetracycline. This acid has also been proven to be a yeast-inhibiting substance (effective for athlete's foot and candida taken internally and applied topically) which also increases the hemoglobin content in the red blood cells and improves both the number and condition of white blood cells. Perhaps by now it comes as no surprise that both fresh royal jelly and pure hydroxydecanoic acid have been shown to prevent the development of transplantable leukemia and abdominal tumors in mice.

Irene Stein, in her book, *Royal Jelly,* does an excellent job in describing all the medicinal, therapeutic and beauty benefits of royal jelly. It's been known for centuries as a remarkably rejuvenating and health-giving substance. A plethora of scientific studies reveal that fresh royal jelly increases mental alertness, aids concentration, acts as a natural tranquilizer and raises energy levels. It has been found to keep skin, hair and nails in peak condition, while also boosting the immune system, thereby providing protection from infections.

While royal jelly has been used for centuries, it came to the forefront in April 1956. At that time Dr. Ricardo Galleazzi Lisi, the personal physician of his Holiness, Pope Pius X11, attributed the Holy Father's recovery from a long weakening illness in large measure to his taking of royal jelly. Soon afterwards, in March 1957, the 88-year-old President of Chile stated for publication that it was the royal jelly he was taking which made it possible for him to develop such tremendous vigor for his most burdensome job. And speaking of royalty (pun intended), it's been reported that Prince Philip of England, his daughter, Princess Ann and Princess Margaret have long been taking royal jelly, as did Princess Diana during her pregnancies.

Royal jelly is available 100 percent pure, or mixed with honey and/or pollen, as a freeze-dried powder and in capsules.

Bee propolis, pollen and royal jelly are available at health food stores. When selecting which products to purchase, read the label and keep in mind the following: look for products that say they are pure, harvested by healthy bees (not disease carrying), are quality controlled and are organic—meaning herbicide and pollutant-free.

It's not difficult to control where the bees fly to collect pollen. Bees' maximum flying range is about four miles. If they are out of range, they begin to lose their sense of direction and will not be able to come back to their hives. Their own instinct keeps them within that boundary. Through this natural behavior beekeepers can control the bee products' "organic quality."

I am always particular about the foods and bee products I include in my diet; I want the very best available. That's why I only select bee products which come from Y.S. Royal Jelly and Bee Farms in Sheridan, Illinois (see Resource Directory). Their wide variety of products are far superior to those of any other bee farm I've ever seen; they meet all the high, rigid standards I described above. The Y.S. Bee Farms beekeepers find areas that have ample uncontaminated flowering crops in the Dakotas, northern Minnesota, and northern Wisconsin. So, naturally, the bees are healthy and strong.

As John Choi, apiculturist and president of Y.S. Bee Farms, told me, when honeybees are gathering their foods (royal jelly, bee pollen, propolis, honey and wax), they instinctively know precisely how to keep all the nutrients alive. I also appreciate that bees are not harmed in the process of creating any of these above bee products.

We were all put on this earth for a purpose, to live in harmony and to learn from one another. Certainly, there is much we can learn and benefit from the incredible honeybee.

And to think, honeybees and their products have been around for 50 million years! That's a reasonable testing period.

SEVEN

Tofu
The Soy Superfood

W hat draws most Americans to tofu is its stupendous versa-
tility. No other food in the world can do what tofu does—
because it can do everything.
—*Mark Messina, Ph.D. & Virginia Messina, R.D.*

What would you do if I were to tell you that I discovered a
natural food that offered the following health benefits:

- It helps prevent ulcers by neutralizing stomach acid.
- It helps prevent breast and prostate cancer.
- It can mimic estrogen's positive effects on the skeletal, reproductive and cardiovascular system while blocking estrogen's
carcinogenic effects on breast tissue.
- It decreases LDL cholesterol and helps prevent heart disease
in many ways.
- It's a good source of calcium and prevents osteoporosis in
several different ways.
- It's low in allergen factors, highly nutritious, rich in vitamins,
amino acids, and free of pesticides and other synthetic toxins
when grown and processed organically.
- It is easy for adults and infants to digest; has no cholesterol, no
lactose, and is very rich in essential fatty acids (EFAs).
- It's substantially higher as a dietary source of protein and iron
than dairy milk.

• It's inexpensive, readily available, virtually tasteless on its own, and easy to add to all of your favorite recipes.

You'd probably want to rush out and buy a case of it, right? What is this incredible product? It's tofu, made from soybeans. This little known food has been referred to as a 'superfood' or 'miracle medicine.'

The most common soybean variety cultivated today is from the botanical genus of *Glycine max. L.*, and is classed in the *Merril Family of Leguminosae* by H. Snyder & T.W. Kwon. The soybean has a venerable history over 5,000 years old, achieving its earliest human cultivation in the Orient. Tofu is a staple of many Pacific Rim countries. According to Dr. T.W. Kwon, Chief Research Scientist of the Korean Institute of Science and Health and Prof. Harry Snyder of the University of Arkansas Food Science Department, the dynastic Chinese developed innovative techniques for processing soybean tofu, and over time have evolved a diverse collection of culinary staples. The result has been the creation of different types of tofu like "bai ye" (pressed tofu), "su-ji" (vegetarian meat replacers), "you-tofu" (fried tofu curd), and "tofu-pi" (tofu milk).

The best quality tofu is made from low oil, high sugar and high protein content soybean varieties. Japanese soybeans tend to be the best quality, with premium regional U.S. varieties following a close second.

The chemical composition of tofu is 88 percent pure water, 6.7 percent protein, 3.5 percent fat, 1.9 percent miscellaneous compounds/carbohydrates and .6 percent ash. Typically, its vitamin constituents include all of the necessary vitamins as well as an exceedingly rich amino acid composition.* All in all, a veritable nutritional arsenal of healing compounds.

---

*Aspartic acid 1.45%, threonine 0.50%, serine 0.65%, glutamic acid 2.28%, proline 0.49%, glycine 9.53%, alanine 0.55%, cystine 0.14%, valine 0.61%, methionine 0.16%, isoleucine 0.61%, leucine 1.04%, tyrosine 0.48%, phenylalanine 0.67%, lysine 0.79%, histidine 0.31%, and arginine 0.94%.

Tofu, Phytochemicals & Women's Health

The two leading causes of death in the United States today are heart disease and cancer. Together they kill over 75 percent of the population. For years, medical research has been looking for the "magic bullet" to prevent or cure these degenerative maladies. The result of their efforts has been mixed.

In the battle against heart disease, for example, the multinational pharmaceutical giants have developed several drugs that lowered cholesterol ratings in the patient. Researchers in the United Kingdom and Finland reviewed these pharmaceutical studies and reported their results in the *British Medical Journal*. They concluded: 1) the death rate actually increased in those trials using drugs to lower cholesterol; 2) drug use should be halted except in severe cases until more research has been done; and 3) dietary changes should be emphasized, since they are safe and effective. In other words, drugs failed to heal at the cellular level, which is where it counts. In fact, the only way to heal a diet-caused disease is to adopt a remedial healing diet!

But what kind of dietary changes are effective? A plethora of scientific studies from all over the world confirm that tofu and other soy products help prevent both heart disease and cancer—among numerous other ailments! This result is attributed to the phyto (plant) compounds found in abundance in the venerable soybean. It is a virtual natural pharmacy in a seed capsule!

In 1982, the National Academy of Sciences, on behalf of the National Cancer Institute, issued a report recommending increased consumption of fruits and vegetables. In support of its recommendation, the National Academy cited the importance of *phytochemicals*. Phytochemicals are components of foods that are not nutrients but do affect health.

In 1983, Dr. Lee Wattenberg, one of the pioneers of the phytochemical research, detailed the many ways in which the phytochemicals may prevent cancer. Over the past decade, study after study has shown how potent the phytochemicals are against cancer and other diseases. Researchers at the University of Minnesota highlighted fifteen different classes of phytochemicals in fruits and vegetables that show anti-cancer activity—and soybeans figure prominently in many of these classes of phytochemicals.*

An impressive number of research papers were presented at the First International Symposium on the Role of Soy in Preventing and Treating Chronic Disease. During this three-day conference, doctors and respected researchers from around the world formally presented ground-breaking work on the apparent significance of soy and soy foods in the prevention of disease. Although all of the biochemical mechanisms are not yet fully understood, every day more is being discovered about the health promoting compounds found exclusively, or predominantly, in soy.

One such component of soy is the isoflavone—a potent phytochemical. The constituents of isoflavone in turn provide hormone-like biochemical regulating properties in the body. *Genistein* is one of the chemical constituents of isoflavone with remarkable biochemical properties if consumed in the proper ratio. More than 200 studies have been published on genistein, including many on its anti-cancer properties.

Genistein has biochemical properties that mimic human estrogen. It functions both as an estrogen agonist and antagonist; that is, it seems to promote the positive actions of estrogen while preventing many of its negative effects. Genistein facilitates maintaining a

---

*The phytochemical classes and their food sources are:
  Allium compounds: onions, garlic, and chives
  Coumarins: vegetables and citrus fruits
  Dithiolthiones: cruciferous vegetables
  Flavonoids: most fruits and vegetables
  Glucosinolates, indoles: cruciferous vegetables
  Glyceritinic acid: licorice
  Inositol hexaphosphate: plants, particularly soybeans and cereals
  Isoflavones: soybeans
  Isothiocyanates, thiocyanates: cruciferous vegetables
  Lignans: flax seeds
  Liminene: citrus fruits
  Phenols: most fruits and vegetables
  Plant sterols: vegetables, including soybeans
  Protease inhibitors: most plants, particularly seeds and legumes such as soybeans
  Saponins: plants, particularly soybeans
Each of these phytochemical classes contains, in turn, many compounds. This list helps us to understand why people who eat a lot of fruits, vegetables and particularly soybeans have a lower risk of cancer.

proper amount of estrogen for homeostasis, that is, a healthy equilibrium. It binds to both estrogen receptors and progesterone receptors in the body. These receptors, when out of balance, promote carcinogenic tumor evolution and growth.

The natural isoflavone genistein seems to mimic Tamoxifen, the synthetic drug most commonly used to prevent recurrence of breast cancer. Genistein's biochemical properties also resemble those of the synthetic drug Premarin in that it lowers the risk of osteoporosis by maintaining trabecular bone density. The isoflavones appear to delay muscle and bone atrophy by providing sufficient estrogenic action to delay aging in humans.

Studies reveal that soy products also play an active role in the prevention of osteoporosis because they are a good source of the minerals boron and calcium. Dr. Kenneth Setchell of Children's Hospital Medical Center in Cincinnati, Ohio, reports that dietary estrogens like genistein may play an important role in preventing hormone-initiated diseases.

Dr. Setchell states, "Recent studies of normally ovulating pre-menopausal women have shown that the dietary inclusion of soy protein (60g/day intake) specifically containing isoflavones, leads to significant positive changes in the menstrual cycle, with the prolongation of cycle length, an increase in follicular phase length, and a marked suppression of the mid-cycle surge of gonadotrophins—luteinizing hormone and follicle-stimulating hormone." Simply translated, when the female body has the right amount of regulating phytochemicals found in soy based foods and other fresh whole foods, the natural regulatory functions of the body become biochemically synchronized and regulated to increase wellness and longevity.

Another way naturally occurring genistein acts like the synthetic drug Premarin is in reducing the painful and debilitating side effects of menopause. According to a recent study in the respected British medical journal *Lancet*, tofu in the diet may reduce the frequency and severity of hot flashes in menopausal females.

Dr. Setchell added that soy foods appear to decrease the risks of breast cancer, ovarian and vaginal cancers, as well as to mitigate hormone-attributed unstable emotions.

The absence of lactase in soy products allows for milk-intolerant individuals to absorb and utilize their rich array of micronutrients. The absence of many contemporary allergens in soy, as compared to dairy milk, makes it a prime replacement and source of calcium, boron, and other trace minerals as suggested in *Soybean: Chemistry and Technology* by Smith and Circle.

Soy products are an ideal source of absorbable calcium to reinforce bone formation and density. A 1988 study by the University of Texas Health Science Center showed that volunteers excreted 50 percent less calcium in their urine when they replaced the animal products in their diets with soy foods. When soy is combined with an adequate intake of essential fatty acids (EFAs) and adequate exercise, calcium is transported to bones and bone density is maintained and increased. This triad relationship of a) exercise, b) EFA intake, and c) calcium from whole foods like soy, is the very best natural prescription for women fearful of or suffering from osteoporosis.

A 1990 study at Guy's Hospital in London found that soy protein after digestion was much easier on the kidneys than animal meats. This discovery may indicate an important and beneficial dietary change for people with kidney disease.

Interestingly, the composition of genistein and other isoflavones in tofu is different from that of whole soybeans, soy flour and soy protein isolates. Some brands of tofu, which I will discuss later in this chapter, according to nutritional analyses, seem to be higher in total isoflavones and genistein. This can usually be attributed to the selection of beans, care in harvesting, length of processing time, and packaging methods. Quality is reflected in the care and attention to details given when handling living foods.

Tofu Helps Fight Cancer

In a study of 8,000 Hawaiian men with Japanese ancestry published in *Cancer Research* in 1989, it was discovered that men who ate the most tofu had the lowest rates of prostate cancer, with other influences factored out. Similarly, a study in Singapore reported in *Lancet* in 1991 found that premenopausal women who rarely ate soy foods had twice the risk of breast cancer as those who ate soy foods frequently. All other food and lifestyle differences were taken into account. In both of these cases it was the *soy alone which made the difference, not the amount of fat.*

Cancer formation is actually a long process in human beings. The time between tumor initiation and outright malignancy generally takes decades. There is a considerable length of time in which the carcinogenic process could be halted or reversed through various strategies based on a whole food regimen.

There are several compounds in soy products that appear to fight cancer according to Earl Mindell in his excellent book, *Earl Mindell's Soy Miracle. Genistein* inhibits the formation of new blood vessels (angiogenesis) by which a rapidly growing tumor feeds itself. *Saponins* are naturally occurring compounds in soybeans, other legumes and some other foods. Saponins significantly reduced the growth and viability of cancerous colon and melanoma cells in laboratory tests conducted by Prof. A. Venket Rao of the University of Toronto. This characteristic of saponins in tofu may also be attributed to the other micronutrients abundantly present in tofu, not the least of these being beta-carotene, thiamin, riboflavin, niacin, pantothenic acid, pyridoxine, biotin, folic acid, inositol, choline and ascorbic acid.

Protease inhibitors present in soy foods are also potent anti-carcinogens. Protease inhibitors are enzymes in the body which act specifically upon the proteins. Enzyme activation or retardation in the body influences many minute-to-minute biochemical actions which contribute to health. A specific protease inhibitor derived from soybeans called Inhibitor BBI is named after its discoverers, Bowman-Birk. BBI has been shown to suppress carcinogenesis in three different species, several organ systems, in different cell types and in different types of cancer.

Phytic acid and lignans are other compounds found in soy products that play a powerful role in cancer prevention.

Tofu Helps Fight Heart Disease

Dr. Cesare Sirtori, at the University of Milan's Center for the Study of Metabolic Diseases and Hyperlipidemia, studied the cholesterol lowering effects of the addition of soy protein to a low-fat diet. One group of volunteers ate soy protein while a control group remained on a low-fat diet. Within two weeks, the serum cholesterol of the subjects eating soy foods dropped an average of 14 percent; in four weeks it dropped about 21 percent. The control subjects who did not eat soy, experienced *no* drop in cholesterol levels despite the fact that they were on a low-fat diet. Some of the soy-eating group were asked to discontinue soy while maintaining their low-fat diet. Their cholesterol levels crept back up to their previous levels in just two weeks. Dr. Sirtoni's conclusion was that soy alone was responsible for the decreased cholesterol levels.

To challenge the results of the first study, a group of volunteers was given a supplement of cholesterol (500mg/day) to see if that would negate the effects of soy. Despite the added cholesterol, these volunteers experienced the same drop in cholesterol as those who were given no cholesterol supplements.

I have reviewed more than 28 studies that have shown that substituting soy for animal protein or simply adding soy protein to the diet significantly reduces cholesterol, regardless of the type of fat in the diet!

Dr. John Potter reported in the October 1993 *American Journal of Clinical Nutrition* that volunteers with only moderately high cholesterol levels (about 240 mg) experienced a 12 percent decrease in cholesterol levels in four weeks when they ate muffins made with 50mg of soy protein each day. In a second trial the soy protein content of the muffins was cut in half, to 25 mg per day, and still those with moderate to high cholesterol had a significant drop. "The more soy people eat, the better. But even moderate amounts have an effect," concluded Dr. Potter. By moderate amounts he meant a couple of servings of soy foods each day, such as some tofu in a stirfry and/or blender drink a day.

Soy protein is a potent dietary tool to reduce the risk of heart disease. Soy protein decreases LDL cholesterol ratios in the blood and is effective in suppressing peroxidized LDL formation, which is the worst form of LDL cholesterol—a major contributor to atheroma formation, hardening of the arteries and congestive heart failure. This type of cholesterol forms when there is a shortage of vitamin E, vitamin C and the carotenes, which act as natural antioxidants—slowing down the chemical reactions in the blood to a safe level.

Soy protein was also consistently shown to elevate plasma thyroxin concentrations in laboratory animals. Thyroxin, manufactured in the thyroid gland, is the primary hormone that regulates metabolism. Increased thyroxin speeds the metabolism, burns fat, and decreases cholesterol. For those of you who are interested in having a fit, lean body, this is great news!

Tofu Protein vs. Meat Protein

Many people consider chicken a healthy protein source. I don't. Three and one half ounces of white chicken meat contain 11 grams of fat; more than three of these grams are saturated fat. Poultry is also fraught with chemicals added to the chickens' feed, which has the potential to increase *Salmonella* in chickens and their eggs. Dr. Virginia Wheeler, the famed independent cancer researcher, asserts that modern chicken breeding conditions promote cancer. Dr. Wheeler has for two decades argued that these cancers may be transferred to humans if the chicken is uncooked or poorly handled. Some insiders in the fowl breeding business have expressed concern that from 20 to 25 percent of fowl may carry malignant cancers. A similar health threat from diseased meat and poor sanitation in meat processing plants was reported on a recent segment of the television program, "60 Minutes."

Meats, including chicken, have been implicated as the primary cause of heart disease. According to Dr. Dean Ornish, in his book *Eat More ,Weigh Less,* meat gives you a quadruple whammy.

Meat is:
- High in cholesterol, which clogs up all your arteries including your heart, and high in saturated fat, which raises your blood cholesterol level.
- High in oxidants like iron, which oxidize cholesterol to a form that is more easily deposited in your arteries.
- Low in healthy antioxidants.
- Prone to be saturated with antibiotics, concentrations of pesticides from feed sources, and many parasites.

In contrast, tofu and other forms of soy products give you more than a quadruple benefit.

Tofu:
- Contains no cholesterol.
- Contains no saturated fat.
- Increases the degradation of LDL "bad" cholesterol, increases "good" HDL levels.
- Is high in naturally occurring antioxidants.

When you consider these healthful advantages, and weigh the exciting new research into the powerful anti-carcinogenic and cholesterol-lowering effects of soy consumption, the conclusion is a simple one: meat harms and tofu heals.

Fortunately, if you eat three times as much tofu as poultry by weight, you will get quality protein (about 25 grams) with half the fat and 42 fewer calories. Also tofu has no cholesterol and its natural oils are full of the healthy essential fatty acids (EFAs) usually deficient in the Standard American Diet (SAD). An even better choice is "lite" tofu which I use, made by Mori-Nu. It has only 35 calories in each three ounce serving and only 0.7 grams of fat.

Soy protein is now officially recognized as a top quality protein. It's finally been given justice. Drs. Mark and Virginia Messina reported in their book, *The Simple Soybean and Your Health*, that over the years nutritionists have used an assortment of methods for assessing the quality of protein. The official method for evaluating protein quality in both Canada and the United States is the protein efficiency ratio (PER), a measure of the weight gain of a growing animal divided by the amount of protein that the animal consumed.

"To determine PER," the authors explain, "rats are fed different proteins and their growth is measured. The more weight an animal gains for a given amount of protein, the better the quality of the protein is and the higher is the PER. Studies measuring PER are expensive and time consuming. Scientists also recognize a much more fundamental problem with the procedure. PER works well for rats but not so well for humans—it undervalues some proteins and overvalues others because rats, not surprisingly, have different amino acid requirements than we do. This is particularly important in the case of soy protein because the PER does not do justice to soy."

Fortunately, things have changed. The Food and Drug Administration has adopted a new method of evaluating protein called the "Protein Digestibility Corrected Amino Acid Score" or PDCAAS, which is now accepted as the method of choice by the World Health Organization. PDCAAS is actually a lot simpler than it sounds. The Messinas explain that PDCAAS simply compares the pattern of essential amino acids in a protein with the requirements that humans have for essential amino acids, then makes an adjustment for how well that protein is digested. In reality, PDCAAS is really a measure of how limiting the limiting amino acid is in a protein.

"The important point about this new scoring method," write the Messinas, "is that soy protein finally receives its due. Under the new system, soy protein has been given a score of one, the highest rating possible, the same rating that is accorded the animal proteins such as milk protein."

Two others researchers provide evidence of the high quality protein available in the soybean. Vernon Young, Ph.D. and Nevin Scrimshaw, Ph.D., at Massachusetts Institute of Technology, reported in the *American Journal of Clinical Nutrition*, 1994, that protein produced in the soybean is of such high quality it is capable of totally supporting the body's daily need for essential amino acids.

How Is Tofu Made?

Many simple processes have been developed over time to create wholesome and inexpensive tofu. Regular tofu has similar methods of manufacture as cheese processing. While cheese is made from animal milk, tofu is made from soy milk. It starts with the whole bean pod which is graded for maturity, quality and freshness. The soy beans are soaked in water from two to five hours, depending on ambient temperatures. The beans are ground in water, centrifuged to eliminate the water, and cleaned. Additional pure water is then added to the soybean pulp, making a white milk-like effluent.

Commercial tofu production uses direct steam to quicken the cooking time. The "steam" or heated soy milk is again screened and filtered to eliminate liquid whey, leaving the now solidifying soy curd. The material is then allowed to cool. As it cools, it forms a soft cheese-like curd or wet cake. In traditional methods, sea water is added to the curd, or more recently, calcium sulfate, magnesium sulfate or magnesium chloride are added, if clean sea water is not readily available. Some commercial processes have evolved even better tofu characteristics with the use of lactates, gluconates, citrates, acetic and citric acids. As the supernatant slurry cools below 70-80 degrees Celsius, the whey is separated from the bean curd.

The soy protein is ultimately transformed into curds and whey. The curd is formed in molding boxes with coarse cloth covers, and holes in the boxes to allow seepage of any remnant supernatant liquids. The remnant liquid is removed by squeezing or pressing the top of the curd boxes. The proteins have a short curing or setting time and the now-stable formed tofu loaf is removed from the molding box. The microorganism responsible for forming a curd is actinomucor or mucor, which renders a creamy somewhat cheese-like mild flavor, and has been described as somewhat salty. (Interestingly, this production technique is similar to the manufacture of cheese where, unlike with the production of tofu the best proteins are often discarded with the whey, leaving a poorer quality protein known as casein.)

Tofu is graded by texture and finish. The majority of these styles are found in the Orient, due to the long history of tofu as a principal food. Tofu flavors and eating qualities are determined by the variety of soybean used and the regional variations in manufacturing techniques.

Tofu styles are differentiated in each country with Doo-bu being the most popular in Korea, Tahu in Indonesia, Tau Foo in Malaysia and Tokua in the Philippines. Each region has its taste, texture and cooking style. Different styles of heat treatment and post processing of tofu create differently flavored and textured tofus ranging from regular tofu which is bland, sometimes slightly nutty tasting, to silken tofu which is milky, almost creamy, used in making pies, protein shakes, etc. Kori tofu, aburage tofu, and su-fu tofu are varieties of fermented soy curd with their attendant spicy, or even cheesy, flavors.

A special Hong Kong delicacy is made by heating regular tofu to create yuba tofu, resulting in a congealed surface film of coagulated proteins. The texture and stiffness of soy milk rendered into a proteinacious film is determined by the amount of coagulating proteins and lipids in the bean. Films are formed when uniform heat is applied to a vat of soy milk and a mechanical stripping rod rapidly separates and lifts the soy film. Yuba Tofu is quite expensive and this edible "fabric" is used as a unique wrapping for other gourmet oriental foods.

Despite 500 years of tofu development, even newer revolutionary processes of tofu production continue. A fresh tofu product developed by Morinaga Nutritional Foods, Inc., coagulates fresh soy milk right in the box. This preserves the whey and produces a smooth "silken style" tofu which is most versatile in the American kitchen. The aseptic packaging method employed by Morinaga requires no refrigeration of the tofu product until opened. Preserving the whey retains some essential health properties normally lost in commercial tofu processing. The aseptic process increases nutrient retention (including important isoflavones) and natural flavor, while ensuring complete safety.

According to Rees Moerman, a member of the International Institute of Food Technologists, the invention of aseptic packaging is "the most significant food science innovation of the last fifty years, preserving vital nutrients and keeping pathogens away from foods. Aseptic packaging techniques allow otherwise easily spoiled foods to be protected in a way that the delicate nutritional properties of fresh foods can be stored for the longest period without the need to add harsh chemical preservatives or stabilizers."

Tofu Is Recipe-Friendly

There are many regional cooking styles in tofu foods. Numerous spices and other flavoring agents create distinctive Chinese, Korean, Japanese, Taiwanese and other oriental dishes.

I used to put up with the sometimes frustrating and old fashioned tofu because I was aware of its health benefits. It was always a hassle to deal with, however, because the tofu was bathed in water to preserve it. I had to change the water every day and it often spilled. To make matters worse, it was high in fat, even though it was "good" fat. Over 50 percent of its calories came from fat.

I now only use Mori-Nu "Lite" tofu in the aseptic package. It's 75 percent lower in fat and has only half the calories of regular tofu. Its smooth texture seems to work better in my favorite dishes, like fresh fruit protein shakes.

The great thing about tofu is that it will take on the flavor of whatever food with which you choose to prepare it. You can marinate it and make shish-ka-bobs, make dips, patés or just add it to anything you are cooking, from pasta to vegetable dishes to smoothies.

Here are some of my favorite recipes using tofu. For more free recipes, refer to the Resource Directory.

- ## Tofu Salad

  1 10.5 oz pkg Mori-Nu Silken
  "Lite Tofu" (Extra Firm), drained
  $^1/_2$ tsp. turmeric
  2 Tbs. celery, diced
  1 tsp. apple cider vinegar
  2 Tbs. onion, diced
  2 tsp. prepared yellow mustard
  1 tsp. parsley, chopped
  scant $^1/_2$ tsp. white pepper
  Dash paprika
  1 tsp. honey

  1. Crumble tofu into small mixing bowl. Set aside.
  2. In a separate bowl, combine vinegar, mustard, honey and turmeric. Mix thoroughly and pour over crumbled tofu.
  3. Add celery, onion, parsley, paprika and pepper. Mix thoroughly.
  Refrigerate approximately 30 minutes to allow flavors to blend.

  Note: Try Tofu Salad in pita bread lined with fresh sprouts, lettuce or other greens.
  Makes 3 servings of $^1/_2$ cup each. Per serving: 57 calories, 1.3 g fat, 6 g protein, 131 mg sodium, 0 mg cholesterol.

- **Vegetable Stir Fry**

  3 Tbs. sesame oil (Spectrum Naturals)
  1 pkg. Mori-Nu "Lite" tofu (Extra Firm), cubed
  2 large cloves garlic, minced
  2 Tbs. fresh ginger, grated
  2 Tbs. "Lite" tamari
  1/2 cup green onion, chopped
  6 cups of fresh vegetables (broccoli, red pepper, mushrooms, carrots, celery, snow peas, etc.)

  1. Sauté garlic, ginger and tofu in oil until lightly browned.
  2. Add remaining ingredients and stir fry until tender-crisp.
  3. Serve over hot brown rice.

- **Sweet and Sour Tofu Cutlets**

  2 10.5-ounce packages Mori-Nu "Lite" tofu, (Extra Firm)
  1 Tbs. soy sauce, low sodium
  2 Tbs. pineapple juice concentrate
  1/2 tsp. chili powder
  1/2 tsp. sweet basil
  1/2 tsp. curry powder
  2 cloves garlic, minced
  1 1/2 tsp. minced ginger
  1/2 cup raspberry preserves (no sugar added)
  1 Tbs. rice vinegar, unseasoned
  scant 1/2 tsp. crushed red pepper
  2 Tbs. lemon juice

  1. Slice tofu lengthwise into four cutlets. Lay the slices of tofu on a baking tray and cover with saran wrap. Freeze overnight.
  2. On the following day, place the frozen tofu fillets into a microwave dish and microwave three minutes on HIGH. Place the tofu cutlets in a shallow baking dish. Combine remaining ingredients and pour over the cutlets.
  3. Bake at 400 degrees F uncovered for 20 minutes.

  Serves 4.

• *Tofu Sour Cream*
$^1/_2$ *pound Mori Nu "Lite" tofu*
$^1/_4$ *cup fresh lemon juice*
2 *Tbs. Spectrum Naturals Extra-Virgin Olive Oil*
1 *tsp. salt*

1. In a blender, combine the tofu, lemon juice, oil, and salt; blend until creamy smooth.
2. Store in the refrigerator.
3. You can add a variety of different herbs and use it on potatoes, vegetables, salads, and for dips.

This will yield about 1$^1/_2$ cups and has about 27 calories for two tablespoons.

• *Basic Fruit Smoothie*
To whip up a fruit smoothie, just throw the following ingredients into a blender and blend at high speed for a minute or two.
$^3/_4$ *cup fresh fruit juice*
$^1/_2$ *cup chopped fresh fruit*
$^1/_2$ *banana (frozen)*
$^1/_3$ *pkg. Mori-Nu "Lite" tofu*
1 *Tbs. honey (or other sweetener), optional*
4-5 *ice cubes*
To make this a great high energy nutritional smoothie, I also add:
1 *Tbs. Omega Fortified Flax*
1 *Tbs. Spectrum Naturals Veg Organic Flax Seed Oil*
1 *tsp. Spectrum Natural Wheat Germ Oil*
1 *Tbs. All One People Nutrient Powder*
1 *tsp. Super All Bee Power (a combination of royal jelly, bee pollen, propolis and herbs in a powder form made by Y.S. Bee Farms).*
Dash of cinnamon, to taste

All these products are described in previous chapters and can be found at your health food store, or see the Resource Directory for more information.

In place of milk, I make nut milks or use Westsoy 100 percent organic non-dairy soy beverages which are available in health food stores. (See Chapter 2 on nutrition.)

A Little Soybean History

According to Drs. Mark and Virginia Messinas in their book, *The Simple Soybean and Your Health*, the history of soybeans began over 5,000 years ago on the windy plains of eastern Asia. The importance of the soybean can be seen in historical records and in the name itself. In China, the word for "soybean" is ta-tou, which means "greater bean." According to the Chinese tradition, soybeans were one of the five sacred crops named by Chinese emperor Sheng-Nung, who reigned five thousand years ago. By 300 B.C., soybeans and millet were always mentioned in ancient texts as the two major food crops in northern China. Tofu was developed in 164 B.C., probably by Buddhist monks, and quickly became a staple of Chinese cuisine. Buddhist missionaries took tofu with them to Japan, where it quickly became a popular item. Today, Japan boasts thirty thousand tofu shops, and the average Japanese eats over fifty pounds of tofu a year.

The man who revolutionized breakfast also gave Americans their first soymilk and meat substitutes made from soy, report Drs. Mark and Virginia Messina. Dr. John Harvey Kellogg was an early champion of vegetarianism. "At his Battle Creek Sanitarium, he invented granola as a substitute for the typical American breakfast of bacon and eggs. At the same time that he was busy inventing new cereals, Kellogg was becoming interested in the health benefits of soybeans. In 1919, he wrote extensively about their usefulness in the diet of diabetics. By the 1920s, he was marketing America's first soy foods. An advocate of a nondairy diet, he developed and championed the first Western soymilk."

In 1932, Dr. A.A. Horvath, known as the Father of the Soybean, published a paper entitled "Soya Flour as a National Food." He made some cogent arguments for making soy an American dietary staple: "When one realizes that these beans are, and have been for upwards of one hundred generations, the principal source of protein in the Chinese diet, and when one further considers the sustained hard manual work that the Chinese are capable of, as well as their mental virility, and the high state of their culture in a period when Europe and America were barbarians, it will be understood that the question of this diet is worth studying to introduce it in the diet of this country."

In the United States, the soybean has been referred to as "the miracle bean." Rarely can a food be found that is more useful or versatile than this little round legume. It is unsurpassed as an efficient and inexpensive source of protein. Its other applications are almost limitless—industry uses soybeans for everything from soap to paint to environmentally friendly ink. Henry Ford once wore suits made out of soybeans.

From the Journal of Chemistry and Industry, 1956, author unknown:

> "Little soybean who are you?
> From far off China where you grew?"
> I am wheels to steer your cars,
> I make cups that hold cigars.
> I make doggies nice and fat
> And glue the feathers on your hat.
> I am very good to eat,
> I am cheese and milk and meat.
> I am soap to wash your dishes,
> I am oil to fry your fishes.
> I am paint to trim your houses
> I am buttons on your blouses.
> You can eat me from the pod,
> I put pep back in the sod.
> If by chance you're diabetic
> The things I do are just prophetic.
> I'm most everything you've seen
> And still I'm just a little bean.

All in all, the soybean has a great concentration of longevity promoters making it both a super food and a miracle food medicine.

EIGHT

Chlorophyll
The Great Cleanser

C hlorophyll, or "solar energy," should become a welcome addition to the menu of those wishing to attain and maintain radiant
health. Its uses are as many and varied as the people who use
and swear by it. —**Paul DeSouza**

All life on this planet is derived, directly or indirectly, from the
sunlight that falls on chlorophyll. Chlorophyll is the green pigment
found in plants, algae and fresh dark green vegetables. Chlorophyll
in all its forms has been receiving a lot of media attention of late.
Some of the best sources of nutrients that prevent disease and
support health are found in plants that are a rich green color—and
one of the reasons is the color itself. If you've ever noticed parts of
the broccoli in your refrigerator turning yellow with age, you are
witnessing the fading of this green pigment. Green plants have been
revered throughout history as efficacious tissue cleansers as well as
effective agents in the treatment of many chronic disorders.

Chlorophyll got its name in 1818 from the Greek words *chloros*
(green) and *phyllum* (leaf). There is a blue-black "chlorophyll-a" as
well as the more familiar dark green "chlorophyll-b." Both of these
chlorophylls are formed in the leaves' chloroplasts—little orga-
nized units of special cells, where stacks of chlorophyll molecules
are stored up until used.

In 1915, Dr. Richard Willstatter won a Nobel prize for discovering the chemical structure of chlorophyll, a network of carbon,

hydrogen, nitrogen and oxygen atoms surrounding a single magnesium atom. Fifteen years later, Dr. Hans Fisher won a Nobel prize for unraveling the chemical structure of hemoglobin, and was surprised to find out it was almost the same as chlorophyll. Hemoglobin is the pigment that gives red blood cells their red color, just as chlorophyll is the pigment that gives plants their green color. When Dr. Fisher separated the heme from the protein molecule to which it was attached, the main difference between it and chlorophyll was a single iron atom at its center instead of a magnesium atom, as in the chlorophyll molecule.

Heme and chlorophyll are fascinating in both their differences and similarities. Both are pigments that carry out their functions in cells, both are vital to the life of the organism to which they belong, both work with carbon dioxide and oxygen, and both have structural similarities. Among their differences, heme has iron at its center, chlorophyll has magnesium; heme takes in oxygen and gives off carbon dioxide, while chlorophyll takes in carbon dioxide and gives off oxygen; heme is red, chlorophyll is green (complementary colors). The iron in blood contributes to the vitality level of the person, while magnesium, as found in chlorophyll, is a relaxant which also acts as a catalyst in the use of protein, carbohydrates, fats, calcium and phosphorus.

Dr. Fisher, excited by the similarity in structure between chlorophyll and heme, immediately began research on possible medical uses for chlorophyll. He was not alone. In laboratories and hospitals throughout the United States, excited researchers and doctors had already begun to investigate the "life blood" of plants.

Healing the Body with Chlorophyll

Not surprisingly, chlorophyll is known to have revitalizing, rejuvenating and detoxifying effects. Foods high in chlorophyll help oxygenate the body, thereby offsetting the deleterious effects of living in an environment polluted with smog and carbon monoxide. Many decades of research have revealed a plethora of noteworthy benefits.

One of the first in-depth medical tests on chlorophyll was reported in the July 1930 issue of the *American Journal of Surgery*. The studies were conducted by Temple University's department of experimental pathology, making newspaper and magazine headlines at the time. Doctors at Temple University used chlorophyll packs, ointments and solutions to treat over 1,200 patients whose ailments ranged from the common cold to a burst appendix with spreading peritonitis. Chlorophyll diluted with sterile water was used to clean out deep surgical wounds, some of them badly infected. Ulcerated varicose veins, osteomyelitis, brain ulcers and shallow open wounds were cleansed with the chlorophyll solution or covered with a chlorophyll salve. Diseases of the mouth, such as trenchmouth and advanced pyorrhea, were treated.

The results were spectacular. The doctors who tested the chlorophyll hailed it as an important and effective therapy. Over 1,000 cases of respiratory infections, sinusitis and head colds were treated under the supervision of Dr. Robert Ridpath and Dr. T. Carroll Davis. They reported, "There is not a single case in which improvement or cure has not taken place." Chlorophyll packs placed on sinuses gave great relief. Head colds were described as being cleared up in 24 hours.

Temple University researchers found that chlorophyll did not kill germs in test tube experiments, but rather that it increased the resistance of cells and inhibited the growth of bacteria.

In another study, Drs. Smith and Livingston demonstrated that chlorophyll caused an "almost immediate growth response" of fibroblasts—the cells the body uses to repair wounds. In the treatment of a variety of types of skin ulcers, chlorophyll was found to have a "stimulating effect" on the supportive tissues, promoting rapid healing.

Similarly, chlorophyll is effective as an external ointment for reducing or removing bad odors from poorly healing wounds. When doctors replaced the chlorophyll ointment with a placebo, the wounds began to reassert their disagreeable odor as well as poor healing. This is because chlorophyll is both wound-healing and inhibiting to bacteria. With all the oxygen contained in chlorophyll, it is easy to see why oxygen-hating microbes would suffer when bathed in this plant juice.

As a topical ointment, chlorophyll has also been shown to be efficacious in the treatment of inflammation that occurs in the skin after radiation treatments for cancer and other conditions. French scientists have shown that chlorophyll can reduce tissue damage caused by radiotherapy. Radiation burns have been repaired by plants that contain significant amounts of chlorophyll, suggesting that this substance may be the common active constituent.

A Cleanser for All Kinds of Things

The common skin disease known as athlete's foot is really the result of fungus infection. As a rule, the fungi responsible for this annoying condition are carried between the toes of the feet, and remain dormant—until the feet become moist or cracks appear in the skin. When this happens, the fungus enters the outer layer of tissue and establishes a place in which to increase its size.

Because fungus is a plant that lives on organic matter, it is not only hardy, but extremely difficult to abolish. That's why athlete's foot has taxed the ingenuity of many doctors. Although there are many salves, solutions and other patented remedies purported to be successful in treating athlete's foot, nothing compares with chlorophyll. In this natural product, we have a healing agent as well as a bacteriostatic; thus it is possible to correct the cause and the effect at the same time.

A podiatrist I know recommends the following: After washing and drying the feet thoroughly, put them in an enamel basin containing a diluted solution of ten parts warm water and one part liquid chlorophyll. Be sure to cover the toes entirely for at least thirty minutes, then dry them well. This treatment should be followed daily for two weeks, then two or three times weekly for two weeks longer to be certain all fungi are destroyed. In obstinate cases, rolls of cotton soaked in full strength liquid chlorophyll, or a chlorophyll ointment, may be put between the toes. Chlorophyll stops the offensive odor as well as the underlying condition.

Chlorophyll has also been shown to be helpful in the treatment of pancreatitis. Pancreatitis is an inflammation of the pancreas that can be very painful and life threatening. It may be caused by excess consumption of alcohol, by gallstones, poor nutrition, excessive calcium in the blood, and excessive blood fat. Chlorophyll-a derivatives (from blue-black colored sources) inhibit proteases, which are enzymes that break down proteins. Protease enzymes support inflammation and are in large part responsible for the harmful effects of pancreatitis.

Chlorophyll has a long history of being effective at deodorizing bad smells. You may be aware of chlorophyll-containing gum for bad breath, and some kitty litter contains chlorophyll. It is also found in mouthwash and toothpaste to help control bad breath as well as skin lotions. Chlorophyll has also been used and documented to act as an underarm deodorant. It is well known among workers in nursing homes, geriatric hospitals and mental institutions that chlorophyll is an important aid in the control of odors from incontinent patients.

In 1990, the Food and Drug Administration determined that the clinical use of chlorophyll taken internally was both safe and effective for reducing body odors. This is especially so for people who have had surgeries such as ileostomies, where the more difficult elimination of bowel or bladder wastes can lead to problem odors.

As documented by research, many diseases are aggravated by poor bowel health. Although not very precise as a diagnostic method, smelling a person's breath is one way of determining if a person is suffering from bowel toxicity. Chlorophyll helps clear bowel toxicity within a few days.

One colon-related ailment is chronic constipation, one of those problems that seem to afflict many people as they grow older. In addition to infrequent and hard stools, constipation may cause bad breath, headaches and has been associated with the development of pancreatitis, hypoglycemia and even cancer (breast and colon). It has been shown that chlorophyll helps relieve chronic constipation problems and also relieves intestinal gas in terms of amount and odor.

The detoxifying and stimulating effect of chlorophyll on the bowel produces an interesting result at times. Many people will release more gases than usual for three to seven days after beginning to use it. Probably the harmful intestinal bacteria are being fermented and destroyed. After this initial adjustment period, the bowel functions better, and the gas problems disappear.

The deodorant properties of water-soluble chlorophyll are dependent on the acid-base (pH) balance of the material that needs to be neutralized. Chlorophyll exhibits deodorant actions on neutral or alkaline material with an optimum pH between eight and 10.5. Chlorophyll also exhibits antibacterial properties on neutral or alkaline material. Bowel toxicity and constipation are associated with a stool pH of greater than seven, with the worst cases having a stool pH of nine. Chlorophyll functions best in treating colons that are suffering from anaerobic bacterial overgrowth syndromes, which are usually associated with a stool pH of greater than seven. Anyone can test their stool by buying pH litmus paper which is available at drugstores, and observing the color changes on the paper.

Many impressive studies too numerous to mention here have noted chlorophyll's ability to nourish the intestines and to have a very soothing or healing effect on the mucous linings. It has also been used beneficially in the detoxification of all the organs, particularly the liver. It can help to wash drug deposits from the body, purify the blood, and counteract acids and toxins in the body.

Besides its tonic effects at improving tissue oxygenation and removing unpleasant internal odors, chlorophyll has been considered as an effective means of removing heavy metal buildup. In her book *Are You Radioactive? How To Protect Yourself*, Linda Clark states that chlorophyll can bind with several toxins, including heavy metals, and help eliminate them. Research done during the last few years has found that chlorophyll can help offset the damaging effects of the environment, radiation, and x-rays, and that chlorophyll cannot induce mutations.

Physicians and dentists have used chlorophyll for years to successfully treat oral diseases, kidney stones, and acute infections of the upper respiratory tract and sinuses. In addition, nutritionists and researchers believe that it may also play an important role in the prevention of cancer. Chlorophyll has also been shown to increase the effectiveness of penicillin by as much as 35 percent.

Chlorophyll's Boost to Immune Functions

Let's not forget chlorophyll's increasing popularity due to its use as an immune-building food supplement. Immunology is fast becoming one of the most exciting and potentially rewarding areas of modern medicine. Immunology is the study of the immune system: the body's mechanisms which fight off foreign invaders, whether they be bacteria, viruses, chemicals or foreign proteins. The body's defenses have a unique way of inactivating or detoxifying each of these types of substances. Chlorophyll has been found to stimulate all the different organs and components of the immune system.

One of the key components of the immune system is *macrophage* cells, which are active against cancer, foreign proteins and chemicals. Macrophages are large cells located in the abdominal cavity, the blood (monocytes), joints (synovial lining cells), bone marrow and connective tissue. They clean the blood, body fluids and cavities of harmful substances (this process is called phagocytosis).

One way to fight cancer is to stimulate macrophage production and activity. This macrophage stimulation causes increased cancer cell destruction and the removal of harmful cancer debris from the blood by this phagocytic activity. *Interferon* is a natural secretion of the body, a protein substance produced by virus-invaded cells that prevents reproduction of the virus. Interferon is thought to be a stimulator of macrophages. Numerous studies show chlorophyll increases the levels of interferon in the body and thereby stimulates the immune system.

Chlorophyll is water soluble and easy to digest. Interestingly, it is also rich in the fat-soluble vitamin K, which is necessary, among other things, for blood clotting. Because of this and other benefits, chlorophyll has been used for women with heavy menstrual bleeding as well as for anemia by holistic doctors, herbalists and other health professionals. Vitamin K also helps form a compound in the urine that inhibits growth of calcium oxalate crystals (common kidney stones), so chlorophyll may be helpful in the prevention of this very painful condition, according to Dr. Amanda Crawford, a graduate of Britain's School of Herbal Medicine and a member of Britain's National Institute of Medical Herbalists.

When the diet is lacking in a sufficient amount of fruits and vegetables, the body tends to become more acidic, and thus a fertile environment for many diseases and ailments. To assist the body's pH balance, chlorophyll can help neutralize the acidifying and stimulating effect of excess protein, sugars and starch. Like vegetables, fruit and nongluten grains such as millet, chlorophyll is alkalinizing and cleansing.

To Sum Up Chlorophyll's Benefits

In general, the salutary action of chlorophyll is subtle, yet remarkable. Here's a brief summary of the healing power of chlorophyll.

1. Strengthens immunity—especially the surface or "mucus" immune system. This is the first line of bodily defense and functions best against allergens, airborne microbes and pollutants.

2. Protects the body from and helps neutralize a wide range of chemical environmental pollutants including low level radiation.

3. Acts as a major detoxifier of metabolic waste products in blood. In a "micro" sense, chlorophyll benefits the body much as green plants benefit our "macro" environment.

4. Stimulates circulation, metabolism and cellular respiration. This attribute has a tremendous application in the recovery phase of debilitating illness and in weight loss.

5. Helps prevent Candida, Epstein-Barr virus, Cytomegalovirus and chronic fatigue syndrome.

6. Acts as an internal deodorant/topical antiseptic. In fact, liquid chlorophyll can be used as mouthwash and as a cleanser for cuts, abrasions and minor burns. Liquid chlorophyll concentrate also reduces urinary and bowel odors.

7. Establishes a healthy intestinal ecosystem by promoting the growth of probiotic (friendly) intestinal bacteria.

There is no toxicity associated with chlorophyll; cramps or mild diarrhea may occur with large quantities, but will disappear on reducing or stopping its intake. A large dose of chlorophyll may turn the stool green, especially if you haven't been in the habit of eating many green foods. This is not harmful and can even be helpful if you are trying to determine your digestive "transit time" (how fast or slowly food moves through the body). Transit time gives some information about how well the digestive process is functioning: too fast, and we can't absorb all our nutrients; too slow, and bacterial changes in a stagnant colon may lead to other health risks. A healthy transit time is between 12 and 17 hours.

How do you take chlorophyll? Eat green plants! Alternatively, you may choose liquids, capsules or tablets of chlorophyll, available in your health food store. I use the liquid chlorophyll and other chlorophyll products by the DeSouza company because of their superb quality, which will be explained in detail in the following chapter.

In the next chapter, I will also explain some major sources of chlorophyll and the special additional properties that they have.

NINE

Greens
Back to the Basics

This is the true joy in life: being used for a purpose recognized by yourself as a mighty one, and being a force of nature instead of a feverish, selfish little clod of ailments and grievances, complaining that the world will not devote itself to making you happy.

—George Bernard Shaw

If you've been looking for an easy way to have more energy, prevent and alleviate disease, reverse the aging process, detoxify your body, improve your skin, and boost your immune system—in short, to create all-round radiant health—then "be sure and eat your greens." Do you remember your mother or grandmother saying this? Now research is supporting their folklore wisdom. The Juiceman, my friend Jay Kordich, author of *The Juiceman's Power of Juicing*, says "All life on earth emanates from the green of the plant." There's no doubt about it. Nutritional scientists have discovered that some of the best sources of nutrients to prevent disease and support health are found in plants of a rich green color—and one of the reasons is the color itself.

Chlorophyll, the green pigment in plants, has long been known as an efficacious tissue cleanser and agent in the treatment of many chronic disorders. Because of its importance to radiant health, I've devoted the entire previous chapter to chlorophyll.

Chlorophyll is found to some degree in every green plant. But nutritionists have found that some of the best sources of chlorophyll are algae, kelp, wheat and barley grasses, alfalfa, liquid chlorophyll and leafy greens. These foods are also prolific storehouses of other nutrients as well.

Alfalfa—A Rich Source of Chlorophyll

Today, the main source of chlorophyll for commercial extraction is alfalfa. Modern processing technology is now able to maximize and optimize the tremendous benefits of this plant that has been of service to humanity for so long.

Alfalfa originated as a wild legume in the dry uplands of western Asia. The Medes of ancient Persia are thought to have been the first to cultivate it, hence its Latin name *Medicago sativa,* which means "sowed by the Medians."

One of the richest mineral foods, alfalfa's roots grow as much as 130 feet into the earth. Concentrated alfalfa is an excellent source of silicon, a mineral that is so important for the development of good teeth, hair, and nails. It also contains calcium, magnesium, phosphorus, potassium, selenium, zinc, and iron, plus all known vitamins. The minerals are in a balanced form, which promotes absorption. Further, it has all of the essential amino acids, making it a complete protein.

Dried alfalfa has been used in teas and pressed into tablets for supplements. Alfalfa is a highly regarded medicinal herb, and is recommended as part of treatment for the following health problems: inflammatory diseases, including arthritis and rheumatism; digestive disorders (alfalfa contains the digestive enzyme betaine that is beneficial to intestinal flora); diseases in which the liver is damaged or functioning improperly.

New processing technology greatly enhances the benefits of alfalfa for human use by releasing and concentrating its great nutritional benefits without diminishing its medicinal qualities. With this method, the juice is first extracted at temperatures below 100 degrees F. The juice is then dried at low temperature to retain active enzymes so important to maintaining good health. By this process one pound of alfalfa is concentrated into one tablespoon of powder.

Liquid Chlorophyll

In 1935, Paul DeSouza investigated, studied, and began the manufacture of chlorophyll products—offering only those products meeting his high standards. DeSouza was one of the pioneer health enthusiasts and avant-garde exponents of the natural, organic farming methods which are in wide use today.

As a young man of 27, DeSouza moved to California and discovered that the fertile farmlands were being destroyed by chemical fertilizers and pesticides which drained the essential minerals from the soil. No effort was being made to return these nutrients to the soil. He searched the world to find an area where the farming methods had not left a depleted, desecrated land as a result of over-production and chemical destruction, and to his amazement he found the answer in Israel. The ancient knowledge of the Hebrews included the wonderful secrets of soil renewal.

He was a true pioneer in this field, and continued to share his vision of "good ground to grow good food." He knew that if the Hebrew agriculturists could renew their lands and keep the thin, poor soil of the desert always productive for more than 6,000 years, it could be done with the rich, formerly fertile lands of California. Thus, the science used today in organic farms came from the great Jewish tradition to DeSouza who carried the knowledge to organic and ecologically aware commercial farmers. DeSouza Liquid Chlorophyll is an essential part of my health program (see Resources).

Kelp

Three-fourths of the earth's surface is covered with water, and a substantial portion of the world's food supply is harvested from its seas, lakes and rivers. It should not be surprising, then, to find that there are other food sources in these waters besides fish. The largest mammal in the world, the blue whale, feeds in great part on seaweed (sea vegetables) and minute sea creatures called plankton.

A particular type of chlorophyll-rich seaweed (which is actually brown) called *Laminaria*—better known as kelp—is definitely one of nature's superfoods. It has been used for centuries as a remedy for respiratory, gastrointestinal, genitourinary and thyroid disorders. It is high in vitamins and minerals, such as calcium, magnesium, potassium, niacin, riboflavin, and choline.

More recently, kelp has gained scientific acclaim as a major source of vitamin C and algin. Vitamin C is one of the antioxidants that helps to boost the immune system. Algin (a colloidal substance found in various kelps) is helpful in pulling out harmful pollutants and heavy metals, such as lead, from the body.

Besides being a source of chlorophyll, kelp is also an excellent source of iodine, an important mineral that comes only from the sea (saltwater fish, sea salt, and seaweed). It is often taken for its iodine content by people who want to improve their thyroid function. Many people rely on iodized salt as a source of this important mineral. However, most Americans consume too much salt (sodium chloride). In fact, the average American consumes between 5,000 and 6,000 mg of sodium chloride per day although the Recommended Daily Allowance is 2,400 mg per day. (Personally, I do not use or recommend table salt.) Regular table salt should also be avoided because aluminum, which is often used as an anticaking agent in table salt, has been strongly implicated in promoting Alzheimer's disease. Therefore, kelp is a better choice for iodine. It's a whole nutrient-rich food provided by nature. Granulated or powdered kelp can be used as a condiment or a flavoring in place of table salt.

Let's digress for one moment to talk about seasonings. Keep a variety of seasonings on hand. My favorite one is Spike (and now also available salt-free) created by the nutritionist, author, and lecturer, Gayelord Hauser. Thirty-nine spices and herbs are blended to create a delicious combination. (For free samples of Spike and other Gayelord Hauser seasonings, see Resources.)

Kelp is not only very high in minerals, but it also provides other superlative benefits: kelp has been shown to reduce blood pressure, cholesterol and the incidence of chemical carcinogen-induced tumors in animals and humans.

One impressive study by Dr. Jane Teas, formally with the Harvard University School of Public Health, found that Japanese women have about one-sixth the breast cancer rate of American women of similar age and economic status. Dr. Teas noted that Japanese women who lived in rural areas of Japan had a much lower breast cancer rate than did Japanese women who lived in urban areas.

Why the differences? The study identified many potential factors, but the one that seemed to be the most consistent was diet. Japanese women living in rural areas of Japan routinely eat sea-weed—a food uncommon in the diets of American and urban Japanese women—and little processed food. Among the urban Japanese and American women, it was reversed: they eat little seaweed and a great deal of processed food. Dr. Teas confirmed her observation by testing her theory in the laboratory. Rats exposed to chemicals known to cause breast cancer and then fed seaweed did not develop cancer.

Although researchers aren't exactly sure how kelp protects the body against cancer, they believe that it boosts the body's own immune system, indirectly allowing it to combat cancer.

Barley & Wheat Grasses

Young barley leaves and wheat grasses are also superfoods. These two greens offer an energy lift and act as a "purifier" and "rejuvenator," probably because of their high chlorophyll and nutrient content.

Both are good natural sources of chlorophyll, minerals (especially calcium, magnesium and potassium), vitamins and enzymes, especially the antioxidant enzymes reputed to slow down the aging process and to control progression of degenerative diseases. Just two tablespoons of barley grass have as much beta-carotene as one serving of spinach. Wheat and barley grasses are rich in vitamin A and beta-carotene, which aids in the formation and maintenance of healthy skin, bones, teeth and mucous membranes and plays an important role in healthy human reproduction. Wheat and barley grasses are packed with vitamins B1 and B2. These vitamins help to maintain a strong nervous system, healthy mucous membranes, and play a vital role in helping to metabolize proteins, fats, and carbohydrates. They are also rich sources of vitamin K, a nutrient that helps maintain normal bone metabolism. Vitamin K also helps the body synthesize the substances needed in order for blood to clot.

Barley grass, in particular, is high in superoxide dismutase (SOD). SOD is an antioxidant enzyme which functions somewhat like vitamin C and the other antioxidants by scavenging free radicals. (See Chapters 2 and 4 on nutrition and fats for more information on free radicals.) These grasses also are an excellent way to help in the elimination of fecal matter and toxins in the colon.

In addition, wheat and barley grasses are high in minerals. Eating these grasses will supply a rich source of calcium (for strong bones, teeth, and muscles), magnesium (for strong bones and good muscle function), potassium (for proper balance of fluids and electrolytes), and zinc (an element found in more than 100 enzymes needed for good health).

Algae

In or near the bodies of water on our planet, there are 25,000 species of algae. Algae, or chlorella, are elementary plants without roots, stems, branches or leaves. They carry on all their functions, including reproduction, at the cellular level. Green algae are among the simplest living organisms. The chlorophyll contained in algae has been estimated by scientists to be responsible for about 90 percent of the photosynthesis that takes place on Earth. Algae form the first link in the series of organisms that make up the Earth's food chain, and they grow just about everywhere.

Spirulina & Blue-Green Algae

Spirulina is the original green superfood, an easily produced algae with the ability to grow in both ocean and alkaline waters. It is ecologically sound in that it can be cultivated in extreme environments which are useless for conventional agriculture. It can be cultivated on small scale community farms, doubling its bio-mass every two to five days, in such a variety of climates and growing conditions that it could significantly improve the nutrition of local populations currently on the brink of starvation. Spirulina alone could double the protein available to humanity on a fraction of the world's land, while helping restore the environmental balance on the planet. Acre for acre, spirulina yields *20 times* more protein than soybeans, *40 times* more protein than corn, and *400 times* more protein than beef. It is a complete protein, providing all 21 amino acids, and the entire B complex of vitamins, including B_{12}. It is also rich in beta-carotene, minerals, trace minerals, and essential fatty acids (EFAs). Digestibility is high, stimulating both immediate and long range energy.

Blue-green algae has been called a perfect superfood. It is naturally soft-celled and does not require that its cell walls be broken, as chlorella does, to render it nutritionally valuable. Its soft or "peptidoglyan" cell wall is virtually identical in structure to the glycogen in the human body and is thus about 95 percent assimilable by the body and easily digested, with no mechanical processing involved.

Blue green algae is rich in neuropeptides, which repair, rebuild and strengthen the neurotransmitters in the brain. This enables the nerve cells of the brain to communicate at peak capacity with the rest of the body. It is high in digestible protein (76 percent), fiber, chlorophyll, vitamins, minerals and enzymes. It is the most potent source of beta-carotene available in the world today. It is also the richest source of vitamin B_{12}—higher than liver, chlorella or sea vegetables. (Super Blue Green Algae is my favorite—see Resources.)

Blue-green algae users report clearer thinking, more energy, a greater feeling of well-being, and improved memory. Therapeutically, it has been used to stimulate the immune system, improve digestion and assimilation, detoxify the body, enhance growth and tissue repair, accelerate healing, protect against radiation, help prevent degenerative diseases and promote longer life.

As a food from the sea, blue green algae is particularly intriguing. In *Energy Agriculture,* Dr. Maynard Murray writes, "Of special interest is the fact that the aging process does not appear to occur in the sea. The comparison between the cells of a huge adult whale and the cells taken from a newly born whale will show no evidence of the chemical changes observed when comparing cells of other adult and newly born mammals."

Chlorella

In 1890, M.W. Beijerinck of Holland, a microbiologist, first developed cultures of *Chlorella vulgaris*, a high-protein single-celled algae. More recently, chlorella-containing fossils over two billion years old have been found. That the genetic structure of this simple plant has remained unchanged over all these years is a testimony to its inherent strength. Not until 1977, with the development of a process that breaks down chlorella's cell walls to create a product that is more digestible and easily tolerated, was it used as a health food in the United States.

The chlorella algae is a single-celled plant which grows larger by maturing and developing its own food, rather than by adding new cells as do most other plants. It is the richest source of chlorophyll on Earth, and therefore particularly valuable for its ability to balance the body chemistry and to raise the level of health of the entire body.

Chlorella is noted for its ability to detoxify pollutants in the body and can remove heavy metals such as lead, mercury and cadmium.

Chlorella provides a plethora of vitamins and minerals. In addition, it is a complete protein because it supplies more than 19 amino acids, including all eight essential amino acids. Ester Lau, M.S., and her colleagues at the University of California at Berkeley, successfully used chlorella mixed with cereal grains as a way to promote growth among laboratory rats. They concluded that chlorella is an excellent source of protein.

Chlorella also helps regulate cholesterol and prevents tumor growth. One of its prime benefits is its stimulation of the immune system. Scientists at California's Loma Linda University School of Medicine found that chlorella stimulates macrophages—the immune cells in the body that kill bacteria, viruses, and cancer cells.

Although chlorella is nontoxic, in large doses there can be a problem with side effects, especially for those whose bodies are extremely toxic and have an overwhelming condition such as yeast infection, according to Dr. David Steenblock in his book, *Chlorella: Natural Mineral Algae*. He says that intestinal gas, irregular bowel movement, nausea, or slight fever may occur for a few days in some individuals as the toxicity in their bodies is neutralized. Likewise, says Dr. Steenblock, "Allergy sufferers sometimes break out in pimples, rashes, boils, or eczema, that, in some cases, can be accompanied by itching. This means that the drive to regain internal balance is being accelerated, and the body is actively working to expel toxins." If this should happen to you, Dr. Steenblock advises that you stop taking chlorella for several days, and allow your system to rest. Then begin taking it again in small doses, working your way up to larger doses.

One easy way to get many of the above superfoods in a daily diet is to get Kyo-Green at your local health food store. (See Resources.) Made by the highly respected Wakunaga of America Company, Kyo-Green is a delicious, nutritious powdered drink mix that blends the concentrated juices of wheat and barley grass, kelp, Bulgarian chlorella (known for its purity), and brown rice. It enhances the immune system, has anticarcinogenic properties, slows down the aging process, neutralizes toxins, helps build the blood, controls progression of degenerative diseases, and much more.

Green & Leafy Vegetables

Green and leafy vegetables should become a part of your daily diet. They add vitamins, minerals, usable calcium and beta-carotene needed for the immune system. They also help ward off diseases such as cancer. Leafy greens are excellent for the gall bladder, spleen, heart and blood, and are a good brain food. Most greens can be cooked or eaten raw in salads or fresh juices. (See Chapter 10 on Juicing.)

To clean them, soak in a sink of cold water for a few minutes and swirl around, then drain the water. Pat dry. Tear the leaves into small pieces, trim the ends of the stems, and chop when necessary. Keep in mind that all leafy greens contain chlorophyll, iron, magnesium, calcium, manganese, vitamin C, potassium, vitamin A, and a bonus of the essential fatty acids, and no cholesterol. The vegetables with the darkest, most intense colors tend to contain the highest level of nutrients.

For dressing on a salad of greens, I usually combine one of Spectrum Naturals delicious vinegars (my favorites are raspberry, mango, peach, garlic and Italian herb) with their organic flax seed oil and some herbs. It's fresh, easy to make, flavorful and healthy.

Here is a brief listing of some of my favorite leafy greens I eat on a regular basis.

- **Arugula**: From the mustard family, this green is peppery and tart, and mixes well with other greens. It is also known as roquette. It adds pizzazz to any raw salad, is high in vitamins A, C, niacin, iron and phosphorus, and is good for normalizing body acid with its high alkalinity.
- **Beet greens**: Best used in juices, they are very high in nutrients, especially iron and calcium. These greens can be used in cooking also. They are known for their benefit in blood disorders, liver function and the flow of bile.
- **Belgian Endive**: Good in a salad with raspberry or mango vinaigrette dressing. I also use the leaves for dipping in place of crackers or chips. It has pale yellow or white leaves. It is kin to chicory with similar healing qualities and nutrient content.
- **Butterhead Lettuce**: Also known as Boston Bibb, this is a very tender leaf, with an almost buttery taste. Makes a good salad when used with spinach, endive, or watercress. Lettuce is said to calm the nerves.
- **Chicory**: A bitter green, with curly leaves, the young leaves are best in salads. High in vitamins C and A, and calcium and iron. Aids in liver function and blood disorders. Try radicchio, often called red-leaf chicory, good in salads.
- **Collards**: A member of the cabbage family. Use only the leaves; they tend to be tough so steam them for 5 to 8 minutes. Collards can be used in salads as a substitute for cabbage and are also great for juicing. No leafy green is more valuable in

the body for disorders of the colon, respiratory system, lymphatic system and skeletal system because of its high nutrition content.

- **Dandelion greens**: The young leaves have a tangy taste. They are good for gall bladder disorders, rheumatism, gout, eczema, and skin disorders. Dandelion is also an excellent liver rejuvenator. They cook the same as any leafy green. Rich in calcium, potassium, and vitamins A and C. These are also excellent to add to juices.
- **Escarole & Endive**: From the chicory family. The leaves are very dark green, with a slightly bitter taste. These make a good salad with a warm citrus-flavored dressing, and can also be steamed. Both are rich in vitamin A, calcium, minerals, B-vitamins, iron and potassium. They're good for most infections, for liver function, and internal cleansing.
- **Kale**: This is the king of calcium. Use only the leaves of this plant. It tastes like cabbage. I often add the juice of kale to carrot and other juices. It's very high in usable calcium and is, therefore, excellent for prevention and care of osteoporosis.
- **Mustard & Turnip greens**: These greens have a nippy taste with flavors varying from mild to hot. They are good sautéed with a little garlic, or steamed. Also, they can be used in juices. They're high in calcium and vitamin C. Good for infections, colon disorders, colds, flu and elimination of kidney stones due to excess uric acid.
- **Parsley**: All types of this plant are rich in vitamin A, B-complex, C, minerals, potassium, and manganese. Parsley contains mucilage, starch, opinol and volatile oil. It is very crisp and tangy. This green has an "odor eating" quality, that helps restore fresh breath after a meal with such foods as garlic and onion. Add to fresh juices or chop to add to salads. Good for digestive disorders, also an excellent diuretic. Try cilantro, a Chinese and Mexican parsley, essential in many Chinese, Spanish, Mexican and Thai dishes.
- **Romaine Lettuce**: This is a wonderful, crunchy green which is highest in nutrients of all types of lettuce. Great in salads. I always keep lots on hand for salads and juicing. This lettuce

is not good for cooking. Being high in chlorophyll, it is a good blood purifier.

- **Sorrel**: This green has a pleasantly sour and slightly lemon flavor. It is easily perishable and best bought fresh or grown in your garden. Try sorrel in salads or as a seasoning in soups and casseroles. Sorrel is a powerful antioxidant with the same healing properties of kale.
- **Spinach**: Its tender bright green leaves are most beneficial when eaten raw. Because of the oxalic acid content, some of the calcium becomes unavailable to the body. Spinach contains many valuable nutrients and is high in iron.
- **Swiss Chard**: From the beet family, this green has a mild taste and is good with walnuts and pine nuts added to a salad. It has the highest content of sodium of all greens. Chlorophyll and calcium-rich, Swiss chard is a natural cleanser and helps strengthen bones.
- **Watercress**: This green has young, tender leaves which should be picked before the plant flowers. The spicy-flavored green goes well with romaine and butterhead lettuce. It's higher in nutrient content than most greens and is excellent for vitamin deficiencies and illnesses of all types. Good added to fresh juices, too.

Aloe: A Desert Succulent

The aloe "cactus," actually a desert succulent, has been touted as one of the "miracle" green plants—and there is now good research to back many of the claims. The leaf gel and whole leaf juices are used for treatment, both internally and externally.

The most common use of aloe vera is the application of its gel (the inside of the leaf) for burns, minor cuts, insect bites, skin irritations and as a skin moisturizer. For more than two decades, I have been growing aloe vera plants in my yard and always have one plant available in my kitchen for quick use.

Recent research shows that the healing benefits people claim are well-founded, and can also be experienced with internal use. Aloe vera has been proven to promote rapid healing of burns, to alleviate ulcers and protect the gastrointestinal lining, to have strong anti-inflammatory properties, and to have antiviral and mild pain-relieving properties. People also report other benefits, such as help in weight loss regimens and help with chronic problems such as arthritis and irritable bowel. However, the type of aloe vera used makes a big difference in whether you will receive the benefits.

I drink Aloe Falls brand aloe juices because they are preservative-free, are certified active, and even taste good (which is rare for aloe vera juices). The Aloe Falls plants are grown without herbicides or pesticides, and they produce the only aloe vera juices I have seen without preservatives. (See Aloe Falls in the Resource directory for more information.)

"Life is feeding everyone." —*John Denver*

TEN

Juices
Radiant Health in a Glass

V*egetable and fruit juices are packed with concentrated nutrients, and simply by drinking a few glasses of delicious juice every day, you supply your body with many of the essential elements that contribute to its strength and general well-being.* —**Jay Kordich**

For centuries, juices from fruits and vegetables have been used to help heal disease and build up the body's natural immunities. For example, it is known that:

Cabbage, broccoli, garlic, onions, leeks and citrus fruit are loaded with antioxidants which suppress the growth of deadly cancer cells.

Apples contain sorbitol, a gentle laxative.

Grapes and blueberries are filled with polyphenols, which kill viruses.

Cabbage is famous for its ulcer-healing properties.

Cantaloupe and garlic are blood-thinners, which can help prevent heart attacks and strokes.

The juices of green vegetables as well as **dark orange vegetables** act as antidotes to the cancer process (a process which continues for years after exposure to carcinogens).

Cherries are a remedy for gout.

Pineapple juice is rich in anti-inflammatory agents to soothe sore throats.

Lemon helps digestion by stimulating the flow of saliva and digestive juices.

Ginger relieves motion sickness.

Sounds incredible, doesn't it? I agree with Bernard Jensen, N.D. who said in his book, *Vibrant Health from Your Kitchen*: "The power and effectiveness of foods in healing and in keeping people well is sometimes astonishing."

You may wonder, "Why not eat the whole fruit or vegetable instead of juicing it?" The answer is that solid food requires hours of digestive activity before its nourishment is finally available to the cells and tissues of the body, whereas juices are easy and quick to prepare and drink, supply an abundance of nutrients, increase the servings of fruits and vegetables in your diet, and are absolutely delicious.

I do not advocate a total liquid diet, because the fibers found in solid foods are important too. While fibers have virtually no nourishing value, they act as an intestinal broom pushed by the peristaltic activity of the intestines. Nevertheless, juices are one of the main ingredients of health.

Eat It Raw!

According the American Cancer Society, the National Cancer Institute, and the National Research Council, Americans do not eat enough fresh fruits and vegetables to prevent disease. Yet these foods have been proven to have powerful protective effects for the body.

Many health professionals are now saying that we need to eat at least seven servings of vegetables and at least two servings of fruit each day. It has also been proven that 50 to 75 percent of our diet should be raw food if we are to enjoy optimal health and abundant energy. Leslie and Susannah Kenton, authors of *Raw Energy*, state that a "vast quantity of evidence . . . exists showing that the high-raw diet—a way of eating in which 75 percent of your foods are taken raw—cannot only reverse the bodily degeneration which accompanies long-term illness, but retard the rate at which you age, bring you seemingly boundless energy and even make you feel better emotionally." I know personally that this is true because for years I have eaten a diet which is at least 75 percent raw.

While cooked foods *sustain* life, they do not necessarily have the power to *regenerate* the cells which furnish the life force to our body. On the contrary, continuous consumption of cooked and processed foods results in progressive degeneration of cells and tissues. You can eat three or four big meals a day, and yet your body may be starved for vital nutrients and enzymes. Very few people in our urban Western culture eat three-quarters raw food.

The addition of fresh fruit and vegetable juices will not only add more raw foods to your diet, but also increase the number of servings of fruits and vegetables you get daily. This will help your body to heal itself and be healthy. I have been an avid juicer for 25 years and know it's one of the main reasons I'm radiantly healthy with an abundance of energy. I've also done extensive research on the healing powers of juicing and juice fasts.

Usually you just can't eat enough raw fruits and vegetables in a day to nourish your body properly. I don't think I could stomach eating five pounds of carrots. But it's easy to drink their nutritional equivalent in a delicious, nutritious glass of carrot juice. That's why juicing is such an important and easy addition to a busy lifestyle.

So now, let's take a closer look at why fresh fruit and vegetable juices are so beneficial. Powerhouses of nutrients, fresh juices revitalize and regenerate your entire body and mind. Juices made fresh and taken immediately send forth cleansing catalysts that penetrate the innermost recesses of your body and help dislodge toxins from your cells. And, at the same time, the abundant nutrients help repair your vital tissues and organs, and give you more energy and health.

Fresh fruit and vegetable juices are an excellent way to get vitamins, minerals, purified water, proteins, carbohydrates and chlorophyll. Fresh raw juices are also full of enzymes. Enzymes are organic catalysts that increase the rate at which foods are broken down and absorbed by the body. Enzymes are found in plant foods such as fruits and vegetables, but are destroyed by the heat of cooking. This is one of the reasons why fresh raw produce should constitute at least half of your diet.

Another benefit is that it takes little energy to digest juice, so you feel the benefits more quickly than when eating the whole food.

It can take many hours to process whole foods, especially when fat is present. But fresh fruit and vegetable juices, which are already separated from the fiber, are easy to digest. Indeed, within moments after you consume a glass of your favorite raw juice, the nutrients and enzymes go to work to create internal rejuvenation. For this reason, you often feel an instant "lift" when drinking a glass of fresh orange juice, as opposed to eating a whole orange.

The juice nutrients speed up the biological process of detoxifying the dead and decaying cells and washing them away. The juice nutrients then accelerate the building of new cells. When the toxic waste products that have been blocking cellular oxygenation and nourishment are washed out, then the juices stimulate metabolic and cell-rebuilding functions.

The extracted liquid portion of fruits or vegetables is a highly concentrated source of super cleaning without compare. Vegetable juices are dynamic sources of alkaline reserve. This helps establish the important acid-alkaline balance in your bloodstream. In addition, abundant supplies of minerals in the juices restore the biochemical and amino acid balance in your bloodstream, cells, tissues, and organs.

And here's a special benefit of juices: minerals provide needed oxygen and nourishment and accelerate the detoxification. With ordinary foods, mineral deficiency often precedes oxygen loss which "chokes" and "starves" your cells and allows waste buildup.

Three Categories of Juices

1. Green juices or "green drinks." Green juices stimulate cells and rejuvenate the body. They also build red blood cells. Green juices contain chlorophyll, which as you know from the chapter on chlorophyll, heals and cleanses the body. "Green drinks" can also be made by adding liquid chlorophyll to the juice. Green juices are made from spinach, lettuce, wheatgrass, celery, cabbage, dandelion greens, alfalfa sprouts, and other similar leafy greens and vegetables. (See Chapter 9 on Greens.)

2. Vegetable juices. Fresh vegetables are restorers and builders. They help remove excesses of protein, fat and acid wastes from the body. Vegetable juices help build the immune system, guard against illness, and are excellent sources of alkaline reserve. Both vegetable and green juices are extensively used in fasting and as nutritional supplements because of their high vitamin and mineral content. But they don't "travel" well because they oxidize quickly, which breaks down the protective enzymes and vitamins, so they should be taken immediately after juicing.

3. Fruit juices. Fruit juices are cleansers. They provide a quicker pick-me-up than vegetable juice because they are almost immediately absorbed, whereas vegetable juices are absorbed within an hour if taken on an empty stomach. Fruit juices also remain stable for a longer period of time and "travel" better than vegetable juices. The juices of different fruits are wonderful combined. I usually have some type of fruit juice combination each morning and another one before lunch as a snack. Since fruit juices have a high sugar content and ferment rapidly in the stomach, I recommend they be diluted with an equal amount of water. People with diabetes or hypoglycemia should be sure to take food with fruit juices

Juicing Made Easy

It's easy to make fresh juices. All you need is high-quality produce and a good juicer. Many different kinds of juicers are available, and I have tried all of them. My favorite and the one I recommend is the Juiceman Automatic Juice Extractor which comes in two sizes (see Resource Directory) designed by the Juiceman himself, Jay Kordich. It's very practical, efficient and easy to use and clean. What I particularly like about this juicer is that it's strong enough to juice skins and all—including pineapples, watermelons and cantaloupes—and vegetables such as cauliflower and broccoli which may look like they're not very juicy. Not so. Their juices are excellent when combined with carrot juice. You're wasting your money and many valuable nutrients if you purchase a juicer that's not designed to juice skins; many of the most important nutrients are in the skins and rinds. However, if you are not able to purchase organically grown, unsprayed produce, I suggest you peel the produce before juicing.

There's one exception to juicing the skins. It's best to peel oranges and grapefruits before juicing, even if they are organically grown, because their skins contain a toxic substance that should not be consumed in large quantities, and because these skins are somewhat bitter. Leave on the white pithy part of the peel, though, because it contains valuable bioflavonoids and vitamin C. Tropical fruits like kiwi and papaya should also be peeled if they have been grown in foreign countries where the use of carcinogenic sprays is still legal. The skins of all other fruits and vegetables, including lemons and limes, may be left on (if grown in the United States). However, if the produce has been waxed, I recommend removing the peel.

When you aren't able to get organic produce, and the produce is not the type that can be peeled, make sure you wash it thoroughly. **Here's a formula for helping remove toxic surface sprays from your non-organic produce**: 1. Fill your kitchen sink with cold water; 2. Add four tablespoons of salt and the juice of half a fresh lemon. This makes a diluted form of hydrochloric acid; 3. Soak fruits and vegetables five to ten minutes; soak leafy greens two to three minutes; and soak berries one to two minutes; 4. Rinse well after soaking.

Never wash or hull strawberries until just before use. They lose their freshness quite rapidly after washing. Leafy greens store better if spun dry after washing. Store greens in zip-lock bags. Celery stores best in the long plastic produce bags with a little water added to the bottom of the bag. For greater freshness, leave the stalks attached until ready to use. Do not juice celery leaves—they add a bitter taste to the drink

Also, make sure you drink your juice right after juicing. Researchers at Stanford University found that in only one minute after the juice is extracted, the therapeutic qualities begin to dissipate. Orange juice, if not consumed within five minutes, loses half of its vitamin C content; if it sits for an hour, it loses all of its vitamin C. So always try to drink your juice when it's fresh. If you want to take juice to work with you, try this: moisten the inside of a stainless steel thermos with water and put it in the freezer overnight. Before going to work, make your juice and put it directly into the cold thermos, filling the thermos to the brim. Juice will stay fresher (less oxidation and vitamin loss) for up to eight hours this way.

Contrary to popular belief, you can get protein from juices. In the cellulose matter of greens lies the finest protein in the world. The strongest creatures on the planet are strictly vegetarian: horses, gorillas, elephants. The only protein that nurtures these creatures is in green plants. Studies reveal that the most disease-free humans are vegans (vegetarians who eat no animal products including dairy or eggs). Humans have the same protein sources available from vegetables, including juices. You may be surprised to learn that one large glass of carrot juice has at least five grams of protein, which is equal to the protein of two eggs.

In general, I do not recommend combining fruit and vegetable juices on a regular basis, with the exception of apple juice. While there's really no known scientific basis for restrictions on food combining, some people—such as those with impaired digestion, multiple food allergies, or severe fatigue—benefit from avoiding combinations of fruit and vegetables. If you experience no adverse symptoms (such as gas or stomach aches) from combining fruit and vegetable juices, let your taste buds be your guide, and make the combinations you like best.

As I mentioned earlier, juicing has been an important part of my health program for 25 years. At least once a month I do a one to three day juice-only diet, and a few times a year I do a several day juice fast. Dr. Elson Haas, a dear friend whose medical practice is in San Rafael, California, uses juice fasts as a form of medical therapy. According to Dr. Haas, he has fasted on juice regularly himself, as have thousands of his patients over the course of nearly twenty years. He told me: "I did my first ten-day juice cleanse in 1975, and the experience changed my life and health. I realized the importance of diet and fasting in preventing disease and maintaining health. I cleared my allergies and back pains, normalized my weight, and felt a new level of vitality and creativity." Dr. Haas finds juice therapy very helpful with colds and flus, recurrent infections, allergies, skin disorders, and gastrointestinal problems, as well as other congestive or chronic disorders.

Every day, I have at least one glass, and often three to four glasses, of fresh juices. I recommend two to four glasses in addition to meals as an excellent nutritional supplement. Drink as much vegetable juice as fruit juice to avoid getting too much fruit sugar. (See contraindications at the end of the chapter.)

Make Juicing a Habit

1. Set a time each day to juice. Be sure to stock up on produce.

2. Produce should be fresh, seasonal, and free of decay. If you notice any signs of deterioration, just cut away that portion and discard.

3. Wash all fruits and vegetables before juicing.

4. In general, don't hesitate to include stems and leaves along with the fruits and vegetables. However, carrot and rhubarb greens contain toxic substances and should be removed.

5. All pits from peaches, plums, etc. must be removed before juicing. In general, seeds (from lemons, limes, melons, grapes, etc.) may be juiced. However, apple seeds should not be juiced because apple seeds contain small amounts of cyanide.

6. Cut up the produce in slices or chunks that accommodate the size of your juicer.

7. Don't get in a rut of having the same juices or combinations day after day. Select a variety of fruits and vegetables and different combinations as this will delight your taste buds and assure a plethora of nutrients to boost your immune system and keep you healthy.

8. Vegetable juices that taste "strong" such as spinach, beet and parsley are high in compounds that should be consumed in small quantities. You can dilute these with milder tasting juices or water. Vegetables like rutabaga, onions, turnips, and broccoli should also be juiced in small amounts; for example, 1/4 turnip would be sufficient per glass. Foods that have a high water content should be your base—like carrots, cabbage, apples and grapes.

9. Always sip your fresh juices slowly—don't gulp them down.
10. Add raw foods and juices gradually to your current diet. Begin slowly so your body can adjust to a new way of eating.

Produce Suggestions & Health Benefits

- **Alfalfa** (sprouts) contains vitamins A, B, C, E, K, and U in addition to B_{12} magnesium, essential fatty acids, selenium, enzymes and much more. It is also one of the richest sources of chlorophyll. It is high in nutrients because alfalfa roots go deep, as far as 250 feet into the clean deep earth. It contains natural fluoride that prevents tooth decay and is used in the treatment of arthritis, mineral deficiencies and many illnesses. Taken with lettuce juice, it also stimulates hair growth.
- **Apples** are a very nutritious fruit filled with vitamins C and A, lots of potassium and modest amounts of B vitamins. They also contain pectin and malic acid. This juice is good for the gall bladder and is known for its cleansing and healing effects on internal inflammation. Apples can help lower blood cholesterol, aid liver function, rid the body of toxins and lessen the effects of X-rays. Apples are also rich in sorbitol, a natural form of sugar and a gentle laxative. Five apples make one large glass.
- **Asparagus** contains high amounts of vitamins A, B-complex and C, as well as potassium, manganese, iron, etc. It contains rutin which contributes to a strong capillary system, and asparagine, which stimulates the kidneys (a natural diuretic). Cancer clinics world wide use three tablespoons of pureed asparagus in their therapies. The high amounts of carotene, vitamin C and selenium make this vegetable excellent for cancer treatment.
- **Beets** provide one of the very best juices for the liver, gall bladder, red corpuscles, anemia, cancer, blood cleansing and stimulation of the lymph glands. Beets are rich in magnesium, beta-carotene, vitamin C and E, potassium, folic acid, and the

antioxidant gluathione. Juice the tips, too. Be sure to dilute the juice with pure water or other juices such as carrot and celery since it is very potent.

- **Berries** of all kinds are delicious as well as nutritious, including blackberries, blueberries, boysenberries, raspberries, and strawberries. They have vitamin C and potassium and are good blood purifiers. Blueberry juice can help prevent recurrent urinary tract infections. This fruit is also a source of polyphenols (an antioxidant) which has been shown to kill viruses.

- **Broccoli** is a cruciferous vegetable high in cancer antidotes like indoles, glucosinolates, and dithiolthiones. It also contains carotenoids (vitamin A). It blocks cell mutations which foreshadow cancer, possibly due to the abundance of chlorophyll. Studies show that people who ate more broccoli, cabbage and Brussels sprouts had a lower risk of colon and rectal cancer. Other studies reveal that women who ate more broccoli were less prone to cancer of the cervix.

- **Brussels sprouts** are also a cruciferous vegetable and very important to health. Countries where Brussels sprouts are frequently consumed have a low incidence of gastrointestinal cancer. Researchers have found there are specific substances in Brussels sprouts that retard cancer. These include chlorophyll, dithiolthiones, carotenoids, indoles, and glucosinolates.

- **Cabbage** is another cruciferous vegetable. It is used in the treatment of colon cancer. The juice heals inflammation of the colon and stomach, and is effective for heartburn. It's also famous for its ulcer-healing capabilities, but should be used only in conjunction with a doctor's prescribed therapy for ulcer treatment. In addition, cabbage has helped eczema, seborrhea and skin infections. It stabilizes chemical reactions in the body, and it makes a good poultice for leg ulcers. It's high in calcium, vitamin C, sulfur, vitamin A and much more. Prepare it fresh and drink immediately, as the vitamin U is destroyed very rapidly by air and cooking.

- **Cantaloupe** has a blood-thinning effect that can help prevent heart attacks and strokes. It's an excellent source of beta-carotene. One of my favorite juices, I have a few glasses each week.
- **Carrots** are an excellent source of beta-carotene. Foods rich in beta-carotene are powerful antioxidants and protect against cancer, boost the immune system and help the body heal itself. Carrot juice also aids in colitis, constipation, all forms of arthritis and skin disorders. In addition, the juice helps to improve eyesight, stimulate appetite, and is good for heart disease. Yellowish coloration of the skin may occur when large amounts are consumed. This coloration is harmless, and will fade when consumption is reduced. I drink carrot juice daily, usually in combination with other juices such as beet, celery, parsley and apple.
- **Cauliflower** is another cruciferous vegetable, rich in vitamin C, potassium, indoles and essential sulfur compounds. It's been found to reduce risk of cancer, particularly of the colon, rectum, and stomach, and possibly the prostate and bladder.
- **Celery** contains vitamins A, B-complex, and C, choline, as well as magnesium, manganese, iron, iodine, calcium, etc. It's also rich in pectin. The juice helps regulate the nervous system and chemical imbalance by having a calming effect. It is also helpful in diseases of inflammation, including arthritis. Further, it's good for reducing water retention, for weight loss, and for stimulating the sexual drive. It's excellent added to other vegetable juices. Celery is a good brain tonic, enhances memory, is good for dizziness, headache and arthritis. Celery juice can be diluted with water and used as a sports drink to replace fluid and mineral loss due to sweating. It contains the same ulcer-healing factors found in cabbage juice.
- **Chard** is high in vitamins A and C, potassium, calcium and iron. It is used to build energy, and as a diuretic and laxative. When the juice of chard is mixed with carrot juice, it helps control urinary tract infections, hemorrhoids, constipation and skin diseases.

- **Cherry** is a traditional remedy for the pain of gout. I love this juice even though it takes extra time to remove all of the cherry pits before juicing.
- **Collards** are a close cousin to kale and an excellent source of calcium and vitamins A and C. Collards improve the nervous, respiratory, skeletal and urinary systems, and aid in osteoporosis, arthritis and colon disorders.
- **Cranberry** juice is commonly known to help prevent recurrent urinary tract infections when consumed on a regular basis. I usually combine it with grape and apple juices for a natural sweetener. By the way, I've never had a urinary tract infection.
- **Cucumber** promotes urination and is good for the spleen, stomach and large intestine. It's also good for acne and as a blood cleanser.
- **Dandelion** is most often known as a weed, but it's rich in many minerals like calcium, magnesium, potassium, phosphorus, sulfur, silicon, iron and chlorophyll. Dandelion greens are good for liver disorders and help cleanse the blood. It also promotes the flow of bile in the liver, removes wastes from the bloodstream and liver and has a healing effect on the kidneys and all infections.
- **Garlic** is a treasure house of healing compounds. It acts as a natural antibiotic and blood thinner and can reduce cholesterol levels. Juice a clove and add it to your favorite vegetable mix.
- **Ginger** root has anti-inflammatory properties and will also protect the stomach from irritation caused by nonsteroidal anti-inflammatory drugs. Migraines and motion sickness can also be relieved by ginger juice. A good digestive aid, ginger thins the blood, lowers blood cholesterol, and reduces fever. Also good as a tonic, for colds, cough, asthma, and relief of vomiting. Ginger contains a substance called gingerol, which may prevent so-called "little strokes." I often combine its juice with a carrot and apple combination or an apple, lemon and wheatgrass combination. A small amount goes a long way; use only one-quarter to one-half inch slice per drink.

- **Grapefruit** is an excellent source of vitamin C. The juice aids digestion and utilization of foods, helps reduce inflammation and is good in weight loss programs. I have grapefruit juice almost every morning, either alone or combined with orange, pineapple or tangerine juices.
- **Grape** juice has long been recommended for healing and cleansing. It's an excellent source of natural sugars, minerals, and vitamins. It's good for edema, cancer, and combats toxins. It's also a good source of the antioxidant polyphenols.
- **Kale** is one of the best cancer fighting vegetables we have on our planet. It's the richest of all leafy greens in carotenoids, which are powerful anti-cancer agents. Kale is rich in vitamin A, C, riboflavin, niacin, calcium, magnesium, iron, sulfur, potassium, phosphorus, sodium, and chlorophyll. A member of the cruciferous family, it is also excellent for arthritis, osteoporosis, and bone loss disorders.
- **Lemon** is a good source of vitamin C and the juice makes an excellent blood purifier. Upon rising each morning, I drink the juice of one lemon in a large glass of very warm water. It helps detoxify the entire body and promotes healing. Lemon juice is a traditional appetite stimulant. Place one or two tablespoons of fresh, unsweetened lemon juice in a glass of water and drink half an hour before meals. This remedy stimulates the flow of saliva and digestive juices.
- **Melons** make delicious juices. Besides cantaloupe, I also juice casabas, honeydews, and watermelon, when in season.
- **Oranges**, one of the most commonly used fruits in America, are high in vitamin C. They also have beta-carotene, which helps fight infections and protects against cancer by supporting the immune system.
- **Papaya** is a delicious fruit high in beta-carotene and vitamin C. It is best known for its digestive support, as it contains the enzyme papain. It's also good for inflammation, heartburn, ulcers, back pain and any disorder involving the digestive system. Chymopapain contained in papaya softens tight muscles which is the reason it is the main ingredient in meat tenderizers. It also has been found helpful in pain relief.

- **Parsley** is a powerhouse of nutrients, which is why I juice it daily and combine it with other juices such as carrot, bell pepper, cucumber and celery. It is very concentrated so you only need small amounts. It helps maintain the thyroid and adrenal functions, is a natural diuretic and aids in digestion.
- **Parsnips** are rich in potassium, and are sweet and delicious. They're one of my favorite vegetables. Though they contain more fiber than most vegetables, they are still juiceable. They help to keep the digestive tract free of cancer causing substances, and they are also helpful in colon disorders, constipation, heart problems, and for reducing high blood pressure.
- **Peppers, Red, Yellow, Orange and Green**, also known as "bell" or "sweet" peppers, contain more vitamin C than citrus fruits. Because of this, they are good for all types of illnesses.
- **Pineapple** is a wonderful fruit containing bromelain, a digestive enzyme. Bromelain also has an anti-inflammatory action in the body. Swish the raw juice around the site of a tooth extraction to reduce swelling, or eat a frozen pineapple juice popcicle to soothe a sore throat. I enjoy this juice by itself or combined with grapefruit, especially after a strenuous weight workout in the gym.
- **Spinach** is an excellent blood cleansing tonic, healing the intestinal tract, hemorrhoids, anemia and vitamin deficiencies. This juice is rich in all mineral and organic substances. However, those who have known liver disease, kidney stones or arthritis should not drink this juice; the oxalic acid content may prohibit the absorption of the calcium found in the spinach.
- **Tomatoes** are high in lycopene, another type of carotene, which possibly gives the tomato its cancer-protecting qualities. A study of 14,000 American and 3,000 Norwegian men showed that eating tomatoes more than fourteen times a month cut the chances of lung cancer. Other studies have shown tomatoes to be a protection against acute appendicitis and other digestive disorders. The juice also aids in cleansing the body of toxins. Fresh, vine-ripened tomatoes are the best.

- **Turnips** produce a juice with twice the amount of vitamin C as oranges or tomatoes. If you have arthritis, you might want to omit oranges and tomatoes from your diet (they have been found to exacerbate inflammation in some people), so use turnips to provide yourself with a source rich in the vitamin C you need. Use the tops, too. Turnip juice is good for the elimination of uric acid and kidney stones derived from uric acid. This is good for people who want to lose weight and for gout sufferers. I like it best when mixed with cabbage and carrot juice.
- **Watercress** is rich in all nutrients including potassium, calcium, sulfur, sodium, chlorine, magnesium, phosphorus, iron and iodine. It also contains vitamins A, B-complex, C and D. Watercress is a powerful intestinal cleanser, blood cleanser and builder. I like to combine it with the juices of carrot, green pepper, dandelion and cucumber for hair, nails, skin, bones, collagen formation, muscle and vitamin deficiencies.
- **Wheat grass** is a treasure-trove of nutrients. Its juice is high in chlorophyll and will stop the development of unfriendly bacteria. It is actually akin to human red blood cells and is excellent as a blood purifier. (See Chapter 9 on Greens.) Wheat grass juice is great for energy and body building. However, it's so potent that it can have a nauseating effect in the beginning if you take too much of it. Start off with an ounce and gradually build up. I usually have it combined with my carrot juice unless I need a powerful energy boost, in which case I'll take two to three ounces by itself.

Important Nutrients in Juices

Nutrient	Juice
Beta-carotene	Carrot, cantaloupe, papaya
Folic acid	Orange, kale, broccoli
Vitamin B$_6$	Kale, spinach, turnip greens
Vitamin C	Peppers, citrus fruit, cabbage
Vitamin E	Asparagus, spinach
Vitamin K	Broccoli, collard, kale
Calcium	Kale, collard greens, sweet pepper

Magnesium	Brussels sprouts, cabbage, turnip greens
Potassium	Celery, cantaloupe, tomato
Selenium	Apple, turnip, garlic
Zinc	Carrot, ginger, green peas

There are several terrific books available about juicing. Here are a few of my favorites:

- *The Juiceman's Power of Juicing*, by Jay Kordich
- *Juicing for Life*, by Cherie Calbom and Maureen Keane
- *Heinerman's Encyclopedia of Healing Juices*, by John Heinerman
- *Fresh Vegetable and Fruit Juices*, by N.W. Walker
- *The Joy of Juicing Recipe Guide*, by Gary and Shelly Null
- *The Complete Book of Juicing*, by Michael Murray
- *Juicing for Good Health*, by Maureen B. Keane

I also encourage you to call Juiceman Juicer for more information. (See Resource Directory.)

For those of you who would like some recipes to use immediately, here are my favorites from Jay Kordich's book.

Carrot/Apple Energizer
6 carrots
2 apples

Liver Mover
2-3 apples
1/2 beet

Potassium Broth
1 handful of spinach
1 handful of parsley
2 stalks of celery
4-6 carrots

Pineapple Special
Pineapple (skin and all)
(I add a few strawberries
for a lovely pink color)

Orange or Grapefruit
3 oranges, peeled
or 1 grapefruit, peeled

Evening Regulator
2 apples
1 pear

Digestive Special
Handful of spinach
6 carrots

Cantaloupe/Strawberry Shake
1/2 cantaloupe with skin
6 large strawberries

Parsley Pick-me-up
5 carrots
1/2 apple
Handful of parsley
Slice of lemon with skin

Waldorf Salad
1 stalk celery
2 apples

Sunshine Lunch
2 apples
4-6 strawberries

Energy Shake
6 carrots
Handful of parsley

Body Cleanser
4 carrots
1/2 cucumber
1 beet

AAA Juice
(Good source of vitamin A.)
6 carrots
1 apple
2 stalks of celery
1/2 handful of parsley
1/2 beet

Jay's Secret
3 carrots
2 stalks of celery
2 cloves of garlic
1 handful of parsley

Ginger Hopper
4-5 carrots
1/2 apple
1/4" slice of ginger

Morning Tonic
1 apple
1 grapefruit

Passion Cocktail
4 strawberries
1 large chunk pineapple
1 bunch of black grapes

Pineapple/Grapefruit
1/2 grapefruit
2 rings of pineapple (with skin)

Alkaline Special
1/4 head cabbage (red or green)
3 stalks celery

Beta-Carotene
4 carrots
3 kale leaves
1/2 apple
Small handful parsley

Tomato Expresso
2 tomatoes
2 stalks celery
Handful spinach
Small handful parsley
1/2 cayenne pepper or
1/2 jalapeno pepper for flavor

Garden Salad Expresso
4-5 carrots
1/2 apple
1/4 green pepper
Handful spinach
Small handful parsley

Lemonade
3-4 apples
1/4 lemon with peel
No need to add water or sugar; the apple acts as a natural sweetener. Add some crushed ice for a delicious, thirst-quenching treat.

There are a very few contraindications to juice therapy. Never drink juices from vegetables or fruits to which you are allergic or sensitive. If you react to sugar (are hypo- or hyperglycemic), dilute high sugar content juices, such as carrot and beet, with other low sugar juices such as celery. You also might want to dilute fruit juices with water 1:1. Consider stabilizing blood sugar with juices of Jerusalem artichokes and green beans. Avoid juice fasts if you are pregnant or lactating. For diabetics, close supervision is required.

Juicing has made a world of difference in my health, and I know it will make a big difference for you, too.

ELEVEN

Exercise
For Your Life!

E ven the best diet combined with the most potent vitamins will never tune up your muscles the way good exercise will.
—Covert Bailey

Fitness is a key to enjoying life—it can unlock the energy, stamina, and positive outlook that make each day a pleasure. Ask almost anyone about exercise, and they'll say "it's good for you." Ask most doctors, and they'll say "it's one of the main ingredients of health." Along with good eating habits, adequate rest and relaxation, and enough sleep, exercise is an important facet of a total program for well-being. It is one of the common sense ways to take responsibility for your own health and life.

Exercise Your Way to Vitality

Let's take a closer look at the latest research on all the salutary effects of exercise on your health—physically, emotionally and spiritually.

Mental Health: Exercise physiologists and medical researchers are now discovering that our sense of happiness and well-being is greatly influenced by the presence of certain chemicals and hormones in the bloodstream. Vigorous exercise stimulates the production of two chemicals, *norepinephrine* and *enkephalin*, that are known to lift the spirit.

A British medical team headed by Dr. Malcolm Carruthers spent four years studying the effect of norepinephrine on 200 people. Their conclusion: "We believe that most people could ban the blues with a simple, vigorous ten-minute exercise session three times a week. Ten minutes of exercise will double the body's level of this essential neurotransmitter, and the effect is long-lasting. Norepinephrine would seem from our research to be the chemical key to happiness."

Fatigue: Inactivity leads to fatigue. According to Dr. Lawrence Lamb, consultant to the President's Council on Physical Fitness and Sports, part of the reason for this has to do with the way we store adrenaline. Lamb reports, "Activity uses up adrenaline. If it isn't used, adrenaline saps energy and decreases the efficiency of the heart." Thus, the downward spiral of energy you feel at the end of the workday will only be worsened if you come home and collapse in an easy chair. "Exercise will get the metabolic machinery out of inertia," says Lamb, "and you'll be refreshed and ready to go."

Stress: "Only when we are in harmony with ourselves physically and mentally can we experience the beauty within and around us and fully share with others," writes Dr. Valerie O'Hara in her excellent, practical book, *The Fitness Option: Five Weeks To Healing Stress.* According to the medical profession, 80 to 90 percent of today's illnesses are stress-related. O'Hara says that each one of us can choose to live productive, energetic lives, based on an inner strength and calmness. Stress does not need to be a way of life. Physical exercise is commonly regarded as an effective means of reducing stress and tension. In fact, a single dose of exercise works better than tranquilizers as a muscle relaxant among persons with symptoms of anxiety and tension—without the undesirable side effects.

In a classic study of tense and anxious people, Herbert de Vries, Ph.D., former director of the Exercise Physiology Laboratory at the University of Southern California, administered a 400-milligram dose of meprobamate, the main ingredient in many tranquilizers, to a group of patients. On another day he had these same patients take a walk vigorous enough to raise their heart rates to more than 100 beats per minute. Using an EMG (electromyogram) machine to measure the patients' tension levels as shown by the amount of electrical activity in their muscles, de Vries found that after exercise the electrical activity was 20 percent less than the patients' normal rate. This means that the body was less tense. By contrast, the same patients showed little difference after the dose of meprobamate.

Heart Health: Regular exercise is one important way to help reduce heart attack risk. It improves blood circulation throughout the body. The lungs, heart and other organs, and muscles work together more effectively. Exercise also improves your body's ability to use oxygen and provide the energy needed for physical activity.

Exercise raises HDL (a lipoprotein associated with decreased probability of developing atherosclerosis) and, in some people, also lowers both LDL (a lipoprotein associated with increased probability of developing atherosclerosis) and triglycerides. It can also lower your blood pressure.

Osteoporosis: This is a condition characterized by decreased bone density. It is never too early or too late to build bone mass. Strength training may be the best exercise for cutting the risk of osteoporosis. Researchers indicate that after the mid-thirties, one percent of our bone mineral mass dissolves each year.

Strength training (weight lifting) workouts tug on the bones, exerting pressure—much more pressure—than non-weight-bearing exercises such as cycling or swimming or even moderate weight-bearing exercises like walking or jogging. That tugging action triggers bone mineralization, stimulating the flow of bone-hardening calcium into the skeleton.

Scientists from the U.S. Department of Agriculture and Tufts University in Boston ran a one-year strength-training test on ten postmenopausal women (average age 67), six of whom worked out, with the other four used as controls. Exercises included double leg press, leg extension, lat (for latissimus dorsi-upper back) pull-down, back extension and abdominal flexion. At the end of the year, body weight and fat mass had not changed in either group. However, while bone density of the lumbar spine of the control group had decreased by 3.7 percent, it had increased by 6.3 percent in the high-intensity strength-training group.

Cancer: Investigations during the past decade at the Harvard School of Public Health and Center for Population Studies showed that risk of cancer was lower in athletic women. Regular, long-term, vigorous exercise established a lifestyle that lowered the risk of breast cancer and cancers of the reproductive system. The study of several thousand women, both athletic and sedentary, found that the less-active women were nearly twice as likely to suffer from breast cancer and almost three times as likely to suffer from cancer of the reproductive system. The incidence of benign tumors of the breast and reproductive system was also significantly lower in athletic women.

The study points up the importance of starting vigorous exercise at an early age. The great majority of the active women in the study started exercising in high school or earlier. Prevention is clearly a long-term effect. Lead investigator, Rose E. Frisch, Ph.D., said the best time to start exercising is about the age of 9, and to keep it up. Those who began exercising young also avoided fatty foods in favor of those foods that supported their activities, namely fresh fruits and vegetables.

Research shows that women who do not exercise tend to become obese, with increased levels of toxic forms of estrogen. After menopause the condition is an established breast-cancer risk factor. Studies at the Norris Comprehensive Cancer Center of the University of Southern California showed that women under age 40 who exercised at least four hours a week could cut their risk of the disease up to 60 percent. Those under 40 who exercised one to three hours a week lessened their risk by up to 30 percent.

Strength and Endurance: Even into the ages of 80 and 90, resistance training (weights) can help or prevent deterioration of muscles and bones and increase energy and strength. A few years ago, Drs. Maria Fiatarone of Penn State and William Evans at the Tufts USDA Nutrition Research Center on Aging engaged 10 nursing home residents, all between the ages of 86 and 96, and asked them to sit on exercise benches and lift weights, extending one leg at a time, three times a week. At the end of just eight weeks, the men and women *tripled* their muscle strength. The absolute weight lifted increased from about 15 pounds on each leg to 43 pounds. The researchers found similar results with a 12-week program of resistance training for 60- and 70-year-old men. Muscle strength of all 12 men increased two- to three-fold. Muscle mass grew by ten to 15 percent.

Just recently, Dr. Fiatarone and associates were able to show just how important these muscle-building efforts were for enjoyment of everyday living. The scientists recruited 100 frail nursing home residents between the ages of 72 and 98 and placed 50 of them in a strength-training program; the other 50, the control group, remained sedentary. Over a 10-week period, muscle strength among the 50 exercisers more than doubled, which resulted, the researchers discovered, in a 30 percent increase in spontaneous physical activity. "The exercise intervention," wrote the researchers, "significantly improved habitual gait velocity (speed of walking), stair climbing ability, and the overall level of physical activity." In fact, several participants who had been limited to using a walker graduated to the use of only a cane, as reported in the *New England Journal of Medicine* (1994).

Weight Control: Food fuels the furnace of metabolism; exercise fans its fire. Exercise that causes sweating and heavy breathing is sugar-burning exercise. Overweight people, however, need fat-burning exercise, which requires slow, sustained activity such as walking. Thirty to 60 minutes of vigorous walking every day will help people lose weight. In addition, lifting weights helps increase lean muscle mass. Sufficient muscle mass is desirable because it burns calories whereas fat stores calories. As a person loses muscle due to inactivity, he or she loses the ability to use calories effectively and usually gains fat and weight even when eating fewer calories. The lack of consistent exercise (both aerobics and weight training) may be the most important factor in explaining why so many of us are overweight.

Longevity: There is no guarantee that exercise will add years to your life, but there's compelling evidence that it might. A study done by Dr. Ralph Paffenbarger, a noted medical researcher at Stanford University, showed that those participants who expended 2,000 calories a week in vigorous exercise such as brisk walking and cross-country skiing lived two years longer than those who did not.

Sex and Libido: If none of the above interests you, maybe this one will. Exercise makes you sexy. A physically fit body is brimming with sex appeal, and exercise unleashes the libido. A recent comprehensive survey showed that exercise increased the sexual confidence of most women; a third of them made love more often, and nearly half of them had an enhanced capacity to be sexually aroused. Studies also show that exercise is a potent stimulus to hormone production in both men and women, chemically increasing desire by stepping up the levels of such hormones as testosterone and prolactin. It is a scientific fact that exercise can dramatically improve your sex life, at any age.

Spiritual Health: Exercise is also very important for spiritual health. A well-exercised and fit body can relax and meditate better. I know my meditations are deeper when I'm exercising every day.

Individualize Your Exercise Program

Several different considerations will assist you in setting up an exercise program in which your time is used efficiently and for maximum results.

Aerobic Exercise

Frequency: Four to six times per week.

Intensity: To find your training rate, subtract your age from 220 and then take 60 percent and 80 percent of this number. This is the target range for your pulse. At the halfway point and at the end of your routine, take your pulse for six seconds and add a zero to the number. You will soon recognize your aerobic training intensity without continually taking your pulse.

Duration: Twenty to 60 minutes of continuous aerobic activity.

Method: Any aerobic activity using the large muscle groups (back and legs) performed continuously in a rhythmic manner is suitable. Fast walking is highly recommended for people of all ages since walking provides all the benefits of aerobic training with a minimum of impact stress on weight bearing joints like hips, knees and ankles.

Resistance Training

This type of training, whether with cables, barbells, dumbbells or machines, or even "free-hand" movements such as push-ups and sit-ups, is an essential accompaniment to aerobic activities in terms of its effects on body composition and appearance, as well as on cardiovascular, musculoskeletal and psychological health and well-being. In addition to developing muscular strength and endurance, one of the unique benefits of resistance exercise is that it helps develop and maintain lean body mass, the majority of which consists of muscle tissue. The importance of muscle is that it burns more calories—far more—than other tissues in the body. (See Chapter 3 on Healthy Weight.) When you increase muscle mass, you increase the number of calories your body is using every moment of the day, not just during exercise, but also at work, at play, and even when sleeping.

The American College of Sports Medicine recommends at least two sessions a week in which the major muscle groups of the body are exercised to fatigue. A sample program might consist of the following:

Exercise	Sets	Reps	Exercise	Sets	Reps
Leg Press or Squat	1-3	10-15	Overhead Shoulder Press	1-3	10-12
Back/Trunk Extension	1-3	10-12	Biceps Curl	1-2	10-12
Lat Pull-Down	1-3	10-12	Triceps Extension	1-2	10-12
Chest Press	1-3	10-12	Abdominal Curl	1-3	15-20
Bent-Over or Machine Row	1-3	10-12	Calf Raise	1-2	15-20

You should strength train at least two, and better yet three, times a week. You should allow at least one day between sessions. An ideal system would be to take two days off between training sessions. If all this seems foreign to you, consult a fitness trainer and ask for help setting up a program geared to your specific needs. (If you want to set up your own home gym, see E·Force® in the Resources.)

Perform at least one set (which consists of a series of continuous repetitions) of each exercise and work up to three sets, time and energy permitting. Use enough weight to cause fatigue in the muscles at the end of each set. When you've finished the set, it should be difficult to perform more repetitions. Rest up to 2-3 minutes as needed between sets.

Remember, as with aerobic exercise, the goal is to enjoy yourself, not kill yourself. Try to make progress in the amount of weight you lift, but remember that the most important thing is to be consistent. Listen to your body and keep the weights and pace within comfortable limits. Learn as much as you can about strength training and bodybuilding. Two excellent sources are *Muscle & Fitness* and *Shape* magazines which are available on most newsstands. And don't forget to always use good exercise form. You *will* progress if you just stick to it and don't overdo it.

Walk Your Way to Radiant Health

Walking is one of the most convenient ways to exercise, but should be done correctly to get the most benefit. The following tips can help make a walking program beneficial and enjoyable.

- Be aware of your posture. Make sure your shoulders are directly over your hips and your hips are moving front to back, not side to side.
- Keep your head up and your chin parallel to the ground.
- Bend your arms at a 90-degree angle to help propel you forward.
- Wear comfortable shoes with good support. Make sure they are suitable for the type and amount of walking you will be doing.
- Keep up a good pace by rotating your hips front to back while pushing off with one foot and pulling the other forward.
- Warm up slowly and establish a pace that is brisk, but not exhausting or painful.

- Make sure your weight rolls through your entire foot, from your heel through to your toes. Be light on your feet.
- Easy does it. Start by walking 20 minutes a day and progressively increase the time.
- Hand weights probably won't help your walk. Increase your workload by walking uphill, walking in sand or against the wind.
- Drink at least eight 8-ounce glasses of water a day. Drink a large glass of water about 15 minutes before you start your walk.

Two formulas are used to compute the percentage of maximum heart rate at which one should work to improve aerobic capacity. One method involves multiplying your estimated maximum heart rate (obtained by subtracting your age from 220) times a percentage (from around 60-80) that's related to your fitness goals and condition. For example, if you're 30 years old, your estimated maximum heart rate would be 190 beats per minute (220-30=190). Multiplying 190 by 60 percent (or 0.6) equals 114; 190 times 80 percent (0.9) equals 171.

The older, the less conditioned or more obese you are, the better it is to start off easier. Work at the low end of your target heart range and keep up the activity for longer periods. As your condition improves, you can up the intensity so that you're working harder, perhaps 70-80 percent (0.7-0.8 times max heart rate, which would be 133-152 beats per minute).

How do you know what your exercise heart rate is? To take your heart rate place your index and middle finger just to the side of your windpipe with a slight pressure toward the back of your neck until you feel the pulse in your carotid artery. Count the beats over a ten-second period and multiply by six (or you can count for 15 seconds and multiply by four) to get your heart rate. Take it about five to seven minutes into your exercise and every ten to 15 minutes thereafter until you learn what the appropriate intensity "feels" like.

Constantly trying to increase your exercise intensity will help burn more calories as well as increase your aerobic power, but what matters in the long run is consistency. When in doubt, always be conservative and go easier rather than harder. The real key is to work at activities that you like and at a pace or intensity that you're comfortable with. You should finish each exercise session feeling exhilarated—not exhausted—and looking forward to your next session.

As an alternative to measuring your exercise heart rate (I recommend that you do so for safety, effectiveness and to enhance your body awareness), you can use the "talk test." If you can carry on a conversation without significant difficulty while exercising aerobically, you're working at a level that's well within your capacity.

See figure 5 on page 190 to help you locate your target heart rate easily and quickly.

I love to walk for exercise and, whenever possible, I find beautiful places in nature to do it. I live a couple of minutes from the magnificent Santa Monica mountains and often go there to delight in the scenery while I work out.

Although I enjoy working at the gym, I think many people get into a rut of only working out indoors. We can feed our bodies and souls more effectively by getting out into nature more. And what a wonderful combination. In nature, you find renewal and inspiration and pure air to breathe. It was Walt Whitman who said, "Now I know the secret of making the best persons. It is to grow in the open air and sleep and eat with the earth."

There are numerous activities I do outdoors such as jogging, skating, cycling, walking and kayaking. I also do my stretching and yoga at the beach after skating or cycling on the bike path in Santa Monica. In addition, I love to kayak and swim in the ocean. Combining different activities (cross-training) assures I'll never get bored and helps me to stay motivated to exercise regularly.

One of the most frequently asked questions is: "If I want to buy one piece of exercise equipment for my home or office that would give me the best all-around workout, what would you recommend?" Well, that's an easy one for me to answer. I use and recommend the E•Force® by CSA, Inc.

It's a great aerobic workout that helps you burn fat and lose weight. It is easy to use and very effective. A twenty-minute

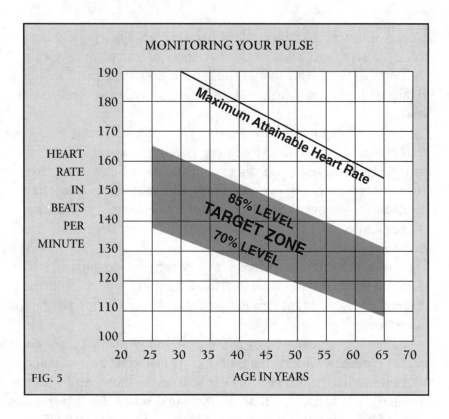

FIG. 5

workout, three times a week, provides the exercise needed to help you achieve your health and fitness goals.

You can quickly change the handlebar position to turn E•Force from an aerobic to a strength training workout. The gravity-based system strengthens your whole body without weights or cables. It is a total body exercise that works on your chest, back, arms, legs, and buttocks.

How to Develop Impressive Abdominals

As a fitness instructor at UCLA and a personal fitness trainer for more than 20 years, I get lots of questions about fitness. One of the most-asked questions is, "Why aren't my sit-ups helping me lose fat around my waist?" Some people mistakenly think they can burn fat around their waists by doing exercises involving muscles in that area, such as sit-ups and side bends. Unfortunately, sit-ups will not reduce observable fat around the waist. Exercises aimed at any single muscle group do not burn enough calories to noticeably reduce fat in that area. In other words, spot reducing doesn't work.

To get rid of undesirable fat through exercise, your body as a whole must burn excess calories by involving as many muscle groups as possible. This means doing exercises like walking, jogging, hiking, rowing, cycling, skating, jumping rope, aerobic dance, or circuit training. Plus, you must do them consistently over a period of time. Fat then comes off from all over the body, not just from the areas being worked.

Like other muscles, your abs (abdominals) thrive on variety and change. And in terms of toning and tightening, they seem to respond best when constantly thrown new stresses.

Have you ever heard someone complain that they've been doing 200 crunches every day for the past six months with no results? Or have you noticed how a new ab routine you could barely finish the first time became pretty easy after a few sessions? That's because muscles adapt to the stress placed upon them pretty quickly. And, in the case of your abdominals, since you're only "lifting" your body weight, you can't really increase the load. Once this happens, they aren't being challenged anymore and you stop making improvements in strength and tone. So what do you do? Get out of the rut. Change your routine. Sneak up on your abs, and they'll respond. Give them a wake-up call. With your abdominals in a perpetual state of surprise, they're always exerting more effort. And because these following exercises work the muscles in your torso from a variety of angles, you recruit different muscle fibers from each of the abdominal muscles.

I've used these six exercises for abdominal strengthening in my UCLA fitness classes for years. They are among the best. They will not place any stress on your back. You should do them in the order listed so you work your lower abdominal muscles before the uppers. If you tire the upper abdomen first, fatigue will limit the amount of lower abdominal work you can do.

1. Knee Lift Reserve Crunch. Lie on your back, feet up in the air and knees bent at a 90-degree angle so they're directly over your hips. Place your hands behind your head in the basic position. (Don't lace your fingers together or pull on your neck; instead, you put your thumbs behind your ears, fingertips just touching. Lengthen your neck. You should be able to see your elbows out of the corners of your eyes.) Keeping your upper body still and flat on the floor, contract your abdominals and lift your buttocks upward 1 to 2 inches, allowing your knees to move slightly toward your chest, then lift your upper torso until your shoulder blades clear the floor. Hold a moment, return to the start and repeat to fatigue. (By fatigue I mean until your muscles are exhausted and it's difficult to do another repetition. A specific muscle fatigue is a different fatigue from a general over-all body fatigue or tiredness.) Your hands function as a cradle to prevent your lower back from arching. Your lower back should remain flat against the floor throughout the exercise.

2. Basic Crunch. Lie on your back, knees bent, feet on the floor, with heels a comfortable distance from your buttocks. Align your spine in the neutral position. (Rotate your hips backward and pull your abs inward so your lower back is in contact with the floor. Not only will this "neutral" position protect your lower back, but it will make the exercises more challenging and effective.) Place your hands behind your head in "basic" position. Curl your upper body upward in one smooth movement until your shoulder blades clear the floor, exhaling as you lift. Hold a moment, return to the start and continue until fatigued.

3. Rotation Crunch. Lie as in the basic crunch. Bend your right leg and place the heel on your left thigh (your right knee will point out to the side). Put your left hand behind your head and your right arm at your side on the floor. Curl your upper body upward and then, leading with your left shoulder, rotate your torso toward your right knee. Return to the start and do several reps until fatigued, then change sides.

4. Continuous Rotation Crunch. Lie on your back as you did in the basic crunch. Curl your upper body up until your shoulder blades are off the floor and then, leading with your right shoulder, rotate your torso toward your left knee. Without rolling down, rotate your torso toward your right knee, leading with your left shoulder. Continue your reps without stopping or rolling down until fatigued. (One rotation left and right equals one repetition.)

5. Double Arm Crunch. Lie on your back with feet in the air, knees bent and directly above hips, so that your calves are parallel to the floor. Extend both arms straight behind your head close to your ears, fingers interlaced. Lift your arms, head, neck and shoulders up and off the floor in a smooth motion. Hold a moment at the top, lower to the start and do several reps.

6. Open Knee Crunch. Lie on your back with your feet in the air, knees bent and directly over hips. Place your hands behind your head in "basic" position. Cross your ankles and turn your knees out to the sides. Curl your upper body upward and forward until your shoulder blades clear the floor. Hold a moment, lower to the start and repeat to complete reps.

When doing these abdominal exercises, exhale when you lift, inhale as you lower. Don't just go through the motions. Think about what you're doing! Research has shown that if you visualize each contraction you may use more muscle fibers. Always work your abs slowly and with control. Don't "bounce" up off the floor between repetitions. You're moving at the right speed if you feel a contraction through your abdominals on the way up and on the way down. Also, when you exercise be sure to wear comfortable clothing that allows you freedom of movement as well as evaporation of perspiration.

How to Attain Optimum Flexibility

Take time to stretch every day. A flexible body, especially for an active person, greatly reduces the chance of injury because muscles that restrict the natural range of motion in the joints are susceptible to pulls, tears, and stress injuries.

For the less athletic, flexibility can provide relief from everyday muscle tension and stiffness, and is also crucial for proper posture.

When we lack flexibility, our bodies compensate in ways that create poor posture, resulting in mechanical imbalances in the back, hip, and neck. These imbalances pull the body out of line, causing stress, strain and even worse posture. Inflexible joints and weak muscles in the shoulder and chest, for instance, can cause rounded shoulders, which can lead to kyphosis (humpbacked spine), a sunken chest and impaired respiratory capacity.

Tight calf muscles can place undue stress on the foot, leading to a variety of orthopedic problems, including painful Achilles tendinitis.

Tight hip-flexor muscles, hamstrings and back muscles can rotate the pelvis forward, resulting in excessive curvature of the lower back, chronic lower back pain, and sciatica.

Drooping your head forward may produce dizziness and chronic strain on the muscles along the back of the neck, resulting in neck and shoulder pain.

The preferred method for enhancing flexibility (which can increase a muscle's length) is through a stretching or yoga program. Muscles exert force by pulling, not pushing. Most muscles attach to bones and cross over one or more joints. When the muscles contract and shorten, they cause a limb or body part to move in a particular direction. The external opposing force can be applied by gravity, by the contraction of an opposite muscle, or by a stretching partner. *The Fitness Option* by Valerie O'Hara, Ph.D., has numerous suggestions and pictures of different stretches and yoga positions to help you become more flexible.

The approach to increasing flexibility in a progressive stretching program is related to the overload principle used to build muscle strength. To increase muscle strength, you must regularly contract the muscle against progressively more resistance with a slightly greater force than that to which it is accustomed. In time, the muscle responds to the overload by becoming stronger. Similarly, to increase flexibility, you must regularly stretch the muscle slightly beyond its normal length. It will adapt to this overload by increasing its length, thereby rewarding you with a greater range of joint motion. To increase a muscle's length, you must regularly pull it about ten percent beyond its normal length: that is the point where your muscles feel stretched enough to be slightly uncomfortable but not enough to cause pain. Typically, you should hold this position for 30 seconds, relax, and then repeat the stretch three to four times. Studies show that you should stretch three to seven days a week, holding the stretch for at least 30 seconds, to increase your flexibility.

For six weeks, 57 men and women with tight hamstrings (back of the thigh) stretched that muscle for different periods. Groups held stretches either 15, 30 or 60 seconds, or didn't stretch at all. Only when the muscle was stretched for 30 seconds or more did it respond by lengthening, thereby allowing more range of motion. Anything less than that was just going through the motions. The surprise was that more wasn't better—the minute-long stretch was only about as effective as the half-minute hold, as reported in *Physical Therapy*, September 1994. This is the first study to test which stretch offered the most benefits over a long period of time.

It's worth tacking those 30 seconds of stretching onto your walking, cycling or other exercise routine, says study leader William D. Bandy, Ph.D., P.T., associate professor of physical therapy at the University of Central Arkansas. Tight hamstrings may force your quadriceps muscles (front of the thigh) to work harder, and that may set you up for knee problems. In addition, tight muscles can be injured by sudden overstretching.

Dr. Bandy feels that people should try to include stretching in their everyday lives. The best time to stretch is whenever you're really going to do it. I teach my fitness clients and students to stretch during commercials while they're watching TV. That's a 30-second to 1-minute period. If I were to ask them to warm up, run and come back and stretch, I don't think they'd do it.

I enjoy doing some type of stretching every day. My rule of thumb is to stretch half the time I've engaged in an aerobic or weight workout. For example, if I cycled, jogged or did a weight workout for 30 minutes, I would devote 15 minutes to stretching. I usually do five minutes of stretching before the aerobic workout and the remainder after the workout. When lifting weights, I stretch before, during the workout—in-between sets—and after the workout is over. Besides elongating your muscles and increasing flexibility, stretching is also a wonderful way to breathe deeply and just relax.

Another excellent book for stretching (includes countless pictures) is *Stretching* by Bob Anderson. If you'd like to start stretching today and want some ideas, here are 5 important stretches. I do these before and after my aerobic or weight workouts.

1. General Flexibility and Upper Thighs. Sitting with soles of the feet together, grasp ankles and pull toward groin area. Then place hands on the inside of your knees and push them out and down toward floor until you feel a stretch. Hold ten to 30 seconds and repeat.

2. Quadriceps. While standing, bend one knee and grasp ankle behind you. Pull ankle toward buttocks until you feel a stretch. Hold ten to 30 seconds. Repeat. Alternate legs. Variation: use a towel to help you stretch if you cannot easily reach your feet.

3. Hamstring. Sit on the floor with one leg straight, the other leg bent with heel against upper part of the other inner thigh. Lean over straight leg and grasp calf or ankle, wherever your extended arms reach, pulling chin towards your knee. Keep knee straight and soft (don't lock knee). Hold ten to 30 seconds. Repeat. Alternate legs.

4. Calf. Stand facing a wall. Using hands against the wall for balance, lower hips by bending knees toward ground and wall until you feel a stretch in lower calf. Do not allow heels to come off the floor. Hold ten to 30 seconds, relax. Repeat. Alternate legs.

5. Lower Back. Lie on back. Raise one knee to chest, grasp with hands and pull in towards chest. Hold the stretch for 30 to 60 seconds. Relax and repeat with opposite leg, then both legs together. End curling your head up toward your knees.

How to Stay Motivated

Every person who exercises regularly, whether an athlete or not, will have to cope with lack of motivation, boredom or burnout at one time or another. Here are a few helpful tips that can keep you motivated to stick to your routine.

1. Make a Commitment. Once you decide to make exercise a part of your life, take precautions that will keep you on the right track. Arrange your personal circumstances so your lifestyle supports your commitment. Make time for exercise. Seek the support of others, but realize the prime reason to exercise must come from within yourself.

2. Define Your Fitness Goals. Write down realistic short- and long-term goals. Your goals provide a path for a specific direction and let you know how you are doing.

3. Repetition. Repetition is the key to mastery. It takes 21 days for the mind and body to create a new habit. During this time, remind yourself that for at least 21 consecutive days you'll stick to your new exercise program. It also helps to share your goals with a friend.

4. Reaffirm Your Fitness Goals Daily. Post your goals where you can see them every day. In addition to a concise list of goals, make a list of your plans for achieving them.

5. Visualize Your Fitness Goals. Visualizing your fitness goals as already completed will increase your motivation, keep you on course and hasten your success.

6. Keep Track of Your Daily Progress. Plan your workouts in advance and keep track of your progress in a diary or on a calendar. Seeing your daily accomplishments is encouraging and increases self-esteem.

7. Be Realistic. Don't set yourself up to fail. If you've just started a walking program and are now up to two miles nonstop, don't make it one of your goals to run a marathon at the end of the month.

8. Exercise with Someone Else. Working out is easier when you have someone to give you support. Many times I've been grateful for friends who got me through workouts I might have skipped if I were working out alone.

9. Use Affirmations. Affirmations greatly enhance motivation. They can be mental, verbal, written or recorded on a cassette for later listening. Keep affirmations positive and in the present.

10. Reward Yourself. You've kept your agreement, you've worked out hard, you've been consistent, and you're seeing positive results. Reward yourself. Rewards increase motivation and create positive associations toward your exercise program.

It's always prudent to check with your doctor if you are middle-aged or older, have not been physically active, and plan a relatively vigorous exercise program.

Like eating habits, exercise is a lifetime commitment. And if you stop exercising, the beneficial effects are rapidly lost; it requires consistent reinforcement.

Will exercise add years to your life? Maybe, maybe not. But you can expect it to improve the quality of your life in the years you have. Being fit will improve your vigor and make you feel good, physically, emotionally and mentally. It gives you a psychological lift and strengthens your sense of accomplishment. The discipline associated with exercise also makes you feel good about yourself. So get started now. The only things you have to lose are some pounds, sleepless nights, and fatigue. Go for it!

TWELVE

Music
Medicine for Body, Mind & Soul

Develop a deeper friendship with great music, and you will see many areas of your life begin to open. —*Steven Halpern*

Few of the main ingredients of health are more effective and enjoyable than listening to music—but not just any music. To be truly health-inducing, it must be music that alters your brain's electrical activity. Let's first look more closely at stress, brainwaves and their association with relaxation, addictions and inner peace.

Stress is arguably the major downside of life of Western-style living in the end of the Twentieth Century. Technological advances have stepped up life's pace (computers now work in nanoseconds, which is a billionth of a second), creating a dizzying abundance of choices (do we really need hundreds of TV channels?) while at the same time eliminating jobs through automation. As a result, a smaller workforce handles a larger workload, often with a cut in pay. We are overstimulated. We receive more information in one day of our lives—from TV, computers, radio, satellites, etc.—than our ancestors of several generations ago used to receive in 1,000 days!

Despite these harsh realities (or perhaps even because of them), Americans are increasingly bent on attaining better health, keeping fit, and reducing stress.

Research confirms that stress debilitates and even kills. Inability to handle stress results in addictive disorders, ulcers, migraines, hypertension, and heart attacks.

The universally recommended remedy for stress is almost too simple to be believed. Relaxation, just plain "chilling out," when practiced regularly, helps prevent many of today's stress-related diseases and helps you live a healthier life. Relaxation provides:

- More energy
- A more robust immune system
- Enhanced concentration, clarity and creativity
- More ease in falling asleep

The emerging field of psychoneuroimmunology underscores the intricate relationship between mind and body, stress and disease. Virtually every month, new studies show the direct effect of psychological and environmental factors on health. For example, people under stress are six times more likely to become infected with the cold virus than those who are not stressed. The more stressed you are, the more the body's immune system shuts down. This cycle of irritation and stress ripples out and has enormous economic and other impacts. The amount of money lost in the U.S. alone to stress-related diseases—absenteeism, illness, and just plain inefficiency on the job—is in the hundreds of billions of dollars per year.

When it comes to the future of health care in this country, prevention and personal responsibility must play a key role. Why wait to get sick before you start doing something to make yourself better?

"Health is not merely the absence of disease, but a state of harmony and well-being that permeates every cell of the body and mind."

—**Dr. Deepak Chopra**

Brainwaves & Relaxation

It is helpful to understand the significance that relaxation and the related *alpha* and *theta* brainwave states can play on your personal health and well-being. Once you do, I think you'll agree how important it is to nurture yourself and to bring more moments of relaxation into your life.

"When people learn to experience inner peace, they are more likely to make and maintain lifestyle choices that are life-enhancing rather than self-destructive."
—**Dean Ornish,** Healing and the Mind, edited by Bill Moyers

In 1993, the prestigious *New England Journal of Medicine* announced the results of a major study that concluded "alternative health care is used by 33 percent of Americans." According to Dr. David Eisenberg of Boston's Beth Israel Hospital and Harvard Medical School, over 60 million Americans now use such alternative therapies to standard Western allopathic medicine. The vast majority seek to achieve more relaxation in their lives.

Recent discoveries in brain science suggest that each of us has a "Minimum Daily Requirement" to have the brain's electrical activity register in the alpha and theta range for at least 30 minutes each day. Most people, however, do not include enough of these brainwave patterns in their daily schedule. Many behavioral problems are now understood to relate to deficiency of this brainwave activity.

Scientists have known for a long time that we have different levels of brainwave activity as measured by different frequencies of electromagnetic wave patterns emanating from the brain. The highest frequency of brainwave activity is exhibited in everyday consciousness, and is called *beta* range (13-39 cycles per second). *Alpha* (8-12 cps) and *theta* (4-7 cps) are associated with deep relaxation, meditation, and mental imagery. The result of achieving alpha and theta brain states is greater control over your mental state, enhanced creativity, increased productivity and general feelings of well-being.

Dr. Eugene Peniston, of the V.A. Medical Center, Fort Lyon, Colorado, and Dr. Paul Kulkosky, at the University of Southern Colorado, conducted sophisticated biofeedback research. According to their studies, chronic alcoholics and children of alcoholics often have lower levels of alpha brainwaves than non-alcoholic individuals. This finding suggests that deficiency of alpha and theta brainwave activity predisposes an individual to the development of alcoholism or other substance abuse addictions.

Even more dramatic was their finding that alcohol enables many of these individuals to achieve alpha wave activity. This is the reason more and more authorities are suggesting that addicts are searching for an experience of attunement, of oneness, of inner harmony and peace, albeit in a dysfunctional manner.

Many unhealthy, compulsive and addictive behaviors such as alcoholism, smoking, overeating, caffeine and sexual addictions are actually the result of our inability to handle stress in our lives.

We are now seeing that the insights from philosophy, religion, biophysics, many spiritual traditions and the emerging field of addictionology all seem to share a common denominator. No matter what the tradition, certain specific patterns of electrical brainwave activity are consistently in evidence when we feel a "oneness" or deep peacefulness. This is true whether described in terms of "mystical experience" or "connecting with one's Higher Power."

Other recent scientific discoveries suggest that there is a biological and electromagnetic reason for brainwaves of deep relaxation and meditation to be in the frequency range that they are. Geobiologist Joseph Kirschvink of the California Institute of Technology has just reported finding tiny magnets (actually, crystals of the mineral magnetite) in human brain tissue. The earth itself has a specific harmonic resonance pulsing at about 8 cycles per second. When we become still, we allow our own electrical receiving apparatus (our neurons throughout the nervous system and brain) to align and attune to the earth's own rhythm—an example of the law of rhythm entrainment. Perhaps this is the fundamental basis for the biblical adage, *"Be still and know."*

Music to the Rescue

Of the many ways to get yourself into a deeply relaxed state, music is one of the best. Thankfully, it's a time-tested way to relax that doesn't require any special training, and is safe, non-addictive, enjoyable and effective.

Most music, from Bach to rock, is intended to stimulate rather than to relax. The music of Mozart, Yanni, and most other composers was never intended to be relaxing in the first place. Most music tends to dominate and override the natural rhythm of your heart by "entraining" it to the rhythm of the beat. When the goal is "attunement" rather than "entertainment," only certain music possesses the characteristics needed to be effective.

In 1969, Steven Halpern, who many consider to be the Father of New Age music, developed an approach to composing that wasn't rock, pop, jazz or classical. It didn't have a dance beat and you couldn't hum the melody. But it had the ability to take the listener into a state of deep relaxation and inner peace.

In an interview, Steven told me, "I created a type of music that allows for a change in the energy fields of the body and also a change in brainwave patterns. My music is not about doing, it's about being. Listening to this music induces a person into a deeply relaxed state—an alpha brainwave state of 8 cycles per second which is associated with feelings of serenity, joy and well-being. When the body gets relaxed there is an attunement to the natural pulsation of the body that also happens to be 8 cycles per second. What happens electromagnetically in the body, around the head, is that you interact and link up with the dominant electromagnetic fields of the planet. Literally, you link up into the larger power source of the planet."

Bringing appropriate music and sounds into your life can help keep your physical and psychological being in tune. You can literally assist your cells and organs to relax and renew themselves, which will add more years to your life as well as more life to your years.

Stringent scientific testing corroborates the positive relationship between listening to this type of music and accessing a relaxation state. Halpern cites a double blind study in which his "Spectrum Suite" was played for one group of subjects and Liszt's "Liebestraum #3" for another. The listeners' brain waves and galvanic skin reaction were monitored, and their electromagnetic energy fields were recorded through Kirlian photography. Listeners to the Liszt piece showed minimal changes; listeners to "Spectrum" showed radical changes in the direction of relaxation. A wide demographic selection of people were used in the study but the response was uniform. Even people who didn't like Halpern's music demonstrated a relaxation response.

Impact of Music on Cells

A variety of scientists and lecturers at the Sixth International Montreux Congress on Stress, founded by Dr. Hans Selye and Norman Cousins, gave testimony to the connection between music and health. Music affects the electromagnetic field characteristics of the membrane of a cell. Traditional medicine is only just beginning to recognize how electromagnetic fields affect the entire body. A microscopic entity like a cell is so small that the amount of energy needed to affect it is minuscule.

Here is yet another way the physical world affects us at a most intimate level. It means that, even though we may not consciously hear a noise, or believe we can "tune out" that discordant, irritating music emanating from one's neighbor (or offspring), our bodies do indeed respond. It's automatic. We resonate physically (i.e. increased blood pressure and emotional distress) as well as on the electromagnetic level.

Dr. Norman Shealy, a world-renowned former neurosurgeon and founding president of the American Holistic Medical Association, conducted a study in which his patients listened to specially chosen music (which included some classical selections, as well as Halpern's "Spectrum Suite"). The patients' levels of beta-endorphins rose dramatically for both. These endorphins are the natural mood enhancers that the body produces. They help us feel good, and seem to produce a drug-free "natural high."

Not only can listening to health-producing music assist you in maintaining sound health, but you can also take responsibility more easily for creating positive moods and feelings. You can then use this renewed and recharged energy state for any other work-related or personal pursuit. (With all the money you saved by not getting sick and by operating at peak performance levels, you'll be able to expand your library of listening choices!)

The Healing or Harmful Effect of Music

From my time spent learning from Halpern about the healing powers of music, I now know that on a physical, psychological, and energetic basis, some music can help promote the healing process and other music is actually harmful. In order to understand how this works, Halpern explained to me four important points.

First, in order for there to be sound, something must vibrate. From atoms and molecules to the strings of a piano, without vibration, there is no sound. The *principle of resonance* relates to the way our bodies respond to the actual frequencies of certain tones or notes, whether high or low. Different parts of our body resonate to different frequencies. Some of the therapeutic effects of sound and music are based on this principle of resonance.

Second, any continuous pulsation which we recognize as rhythm causes our heartbeat and pulse to synchronize with it. This phenomenon is known as the *principle of rhythm entrainment.* Most importantly, says Halpern, some rhythms are in harmony with the natural pulsations of the body while others are not. Many of the more prevalent rhythms of today's music scene are not part of any organically-based model and may produce negative effects, as Dr. John Diamond has demonstrated in his landmark book, *Your Body Doesn't Lie.*

Third, there seem to be *psychological constructs* that can be encoded into composition. These constructs tap psychological and emotional responses in listeners. However, people's responses are quite idiosyncratic and vary widely among listeners. Halpern believes the pleasure principle and the endorphin response to music we enjoy comes into play in this regard. Some people feel pleasure with rock music while others feel pleasure while listening to Beethoven.

A fourth principle which Halpern says is an overlying principle, is that of attunement. Are the sound stimuli assisting listeners to move into more attunement, more complete harmony with themselves as physiological/emotional/spiritual beings?

Each of these principles, states Halpern, must be considered when we try to understand how sound and music promote or deter healing. Every style of music, be it New Age, classical, chant or other, has a purpose and viability. Our job is to learn how to choose most wisely.

Choosing Music Wisely

Traditional music therapy labels music as sedative or stimulative. These are broad categories, but what is not generally known is that these do not hold true for a significant percentage of the population. For instance, according to the Music Research Foundation's landmark studies, only about 55 percent of those who listened to a sedative and relaxing composition such as Liszt's Liebestraum #3 found it to be sedative and relaxing. What about the other 45 percent? They might find it stressful or stimulating. The problem is that there is no way to know beforehand. This is one of the big problems in using existing classical music in therapeutic situations.

Another very important consideration in choosing music wisely was identified by Dr. John Diamond. After studying over 20,000 recordings, he found that different versions of the same composition might have radically different effects on listeners, due to the mood or energy imparted to the recording (or live performance) by that performer. It's therefore meaningless to say, states Halpern, "For relaxation, get some music by Mozart," as many writers do. You need to designate which piece, and who performed it.

Another important point in regard to choosing music is that, what you think you get is not necessarily what you get. In other words, many people think they get relaxation from watching TV or listening to Mozart or Yanni. (I enjoy Yanni's music but it's not what I listen to when I desire total relaxation.) Biofeedback measurements prove that they are mistaken. In this case, belief does not equal fact.

There's a school of thought that suggests that patients will receive the greatest relief from anxiety, for instance, when allowed to listen to their favorite music, no matter what it is. Halpern has seen similar claims made for choosing music to use during childbirth, or during surgery. There's absurdity and danger in this approach, according to Halpern. Let's look at an example. When it comes to choosing music for relaxation, which is a fundamental cornerstone of health and well-being, the music chosen may ignore the well-established physiological parameters of relaxation. One of these is that relaxation means having a relaxed heartbeat in the range of sixty beats per minute or less. Most music is faster than sixty beats per minute. Patients who choose "Chariots of Fire" or selections from Bruce Springsteen for relaxation are fooling themselves, or are caught in a musical habit the impact of which they do not appreciate.

In his book, *Tuning the Human Instrument,* Halpern reported that more surgeons were starting to use specially composed relaxation music, such as his "Spectrum Suite" in surgery. Recently, some surgeons have stated that they like to operate with music, but only of their choice. One of these surgeons chooses country and western, another favors heavy metal. Remember rhythm entrainment? That means the blood of the patient would be pumping faster than normal—not what I would want if I were on the table. Clearly country and western and heavy metal are not designed for this context because the physiological effects of the music will conflict with the natural needs of the body.

Similarly, consider music during childbirth. The mother might like Springsteen's "Born in the USA," because the pounding rhythm helps her push. But research by Dr. Chamberlain, reported in his keynote address at the International Pre- and Post-Perinatal Psychology Conference, has shown that it's terrible for the baby.

No matter what one's musical taste, therapeutic music is that which enhances the built-in healing modalities of the body. You're just fooling yourself and wasting your time, says Halpern, with anything else. The problem is that there are very few truly relaxing and healing albums that ever make it onto the best-seller lists. If all you have access to is classical or contemporary instrumental (and not intended-to-be-healing) recordings, you are not working with a full deck (pun intended).

If you pay attention to the feedback from your body/mind, and are experienced in identifying therapeutic and positive effects, and if you've done your homework, you can trust your instincts. If not, trust the professionals—the artists and therapists who devote their lives to the work of producing music with therapeutic effects. The truth is, most people have not had any training in accurately identifying what a true relaxation state really is. What they think is relaxing is only relatively relaxing compared to being caught in rush hour traffic.

Meaningful states of relaxation are a breed apart from not being stressed. In a state of deep relaxation, a whole host of beneficial psycho-physiological responses occur that simply do not happen by themselves.

Relaxation: A Key to Healing and Attunement

As I mentioned earlier, recent discoveries in brain science suggest that each of us has a Minimum Daily Requirement to spend at least thirty minutes each day during which the brain's electrical activity registers in the alpha (8-12 cps) and the theta ranges (4-7 cps). Listening to appropriate music is one of the easiest, most effective and enjoyable ways to ensure that you're getting your Minimum Daily Requirement. But, once again, not just any music will do.

The popularity of Gregorian chants, to which I listen often, may touch on this basic requirement of health and happiness. These chants didn't come about by chance; the elements of positive intent and conscious performance resulted in centuries of proven effect. New Age healing recordings should be understood as akin to the tradition of Gregorian chant, that is, as a contemporary expression of an ancient art.

Am I recommending that you omit listening to all music that doesn't elicit a relaxation response? Absolutely not! I enjoy listening to all kinds of music including rock, easy listening, country and western, and classical. In fact, there's even benefit to these more complex types of music, according to psychologist Frances Rauscher, Ph.D. and neuroscientist Gordon Shaw, Ph.D., of the University of California at Irvine. They say that complex music enhances your spatial intelligence (the ability to view the world accurately). They've shown that spatial IQ scores of college students go up after hearing 10 minutes of a Mozart sonata and that musically-inclined preschoolers' puzzle-building skills improved also. So enjoy whatever music you wish, but choose wisely when it comes to relaxation and attunement.

Recently Halpern began composing music for children. He explains, "I was horrified to read that by the time a child is 18, he has already witnessed 20,000 TV murders. I believe we need influences that balance that stuff out. If a parent provides a more harmonious, nurturing, soothing environment at home, even if you only play music at night when the children are sleeping, it helps." Parents have reported to him that their babies cry a lot less when they play his music.

Sound into Silence

No special effort is involved when listening to music that relaxes. You may listen as background while you go about your work, at home or at the office. Many people find it especially useful as a way to get centered at the start of the day, and as a way of de-stressing after work, either during the commute or upon reaching home. Others play the music during meals, while eating, reading, stretching or relaxing, or while enjoying intimate moments with loved ones. Many people find that it's easier to merge with the music when they use headphones. Close your eyes, listen deeply and become the music.

A catalog of Steven Halpern's music is available; see the Resource Directory. I also suggest you look into other composers. Visit your local music store and see what they offer; give preference to music stores that let you listen to anything available in the store (usually with headsets) before purchasing.

We now recognize that there is an innate drive in each of us that seeks an experience of oneness, of attunement, of inner harmony and peace. The better able we are to achieve that state on our own, the less we'll need to resort to alcohol, drugs, caffeine, or other forms of addictive behavior as distorted expressions of that search for serenity.

True healing involves an integration and attunement with oneself and one's world. What has been forgotten in much of the criticism of New Age music is that the true exponents of this genre focus on this goal: how to use sound and music as a vehicle to bring us into a state of inner peace and harmony. Using music as the gateway to silence and stillness is perhaps the most ancient of all uses of music. In this state we are reminded who and what we really are.

Unlike most music, which evokes a culturally-conditioned response of intellectual analyses, emotional and memory activation or knee-jerk reflex, certain music, such as Gregorian chant or New Age, can allow the human instrument to play itself more effectively.

When we become still, as we do in a state of deep relaxation, meditation, or prayer, we allow our own electromagnetic receiving apparatus (our body, mind and spirit) to align and attune to the fundamental frequency of the earth itself.

This is in the precise range of deep alpha brainwave activity. The electromagnetic fields created by our electrical nervous system entrains to the electromagnetic field of the earth. What can be more natural than that? The appropriate music that assists in attaining alpha or theta frequencies can help each of us, on an individual basis, experience a greater sense of wholeness, oneness and attunement.

In addition, when two or more of us are tuning into this vibration of love and light, we help amplify others' entrainment to this state. Individual entrainment thus enhances collective entrainment. In other words, as we experience inner peace and harmony within ourselves, we are able to establish and emanate a harmonic vibration with which others can resonate. This may ultimately be the greatest gift that music has to offer. The right music can help each of us to take responsibility for ourselves and do what we can to create more relaxing, peaceful, happy lives.

THIRTEEN

Massage
The Healing Touch

T reat yourself to a massage. It can be equivalent to a long nap, in terms of refreshment; it not only gives you energy, it calms your nerves, releases stress and makes you glow with a feeling of well-being. —*Alexandra Stoddard*

Massage, one of the earliest and most basic forms of healing, has been used successfully throughout history as a means of restoring and maintaining well-being. From the ancient Greek gymnasia and Roman baths to modern day spas and health clubs, massage has been recognized for its health enhancing effects. In fact, this age-old healing practice has experienced a great resurgence in popularity in the last quarter century. Today, massage is a flourishing art form.

Athletes, dancers, over-stressed executives, weary housewives or househusbands have all discovered its pleasure and benefits. From infancy to old age, massage has been found to enhance general health and well-being. Because it is used for health promotion as well as for its curative aspect, it can truthfully be said, "If you have a body, you can benefit from therapeutic massage." Once experienced, massage often becomes a regular part of maintaining wellness. Therapeutic massage is truly one of the most pleasurable and salutary treatments life has to offer.

As a result of its acceptance, both as a healing tool and relaxation vehicle, many schools have been founded which emphasize various techniques. Therapeutic massage has many applications and variations. Many of the therapeutic effects of massage recognized by personal and clinical experience over the years have been supported by scientific research. In addition to the commonly known benefits of relaxation and stress relief, new applications for therapeutic massage are surfacing in areas related to mental and emotion well-being, infant care, aging, athletics, and other special situations. Exciting new discoveries link touch in general, and therapeutic massage in particular, to improved immune system functioning.

Proven Effective

Why include massage as part of your life? Consider the numerous benefits. Therapeutic massage reduces stress and tension, improves circulation, aids in removing cellulite, relieves muscle spasms, and helps to rid the body of toxins and extra retained fluids. It also helps improve the skin. Of course, it feels fantastic, but the therapeutic benefits of massage have largely been relegated to intuition and ancient wisdom—until now. The University of Miami's School of Medicine opened what they call "the first institution in the world for basic and applied research on the sense of touch"—The Touch Research Institute. Their projects have included researching the impact of massage on the immune functioning of AIDS and cancer patients, the effects of touch on patients with addictions, and the effects of touch on physical and emotional development.

The Institute reported some impressive initial results.

- Premature "crack babies," each given three 15-minute massages a day for ten days, suffered fewer complications, displayed markedly more mature motor behavior and gained an astounding 28 percent in weight by the end of the 10-day period.
- Abused children living in a shelter became more sociable and active with regular massage.
- Preschoolers were more focused when given massages.
- Adult office workers were more alert when given regular massages.

• HIV-positive males who received five massages a week for a month showed improved immune function and significantly reduced anxiety and stress.

Massage is clearly therapeutic.

At Cascade Institute of Massage in Eugene, Oregon (one of over 300 such schools in the nation—see Resource Directory) these therapeutic aspects of massage are emphasized in their student Community Outreach program. As part of their 500 hour training program, students work with clients from a wide variety of social service agencies, including abused women's shelters, nursing homes for the elderly, half-way houses for the handicapped, an AIDS hospice and a Free Clinic for low-income and homeless people, among others. Out of this experience, the students come away with a deep appreciation for the benefits of massage and a sense of how rewarding this work can be.

Massage in Your Fitness or Sports Program

Why are so many sports and fitness enthusiasts including regular therapeutic massage as part of their conditioning programs? There is a growing awareness that a complete workout includes not only the exercise itself, but also caring for the wear-and-tear and minor injuries that naturally occur with strenuous movement. The physiological and psychological benefits of massage make it an ideal complement to a total conditioning program.

Who can benefit from regular massage? Anyone who routinely stretches their physical limits through movement such as running, cycling, hiking, swimming, dancing, tennis and other racquet sports, strength training and aerobics. In fact, anyone who experiences regular physical stress like mothers with small children, carpenters, gardeners, or those who use their bodies strenuously in their work will find relief with therapeutic massage.

Massage is beneficial when starting a conditioning program, because it helps you get into good shape faster, and with less stiffness and soreness. It helps you recover faster from heavy workouts, and relieves conditions which may cause injury. Did you know that a muscle which as been worked to its maximum will recover only 20 percent after a thirty-five minute rest, but will recover 100 percent after a five minute massage? Needless to say, massage is especially effective for athletes when given before and after strenuous workouts or competition. And it can be something to look forward to after a workout—a healthy reward.

Regular exercise increases vigor and promotes a general sense of well-being. If done in moderation, exercise can help relieve the effects of stress, and has been linked to decrease in psychological depression. The fun of sports and physical activity is a "healthy pleasure" and greatly improves the quality of life. Regular exercise produces positive physical results, like increased muscular strength and endurance, more efficient heart respiratory functioning, and greater flexibility. Exercise, along with a healthy diet, also results in less body fat and greater lean body mass. These are the components of health-related fitness. (See Chapter 11 on Exercise for more detail.)

These positive physical changes occur as the body gradually adapts to the greater demands put on it by regular exercise. Conditioning has been described as a process of pushing the physical limits (tearing down), recovery, and then building up to meet the new demands. Recovery is often overlooked, but is essential for the rebuilding phases, and to realizing the benefits of a conditioning program.

The "tearing down" phase of the adaptation process often involves stiffness and soreness, especially when the amount of movement is significantly increased from what the body has been used to in the past. Referring to post-exercise soreness, people often comment about finding muscles "I didn't even know I had."

Delayed muscle soreness (24-48 hours after exercise) may be caused by any of a number of different factors. Some possible causes are minor muscle or connective tissue damage, local muscle spasms that reduce blood flow, or a build up of waste products (metabolites) from energy production.

Trigger points or stress points may also cause muscle soreness and decreased flexibility. These points are specific spots in muscle and tendons which cause pain when pressed, and which may radiate pain to a larger area. They are not bruises, but are thought by some to be small areas of spasm. Trigger points may be caused by sudden trauma (like falling or being hit), or may develop over time from the stress and strain of heavy physical exertion or from repeated use of a particular muscle.

Heavily exercised muscles may also lose their capacity to relax, causing chronically tight (hypertonic) muscles, and loss of flexibility. Lack of flexibility is often linked to muscle soreness, and predisposes you to injuries, especially muscle pulls and tears. Blood flow through tight muscles is poor (ischemia), which also causes pain.

How Massage Helps

Recovery: Therapeutic massage helps the body recover from the stresses of strenuous exercise, and facilitates the rebuilding phase of conditioning. The physiological benefits of massage include improved blood and lymph circulation, muscle relaxation, and general relaxation. These in turn lead to removal of waste products and better cell nutrition, normalization and greater elasticity of tissues, deactivation of trigger points, and faster healing of injuries. It all adds up to relief from soreness and stiffness, better flexibility, and less potential for future injury.

In addition to general recovery, massage may also focus on specific muscles used in a sport or fitness activity. For example, areas of greater stress for runners and dancers are in the legs, for swimmers in the upper body, for tennis players in the arms. These areas are more likely to be tight, lose flexibility, and develop trigger points.

Overtraining: Adequate recovery is also a major factor in avoiding the *overtraining syndrome*. Overtraining is characterized by irritability, apathy, altered appetite, increased frequency of injury, increased resting heart rate, and/or insomnia. It occurs when the body is not allowed to recover adequately between bouts of heavy exercise. Therapeutic massage helps you avoid overtraining by facilitating recovery through general relaxation, and its other physiological effects.

Trouble Spots: You may also have your own unique trouble spots, perhaps from past injuries. A massage therapist can pay special attention to these areas, monitor them for developing problems, and help keep them in good condition. An experienced massage therapist can also complement treatment received from other health care professionals for various injuries.

For the Competitor

During competitions, such as tournaments and races, athletes push themselves to their limits performing at maximum effort. At these times, explains chiropractor Joel Bienenfeld of Pacific Palisades, California, sports massage is used to prepare for and recover from the stresses of all-out effort.

Pre-event: Pre-event sports massage is given within the four hours preceding an event to improve performance and help decrease injuries. It is normally shorter (10-15 minutes) than a regular conditioning massage, and focuses on warming-up the major muscles to be used and getting the athlete in a good mental state for competition. Certain massage techniques can help calm a nervous athlete, and others can be stimulating.

Inter- /intra-event: Inter- and intra-event massage is given between events or in time-outs to help athletes recover from the preceding activity, and prepare for the activity coming up. It is also short, and focuses on the major muscles stressed in the activity.

Post-event: Post-event massage is given after a competition and is mainly concerned with recovery. Recovery after competition involves not only tissue normalization and repair, but also general relaxation and mental calming. A recovery session might be 15 to 90 minutes in length.

Some tournaments and races provide sports massage for competitors, or you may want to schedule an appointment before and/or after an event with your own massage therapist. You don't have to be a professional athlete to benefit from therapeutic massage.

Traditional Western (Swedish) massage is currently the most common approach used for conditioning programs. It is frequently supplemented by other massage therapy approaches including deep tissue, trigger point work, and acupressure. Some massage therapists have special training in sports massage and greater experience working with athletes. Discuss your conditioning program with your massage therapists to choose the approach best suited for your needs.

Making the Most of Your Conditioning Massage

- Schedule your conditioning massage (30 to 90 minutes duration) for after your workout or on a rest day.
- Cool down completely after your workout before getting massage.
- Take a shower, sauna, steambath, or Jacuzzi before a massage, if available. This will give a head start to the recovery and relaxing process.
- Tell the massage therapist about your current activity, workout and/or sport participation so she or he can tailor the massage to your unique needs. The massage therapist may want to talk to your personal trainer, aerobics teacher, or coach to confer about your situation.
- Let the massage therapist know about upcoming competitions or events. It might affect their approach to an individual session.
- Tell the massage therapist about past or recent injuries which continue to cause problems or pain. The massage therapist may want to talk to your health care provider about your injuries, either to help the healing process or to avoid further damage.
- Give the massage therapist feedback on painful areas that may need special care or attention.
- Depending on your general physical condition, first time massages may leave you slightly sore. It's like exercise—your body may have to adjust to it. As tissues become healthier, you will appreciate deeper and more vigorous massage.

• Just like your regular exercise or training schedule, plan ahead for regular massage appointments. "Regular" means once-a-week to once-a-month.

More Closeness and Intimacy

Massage is also an excellent way to become comfortable being touched by another person. This may sound elementary; however, for many of us, being touched in a nonsexual, caring fashion is not an accepted part of our daily lives.

Dr. Barbara De Angelis, world renowned relationship expert and author of several best-selling books, including *Are You the One For Me?* and *Real Moments,* feels that massage is a terrific way to foster closeness and intimacy. She says that "one of the biggest problems between couples is the lack of real intimacy. In my workshops, I teach people that every moment is an opportunity to make love, whether we express that love sexually or not. I suggest scheduling what I call 'planned intimacy'; a time when you plan to be together with someone you feel close with, without specifically planning to be sexually intimate. This is a perfect time to give and receive a massage with your partner."

Dr. De Angelis explains that massage is an ideal way to express one's love and caring for another person through the hands. To be touched lovingly, without feeling like someone is trying to "turn you on" can create a great deal of trust and intimacy between two people. She adds that one of the most common complaints from women about loving relationships is that they don't get enough non-sexual touching and caressing. Massage is not only a wonderful way to receive that healing touch, but also a way to teach your partner how you would like them to touch you.

Variations

In massage, one person uses his or her hands to touch and manipulate either one's own body or the body of another. There are many types of massage.

Acupressure is a traditional healing treatment used in China, and consists of pressing on certain points related to all parts of the body and to different health problems. For example, the Chinese claim that a toothache can be relieved by pressing certain points underneath the eyes. *Shiatsu* is a more modern version of acupressure, developed in Japan. In this form, the ball of the thumb is usually used. *Kum Nye* is a Tibetan form of massage only recently introduced in the West.

Polarity Therapy is said to be derived from yogic and spiritual practices in India. Often, the therapist's hands are held far apart while applying pressure and rocking motions to specific "poles of energy" in the body.

Trager massage usually involves vibratory and shaking motions, and, like Polarity, may be performed while clothed.

Zone Therapy or Foot/Hand Reflexology is not really a complete massage because only the feet or hands are treated. The technique claims to affect remote parts, such as the eyes, for example, by massaging the junction between the second and third toes. Its practitioners believe that every part of the body is mapped into a specific part of the feet and hands, and that by massaging the hands or feet only, effective benefits are obtainable.

Reichian massage is intended to dissolve "body armor," which is said to be formed as a defense against releasing emotions and built-up tensions. Much attention is paid to breathing and verbal analysis.

Proskauer massage also works with breathing, and is usually light and subtle. The more advanced techniques such as deep tissue and lymph massage and Rolfing should not be attempted by people not specially trained in these methods. It is important for the massager not to work beyond his or her understanding.

Of course, the easiest way to be massaged is to pay a professional masseuse for a therapeutic massage. But it's not always necessary to pay for such a service if you have thoughtful friends who wish to share in the experience. Often, it is more enjoyable to have a friend massage you rather than a stranger, even though your friend may not be a professional therapist.

If you want to learn more about the technique of massage, check in your community for classes. You may look into your local YMCA, hospital or community centers. Often times they offer massage classes. Look in the Yellow Pages under "Massage Schools." You might also consider reading books and gathering information on the topic.

For those of you who would like some pointers so you can get started right away, consider the following.

The Main Ingredients for Good Massage

The only good way to do massage is with oil. Your hands cannot apply pressure and at the same time move smoothly over the surface of the skin without some kind of lubricating agent. Oil fulfills this function better than anything else. The skin will absorb most of the oil; thus I don't recommend petroleum products like baby oil. If you can eat it, it's probably okay to use on your skin. I personally like to use cold-pressed almond or canola oil by Spectrum Naturals which is available in health food stores.

What about a massage table? Its advantage is that it eliminates some bending and stooping as you work. This means that if you are giving a long massage, your own back is less likely to get tired. A table also makes it easy for you to change your position around the person you are massaging—from head to leg, from one side to the other side, etc.—without a break in the flow of your massage.

When looking for tables, take a number of things into account. Tracy Wise, co-owner of Cascade Institute of Massage, advises that the standard 27" wide table is wide enough for most people although he prefers using 29" wide ones in the school. The price of portable tables runs from as low as $250.00 for a 24" wide table with no head rest (face cradle) to about $650.00 for a wide table with good covering and a headrest. He considers a headrest essential for people with neck tension and/or injuries because it permits lying face down without twisting the neck.

Look for a table that is strong, stable, and silent even under vigorous massage. It should not rock, wiggle, or squeak. It should be comfortable and secure to lie on, and should easily support two or three adults.

Adjustable height is another added bonus on tables. Look for those with at least a five-inch range, preferably nine or twelve. Adjustable height allows you to find your best working height by trial and error, allows people of different heights to use the same table, and gives a larger resale market.

Before buying, find out if the warranty covers both faulty materials and workmanship and for how long the builder has been in business. (See Resource Directory)

That Special Touch

A person receiving a massage enters a universe where the sense of touch alone is important. For this reason, any outside noise and bustle can be extremely disconcerting. Make the room as comfortable as possible. Dim the lights. Some people might also prefer tranquil, soothing music.

The next thing to consider is warmth. Nothing destroys an otherwise good massage more quickly than coldness. The temperature in the room in which you give a massage should be about 70 degrees F. or slightly more, and be free of drafts.

It is insignificant whether you start at the top or bottom of the body. Your choices are as varied as your creativity. Your choice basically comes down to whether you wish to work across the body or to proceed up the same side. As long as you have some methodical way of covering every part of the body that is to be massaged, the massage will be complete with no obvious omissions.

Allow the person being massaged to choose whether to first lie face down or face up. It's helpful to have a clock or watch placed so that various areas of coverage can be conveniently timed. If you are giving a 30 minute massage, ask the receiver to turn over after 15 minutes. At this halfway point, make sure that you, the massager, are relaxed. Oftentimes, there is a tendency to neglect any discomforts you might have if you are giving a good massage. During all phases of the massage, check your posture and make adjustments for any difficulties you are experiencing.

Make sure that you feel good before you work on another person. If you're rundown physically or emotionally, you should be receiving, not giving. Feel free to re-schedule the session, if necessary. Otherwise, your "burn-out" state might be transmitted to your partner.

Birthday Suit?

What should the person wear or not wear? Here is what Ruth Wise, a licensed massaged therapist, co-owner and Director of the Cascade Institute of Massage says: "I think draping is necessary most of the time, except if you know someone very well. Never assume because you are 'dressed' friends that you are also 'undressed' friends. Issues of abuse, boundaries, sexuality, being able to say what your needs are and self-image can all arise."

She suggests to always tell a person to take off as much as they are comfortable taking off. If they are nude because you told them to take it all off, they may be unable to relax and feel safe, which are primary considerations in therapeutic massage.

Your nails need to be trimmed as short as possible and filed smooth. Otherwise, acupressure becomes acupuncture! Remove all jewelry. Avoid loose clothing or long hair that will trail over their body. The recipient should also remove contact lenses and jewelry.

Ask about cuts, bruises, other injuries and recent operations, in order to avoid touching these spots. Find out about which areas are the most tense. These are the areas where you can spend the most time. Ask your partner about past and present health. If in doubt, wait until after a physician has been consulted before massaging. If there are any serious medical problems such as cancer or heart disease, check with a physician before proceeding.

Be very careful with senior citizens as they tend to bruise more easily, with bruises that can sometimes last for days or even weeks. Their ability to repair damaged tissue is diminished with age. Deep tissue work is contraindicated in treating the elderly; however, gentle massage can be most beneficial. Atherosclerosis is a common condition among senior citizens so care must be taken to stay away from the carotid arteries located on each side of the neck.

Be sure to establish a communication code for pain. You'll want to apply pressure to the "edge of pain," not past it. Ask the person to say 'good' when the pressure is best and don't press any harder. To help you feel relaxed while massaging, make sure your center of gravity (two inches below the navel) is directly over the area you are massaging, whenever possible. Position yourself right next to the body part you are massaging. Move your entire body, not just your hands. Let your legs—not your lower back—support and move you.

If you have never given or received a massage, you might consider first giving a massage to those areas on your own body which you can reach comfortably without straining. See what feels good to you. Do you like movements to be fast or slow, soft or hard? A good area for practicing on yourself, as well as your first attempts with another person, is the foot.

Here are some simple guidelines from Ruth Wise: "Steady the left foot with your left hand. Stroke the knuckles up and down from just below the toes to the heel pad. Move your knuckles in small circles; press firmly yet gently. Be sure to cover the entire sole, including the bottom of the heel. Next go over the sole with the thumbs of both hands. Hold the foot in place with your fingers and work both thumbs at once in small circles. Again cover the entire sole. Go slowly. Be thorough. Remember those thousands of nerves connecting the foot with the rest of the body."

Getting Started

Two of the best overall how-to-get started books on massage are *The Book of Massage* by Lucinda Lidell and *The Massage Book* by George Downing. Another book that is effective in summarizing the importance of being touched for our development and well-being is Ashley Montagu's *Touching*. For massaging young ones, I recommend *Loving Hands: The Traditional Indian Art of Baby Massage* by Frederick LeBoyer. There are also numerous videos available in libraries, catalogs and bookstores you may want to consider.

In *The Massage Book,* Downing recommends that for couples, or for others sharing the same life and the same home, the ten-minute massage can open the door to something extraordinary: doing massage together every day for ten minutes each. When a day comes along in which you have the time and inclination, trade a full massage. Even ten minutes every day may sound hard if your life is a busy one. It is often difficult until you get in the habit of it. Yet, I assure you that nothing else in the world requiring so little effort will as effectively change, over the course of time, the mood and tempo of your entire life.

If you follow some of the simple guidelines included in this chapter, you can give a friend or family member as much joy as you will receive from the massage. What could be a nicer gift for someone you love? And with loving intentions, your therapeutic touch can truly be a magical one.

> *Life is a song—sing it.*
> *Life is a game—play it.*
> *Life is a challenge—meet it.*
> *Life is a dream—realize it.*
> *Life as a sacrifice—offer it.*
> *Life is Love—enjoy it.*
>
> —*Sai Baba*

FOURTEEN

Gravity
Learning to Co-Exist

G*ood posture and a well functioning spine contribute toward a proper foundation in the pursuit of optimal health.*
—*Joel Bienenfeld, D.C.*

We can't see gravity. We can't hear gravity. Nor can we touch, taste or smell gravity. Our insensitivity to gravity, and its constant influence on our mental and physical well-being is truly monumental. Nevertheless, gravity is at the heart (or the bottom) of all weighty matter on this planet. On the surface, gravity may seem to be an irrelevant consideration to health and happiness. Below the surface, however, gravity is a tremendous undermining force, the source of numerous pitfalls, an energy that tirelessly works to run down our health, fitness and beauty.

All upstanding people are victims of gravitational abuse. This force dominates every activity—breathing, eating, moving, even sleeping. We can avoid unhealthy foods, contaminated water and polluted air, but we cannot get away from gravity. It never lets up!

Gravity alone causes our bodies to be out of shape. Sometimes trying to shape up our bodies with certain exercises merely compounds the matter. For example, the harder we run, the higher we jump, and the heavier the objects we lift, the greater the gravitational shock created on our already well-grounded bodies. The earthly impact on our bodies from just walking is over twice that of our static physical weight, thanks to gravity. Good posture helps to prevent the negative effects of the gravitational pull on our bodies and spine. My chiropractor, Joel Beinenfeld in Pacific Palisades, California, is always reminding me of the importance of good posture whether sitting, standing or walking. For years I have gotten chiropractic adjustments every couples of months to prevent as well as take care of problems.

Gravity is our sole connection to earth. In fact, we're all stuck to this planet because of it. No matter what we do, or where we go, we can never get away from gravity. To be sure, it is always underfoot.

Just sitting and standing all day, and sleeping with our heads propped up on pillows all night, enables gravity to work against us 24 hours a day. Just as gravity keeps water from flowing upward, it also keeps our blood from flowing freely upward and into our heads. Thus, our eyes, ears, gums, scalps, complexions and brains—all areas above the heart are where blood circulates least— are the first to deteriorate in our heads-up lifestyle.

Gravity Pulls You Down

Medical professionals have made the connection between gravity and health. Martin Jungmann, founder of the Institute for Gravitational Strain Pathology, says, "It is generally accepted that the force of gravity, which is part of man's natural habitat, has bearing on his health." Moreover, the relentless, downward pull of gravity affects our faces, necks, shoulders, backs, chests and abdomens. It is gravity, and not old age, which is the underlying cause of shrinking stature.

Robert M. Martin, founder and author of *Gravity Guiding System*, cites drooping, sagging stature, bulged out mid-sections and unsightly posteriors as examples of the "devastating effects of gravity." He goes on to say, "Lack of blood flow to the brain no doubt plays an important part in geriatric degeneration and premature aging. When the brain lacks a sufficient supply of blood, the natural results will be slow body reactions and sluggish mental and physical reflexes. It is impossible to overestimate the importance of maintaining continuous free-flow of blood in the body. In the inverted position, one will definitely feel a rush of blood to the head. And the easiest way to invert the body is to lie on an inclined plane, with the head downward, and the feet upward."

As fetuses, we all begin life in water, that is, in the near-weightless environment of our mother's womb. While there, most of us turn upside down to prepare for our head-first entrance into the world. As infants, we spend much of our sleeping time in the bottoms-up position. By keeping our heads lower than our hearts, we naturally maintain proper blood circulation to the brain. As children, we eagerly seek ways of freeing our bodies from gravity's restricting hold. Hence, our innate fascination with such activities as bouncing on beds or trampolines, swinging on swings, sliding down slides, rolling down hills and jumping on and off of higher and higher objects.

As adults, we mostly alleviate the gravitational pull on our bodies with a recliner chair or by elevating our feet on the nearest table or chair. And if we're really hurting, we may even put our legs up on a wall. As earthlings, consciously or unconsciously, we regularly confront our inborn fear of falling with such popular gravity-defying (and death defying!) activities as flying, climbing, jumping, diving, skiing and bungee jumping—all of which I've experienced.

We must learn to work with the law of gravity instead of allowing gravity to work against us. There are a variety of different yoga positions where the legs are elevated higher than the upper body, achieving this increased circulation to the upper torso. For more than twenty years I have practiced lying on a slantboard, which puts the legs higher than the heart and the head lower than the heart. In this position, the pull of gravity on your face, neck, back, internal organs, legs and feet is naturally and effectively reversed.

Using Gravity to Your Advantage

When I was introduced to the slantboard by Dr. Bernard Jensen, I never dreamed that such a simple device would not only improve my physical appearance but would also have a tremendous impact on my overall state of health. He was right. "Every patient of mine uses a slantboard, or he or she is not one of my patients," Dr. Jensen plainly states.

Using a slantboard has made a very positive difference in my life—improving my complexion, giving me energy, relieving back and shoulder strain and helping me to relax. I have since been recommending the slantboard in my counseling and all my workshops on health and healing. I have seen use of the slantboard reduce or eliminate headaches, insomnia, varicose veins, chronic fatigue and neck, back and shoulder tension. I have also seen it improve posture, complexion and circulation and foster relaxation and peace of mind. (Always check with your doctor before slanting, especially if you have high blood pressure.)

A number of other well-known personalities in the natural health field have also actively advocated the use of a slantboard in their holistic programs and practices.

Gayelord Hauser in his book, *Look Younger, Live Longer*, states: "In the slant position, the spine straightens out and the back flattens itself. Muscles which are ordinarily tense, are relaxed and at ease. The feet and legs freed from the customary burden and the force of gravity, have a chance to release accumulated congestions in the blood stream and tissues, and thereby reduce the possibility of swollen limbs and strained blood vessels. Sagging abdominal muscles get a lift, and the blood flows more freely to the muscles of the chin, throat and cheeks, helping to maintain their firmness. The complexion, hair and scalp benefit from increased blood circulation, and the brain is also rested and cleared."

In his popular book, *Become Younger*, Dr. Norman Walker has this to say about slanting: "I consider the slantboard a most excellent means to help prolapsed organs to relax, to help the functions of the colon and as an aid to give invaluable exercise to many parts of the anatomy which we are so apt to neglect in our daily routine of life. By all means, use the slanting board as a aid to become younger."

Dr. Marsh Morrison, author of *Doctor Morrison's Miracle Body Tune-Up*, tells us: "Living vertically in a straight up-and-down fashion and balancing oneself on two little feet, one suffers such gravitational conditions as drooping eyelids, sagging colon, dropped stomach, prolapsed uterus, rounded shoulders, sunken chest, hemorrhoids, hiatus hernia, hanging jowls, varicose veins, and fallen arches. Unfortunately, not one of the existing doctoring or healing professions has yet come to fully understand this or deal with it adequately. Yet I have found the above mentioned conditions, and many others, can be corrected by the slantboard."

The most comprehensive work on the subject is the book, *Slanting*, by Sharlin Leslie. "Initially, the notion that gravity plays a significant role in the cause of conditions normally attributed to the inevitable aging process, was relatively new to me," confesses Ms. Leslie. "However, the more I thought about it, the more it began to make sense to me. Moreover, when I was first introduced to the slantboard, I never dreamed that such a deceptively simply device would improve not only my physical appearance, but would have a tremendous impact on my overall health.

"While the slantboard has been in use in exclusive health spas and exercise salons for many years, it still remains, for most people, one of the best-kept secrets for the enhancement of mental, physical and emotional well-being. If we view gravity as part of the problem, then I believe we can look to the slantboard as part of the solution. And, perhaps, the most salient feature of the slantboard is that it enables us to participate more fully in our own health maintenance program. To be sure, slanting has something for everyone; and the slantboard is definitely an idea whose time has come."

When describing her first time on a slantboard, Leslie says, "The unfamiliar rush of blood to my head made me feel slightly dizzy and my heart sounded as if it was pounding between my ears. The initial reaction lasted only a few moments, though, and quickly gave way to a feeling of pleasant, soothing relaxation."

Leslie experienced back problems, felt tired, wanted to lose a few pounds, and have a healthier complexion. She began using the slantboard on a regular basis for fifteen minutes, twice a day. After just two weeks, she noticed a more glowing complexion, healthier-looking hair and the loss of several pounds with no effort. At the end of two months her chronic back pain had subsided enough for her to discontinue her weekly visits to the chiropractor, and the dull, aching sensation in her lower legs was greatly reduced. She had also found a new state of well-being.

I have a slanting session daily as part of my health program. It's also a great way to practice deep breathing, concentration, visualization and meditation. My visualizations on the slantboard are always very deep and relaxing; my spine stays straight, which is an important aspect of meditating properly. After ten to thirty minutes of slanting, I always feel refreshed, rejuvenated and relaxed.

Here's what you can expect while lying on the slantboard.

- An immediate and pleasant change of direction in gravity's pull on the face, neck, shoulders, back, chest, abdominals, hip, legs and feet.
- A flow of fresh blood to the head, increasing the supply of oxygen to the brain, and literally the washing away of tension, depression, headaches, fear and fatigue.
- The realization of being head-over-heels, and in a wonderful new position for literally overturning gravity's force in our earthly lives.

According to the above authorities, there is no one proper height our bodies must assume to benefit from lying in the slant position. However, give or take an inch or two, a 14 inch elevation, at the feet end, is a good average. There are also a number of alternative ways of achieving the slant position: Elevating the end of your bed, putting an ironing board up on a chair, or lying in the head-down position on the side of a hill. Purchasing a light and collapsible slantboard, of course, is the easiest and most popular method to obtain the slant position. For more than 20 years, I have been using (and highly recommending) The BodySlant® (see Resources). Resting in the incline position on the BodySlant is as easy, safe and comfortable as resting on a bed. I especially love using it after heavy physical and mental activities. The calm, peace and relaxation it provides is wonderful.

From any angle you look at it, slanting is beneficial to your health and is guaranteed to go to your head. The slantboard is designed to help us co-exist with the law of gravity, naturally and gracefully. Let gravity work for you and not always against you.

FIFTEEN

Clothing
It Can Affect Your Health

T he secret is to be a professional person with yourself, and give yourself the same attention, thought, and care you give your clients and family. —*Alexandra Stoddard*

Feeling vibrantly and radiantly alive is more of a priority these days, consequently more people are becoming aware of the foods they eat and drink. Yet few are aware of the health effects of what they put on and around their bodies. The clothes we wear, as well as the fabrics in our environment, can have adverse or beneficial effects on health.

Let's begin with the color of material. My grandmother used to say, "Dress in darker colors in the winter, lighter colors in the summer, and with the colors of the forests in the months between." In other words, dress with the seasons. Her advice has its scientific basis in the fact that black or darker colors absorb heat and so help keep the wearer warm during the cold winter months; white, or lighter colors, reflect the light and thus the heat of the sun, and so keep the wearer cool in the summer.

Clothes colors can elevate or depress feelings. They affect people's energy levels. This is not merely anecdotal. On a scientific level it is known that colors have the power to excite or depress. Though it is a subtle thing, color should certainly not be overlooked.

Color is vibration and different colors produce different vibrations which can be used to elicit specific energy levels that the body might need. Colors such as red, orange and yellow tend to stimulate and energize. Blues, greens and purples are more conducive to relaxing and cooling. Colors themselves can express something about the wearer. Numerous studies show that color affects mood. Warm colors are considered energizing; cool colors are relaxing. Color has also been associated with personality traits:

Blue: peaceful, cool, soothing
Green: calm, restful
Orange: cheerful, energetic
Purple: sensuous, showy, regal
Red: passionate, bloody, vigorous
Pink: gentle
Violet: spiritual
Yellow and Gold: wealthy, uplifting

The color and weight of clothes are obvious factors in keeping the body warm. In addition, the texture and chemical makeup of clothes, as well as the way they are washed, affect a person's skin and health. In fact, patient visits to doctors are frequently caused by a patient's choice of clothing. The common medical complaints that can very often be traced to clothing are: heat rashes from clothes that are too hot; allergies related the perfumes and other chemicals in detergents and softeners; chafing from elastic or tight clothes; "jock rash" from wearing tight pants and fabrics that don't breathe; vaginal infections from wearing nylon underpants; and rashes and/ or chafing from coarse-textured clothes on delicate skin surfaces (e.g., genital areas, underarms, breasts and neck).

Clothes and the Weather

Clothing insulates the body from its surroundings. It may reduce radiant heat gain in a hot environment or retard conductive and convective heat loss in the cold.

In providing insulation from the cold, the mesh of the cloth fibers traps air that then becomes warm. Cloth provides a barrier to heat loss because both cloth and air are relatively poor heat conductors; the thicker the zone of trapped air next to the skin, the more effective is the insulation. For this reason, several layers of light clothing, or garments lined with numerous layers of trapped air—such as those lined with feathers, fur, or other fabrics—provide much greater insulation than a single bulky layer of winter clothing. When clothing becomes wet, through either external moisture or condensation from sweat, it loses its insulating properties and actually facilitates heat transfer from the body, because water conducts heat much faster than air.

When you are active in the cold, the problem is usually not one of adequate insulation but rather the dissipation of metabolic heat through a thick air-clothing barrier. Cross-country skiers alleviate this problem by removing layers of clothing as the body becomes warm. In this way, core temperature is maintained without reliance on evaporative cooling. The ideal winter garment in dry weather insulates the body from heat loss while permitting the escape of water vapor from the skin through the clothing if sweating should occur. Wool clothing is an excellent example of this type of efficiency.

How about dressing in warm weather? Dry clothing, no matter how light, retards heat exchange compared to the same clothing soaking wet. The practice of switching to a dry tennis, basketball, or football uniform in hot weather makes little sense from the standpoint of temperature regulation. Evaporative heat loss occurs only when the clothing becomes wet throughout.

Different materials react to water in different ways. Cottons and linens absorb and retain moisture readily. Unlike cotton, wool is efficient at transporting moisture away from the body. On the other hand, heavy "sweat shirts" (other than pure cotton) and clothing made of rubber or plastic produce high relative humidity close to the skin and retard the vaporization of moisture from the skin surface; this significantly inhibits or even prevents evaporative cooling. Warm-weather clothing should be loose fitting to permit the free circulation of air between the skin and environment in order to promote water movement away from the skin. Natural fibers will permit your skin to breathe more efficiently.

For active wear, I like fabrics which incorporate Cool Max fabric. It's lightweight, breathes well and wicks away moisture from the body. It also dries three times faster than cotton which is a bonus when sweating while exercising.

Harmful Synthetics

Synthetic fibers cause many people problems without them realizing it. Possibly you have heard someone say, "I have a headache every time I wear this dress" or "It seems my sinuses act up every time I put on this shirt." Studies now show synthetic clothing and synthetic bedding can be as harmful as some of the synthetic food ingredients that many people try to avoid. The adverse effects of synthetic fabrics become even more dangerous because they are so subtle that few people realize their origin.

Some of the synthetic-caused difficulties include allergies, respiratory problems, depression, distressing heart responses, slowing of the mental responses, slower healing of irritations and wounds, poor sleep patterns, and distress intensified by magnification of air pollution.

Many synthetic fabrics have undesirable effects due to electrical forces known as ions. These ions are created largely by natural forces: wind or cosmic rays, radioactive gases escaping from earth, lightning and falling water—any phenomenon with sufficient force to coax air molecules to "dance." The molecule may be likened to a small golf ball. At its core are positively charged protons. Encircling these is a single negatively charged electron which weighs about 1,800 times less than the protons.

When jostled by wind or other atmospheric friction, the electron—an unstable character at best—detaches itself and goes in search of a new home. Once it has departed, the original molecule assumes a positive charge, becoming a positive ion. The electron, meanwhile, merges with another molecule, and in so doing imparts an additional negative charge. That molecule then becomes a negative ion.

We inhale ions when we breathe, and also assimilate them through our skin. Thus, ions in the environment affect our bodies, although until recently scientists haven't been able to understand how or why.

Much of the research on the effect of ions on health has been conducted by Dr. Albert Krueger, physician-turned-biometeorologist and professor emeritus at the University of California at Berkeley. His findings are reported in the book, *The Ion Effect*, by Fred Soyka (Bantam Books, 1977). Krueger discovered that ions affect humans by altering the level of serotonin—a neurotransmitter in the blood—in the brain and body tissues. Positive ions increase the serotonin level; negative ions lower it. Serotonin has been dubbed "the ultimate downer." When serotonin levels are high because of the presence of positive ions, the following have been reported: aching joints, insomnia, irritability, tension, tremors, migraines, suicidal impulses, dry throat, nausea, hot and cold flashes, diarrhea, vertigo, respiratory ailments, hyperactivity, fatigue and depression. Pain is also felt more intensely.

But when serotonin levels drop because of the presence of negative ions, a sense of tranquil well-being occurs. Pain sensations are reduced and spirits are lifted. A full moon and certain winds, (such as the Santa Ana winds in Southern California and the Chinook winds) create a preponderance of positive ions. These winds (also called the "Witches Winds") are both hot and dry and carry a positive charge, unlike most other winds. Studies have shown a higher incidence of crime during these times.

By the same token, rain, waterfalls, waves, lakes and the forest foster a more peaceful and calm state because of the abundance of negative ions they produce. Generally, spend as much time in nature as possible to improve your moods and lift your spirits.

Your clothing carries electrical charges which impact the charge of the ions around you, depending on whether the clothing is conductive or non-conductive. In some materials small electrical charges can move around freely, that is, they are conductive. Other materials restrict and trap the charges' movements and they are known as non-conductive. When one or more particles of the same charge are trapped on a non-conductive object and cannot escape, the object is said to have an electrical charge.

Synthetic fabrics are non-conductive because they are woven from man-made fibers which under a microscope appear as solid plastic rods. They do not allow charges to escape and have what is called a positive potential.

On the other hand, the fibers of natural fabrics such as cotton, wool, linen or silk are tubular, with a hollow core rather than the solid-rod structure. Here is the secret: cotton fibers can absorb and hold small amounts of moisture. Water is conductive, and this small amount—even the amount absorbed from your body—gives cotton the ability to drain away and rapidly lose any charge that might otherwise be trapped. Cotton fibers become neutral in the battle of the charges.

Static electricity consists of charged particles, both positive and negative, but the life span of positive ions is very long and the life span of negative ions is very short. Therefore the preponderance of static is positive. When static electricity clings to clothing, it is due to an active electrical charge. If clothing has a positive charge, it attracts the negative ions in the air to itself, thus diminishing the number of negative ions available for inhalation.

Whenever possible, wear natural clothing fibers such as cotton, linen, wool or silk. Avoid synthetic products, since they promote the storing of static electricity. Some common synthetic fabrics include nylon, dacron, acrylic, polyester fibers, man-made fibers, and almost anything that isn't cotton, wool, silk or linen. Many clothing manufacturers now blend synthetics with cotton or other natural fibers so that the clothing can "breathe" and be absorbent. The standard seems to be 50 percent cotton and 50 percent "man-made fiber." Half a loaf is better than none.

Negative Ions Are a Plus

Various other environmental factors can cause a depletion of negative ions in the air, creating an unhealthy imbalance and leading to problems. To counterbalance these factors, furnish your home and workplace with items made of natural materials. Select furniture made of wood rather than plastic; lay wool carpeting on the floor; hang natural fabric draperies and curtains.

Most people are totally unaware of any effect, but asthmatics or people with emphysema and other respiratory ills often suffer additional agonies because of the clothes they wear. Dr. Bernard Watson, professor of medical electronics at Britain's St. Bartholomew's Teaching Hospital in London, says: "Changing the immediate unhealthy ion environment to help an asthmatic means changing everything including clothes, sheets, and furniture."

To increase the negative ions in my home or office, I use the Elanra Therapeutic Ionizer and have seen positive difference in my well being. Studies show the ionizer helps to reduce and reverse the serious effects of positive ion poisoning, other environmental sensitivities, and promotes many other health benefits. For more information, please refer to Bionic Products in the Resource Directory.

Also, there are health hazards associated with detergents and other chemicals such as formaldehyde that are sometimes left in clothing. Allergies can develop if people are sensitive to these substances. If you find large patches of skin anywhere on your body which are red or sensitive to the touch, this may be your reaction to a laundry detergent. If you suspect detergent reaction, change to pure laundry soaps.

Give more thought to your clothes than only color and style. The more natural the selection, the healthier you will feel.

SIXTEEN

Living Your Highest Vision
Turning Dreams Into Reality

T*he way for you to be happy and successful, to get more of the things you really want in life, is to get the combinations to the locks. Instead of spinning the dials of life hoping for a lucky break, as if you were playing a slot machine, you must instead study and emulate those who have already done what you want to do and achieved the results you want to achieve.* —**Brian Tracy**

Positive thinking became almost synonymous with success in the 1970s. In its early use in organizations such as Dale Carnegie's success courses, positive thinking meant using willpower and conscious, positive thoughts to achieve goals. Napoleon Hill's maxim of success, "What you can conceive and believe, you can achieve," is a popular positive thinking slogan. Never underestimate the divine potential of positive thinking. If it's rightly employed, this power of the mind is a catalyst that makes possible a wondrous transformation in our lives. It was Ralph Waldo Emerson who said: "The good mind chooses what is positive, what is advancing—embraces the affirmative."

Positive thinking is the belief in our *own* self-worth—and in the value of everyone else and every circumstance. That positive belief leads to self-confidence, respect for others and a lifestyle based on strong values. Sometimes you slip into the habit of negative thinking because you feel discouraged, depressed, lonely, isolated or stressed. You want results fast and easy. But life isn't like that. Life is meant to be a challenge. When our minds are full of fear, doubt and clutter, good ideas can't get through. You get your best ideas and make your best decisions when you're relaxed, open to impressions and responsive to them. Find a way to link the present situation with wonderful opportunities to learn and grow. You can't just sit at a desk and think positively about something and expect it to happen. You have to make it happen—or at least help make it happen. Keeping alive a goal or dream, or even hope, requires action.

For me, the best action I can take is to look for the hand of God in every situation—finding in happy experiences glimpses of His infinite kindness, and in painful ones His guidance and blessings to help me win new victories over my limitations. In other words, I try to behold the Divine in everyone and everything.

Take Charge of Your Mind & Life

It's curious to me that no one ever taught me how to use my mind in school. I was taught mathematics, history, science, social studies, and English, but no course was offered on the science of mind so that I could learn more effectively. If I had my way, I would require all students, each year of their education, to take a class I'd call "mind power." This would be the science of mind and would cover a variety of topics, including mind strength and clarity—how to be alert yet relaxed. A special section would be devoted to awareness, or mindfulness, and how it affects all areas of our lives. Finally, students would be shown how to choose effective, positive thoughts—to be in control of thinking at all times, instead of allowing thoughts to be in control.

Control of the mind is essential if we are going to be happy and healthy. Be loving but firm with your mind, for it is like the reins that control the horses—the emotions and the body—and guide them to safety along the road of life. Train the mind always to be loving and kind and to see the best in others and in everything. When the road of life is steep, keep your mind even.

Making your dreams a reality doesn't happen by luck. Success is not an accident. You can choose to be active and create what you want, or simply respond to whatever happens around you, hoping for the best. Successful people are very deliberate about making the choice to be in charge of their lives. They don't get up in the morning and hope that they'll have a good day. High-achieving people take full control of their lives and if they don't find the circumstances they want, they make them.

Successful people make a choice to begin working on some dream. Nothing will ever happen without your having the courage to begin. Yes, this means taking risks, being vulnerable, making mistakes, and even failing. But life can't be lived on the sidelines if you want to be successful. The fun is challenging yourself to something you've always wanted to do.

Are you living your highest vision right now? Our lives reflect our thoughts, dreams, expectations, beliefs, hopes, feelings of self-worth and desires. Knowing this, you can consciously modify your inner states to create and live your highest potential and vision. You are not the victim of circumstance; you are the architect of your life. Your conscious thoughts create an unconscious image of your life, yourself, your feelings; your unconscious image reproduces itself perfectly in your circumstances.

Each of us is given free will, and we can create our own happiness and our own heaven or hell. You can do it by choosing your thoughts. Choose negativity and you will get unhappiness and hell. Choose confident living and positive thoughts and you will produce a heaven of happiness. Thoughts can imprison you or set you free. Complications, conditions or people do not upset you—but the way you think about them causes your upset. Freedom is not possible until you discipline and retrain your mind. Inevitably, your beliefs and thoughts create your reality. Right this moment, you can choose to see things differently, to live life from love, peace, and joy instead of from fear.

My Ocean Swim

A few years ago I had a glorious experience that showed me the tremendous power of thought. It also reminded me to "be here now" and to celebrate living each day. It was a splendid morning and I was accustomed to going to the beach for an invigorating swim a few times each week. It was very early, just before sunrise. After some stretching exercises and a short run, I was ready for my swim. Because it was the end of summer, the water was still comfortably warm. But this morning there was something in the air that I couldn't quite put my finger on. I felt it deep inside me—a joyful anticipation, a faint knowing that today would be different, that this day would be one I would celebrate the rest of my life. I went out into the ocean, rode a few waves, and then swam past the swells.

I was aware of the peacefulness of the water. Glassy, sparkling, and clear, it rejuvenated my body and soul with each stroke. A few minutes later some old friends joined me, a group of pelicans who seem to enjoy escorting me. They were gliding flawlessly a few feet above my head when suddenly they flew away. Surprised, I waved good-bye as I turned over to begin the backstroke. It was then that I saw something that made my heart plummet.

A large, dark, frightening fin was heading straight for me. Shark! I quickly looked toward the beach. No one was there. I had always taken for granted that I would stay calm in a life-threatening situation. But not this time! I can laugh now, but you should have seen me that morning. As the fin continued in my direction, I simply froze and treaded water. I was so terrified, I couldn't even cry or swim away. And then it happened, a sight that will forever warm my heart and soul. The fin danced out of the water. It was a dolphin followed by a school of about two dozen more!

About two weeks before this swim I had watched an incredible PBS special on sharks. The images and feeling from that program were still vivid in my mind. Then a few days after that, I had watched a moving Jacques Cousteau special about dolphins. For as long as I can remember, I have had a deep love for dolphins and whales. Following the dolphin show, during my evening meditation, I visualized myself swimming and playing with a school of dolphins. I accepted and affirmed that that was my desire and reality. I then thanked God for this wonderful experience.

There in the ocean that morning the dolphins stayed with me for the next half hour, swimming, jumping out of the water, and jumping over me. I swam under-water with them, listening to their beautiful sounds, touching their skin, feeling a connection and an exchange of love. For what seemed like hours, nothing else existed except my world of dolphins. I was oblivious to any thought of the past or future. Being right in the moment, I rejoiced in the joy of discovery.

Then, as quickly as they had arrived, they swam off, and I was left alone and immensely grateful. I swam back to the shore, where there was now a group of people who had gathered and watched my dance with the dolphins. I answered many questions and tried to share what the experience had been like for me. I found it was very hard to put my feelings into words. Experiences that speak directly to your heart are often difficult to express clearly.

The others left and I just sat there, enveloped in wonder at this truly remarkable experience. All I could do was cry—what had happened touched me so deeply, so lovingly. The experience was a beautiful lesson in living in the present and appreciating each moment. And because of that experience and so many others, I will never doubt the power of belief and thought to create any reality we choose.

The Principle of Choosing

Let's look at an all-too-common example of how the principle of choice works: weight control. Let's assume that you've always had difficulty controlling your weight. You've tried all kinds of diets and they've never worked, so you have negative feelings about diets. You've tried to limit the amount of food you eat without much success, so you don't have much faith in your self-control. You get on the scale every morning and the figures reinforce your image of yourself as overweight. It really is a vicious cycle. In order to better understand why you keep repeating the same patterns, let's look at the way your mind works.

Brain researchers see the mind as composed of three primary parts: the *conscious, subconscious* and *superconscious* minds (I'll discuss the superconscious later in the chapter). As the window to the world, your conscious mind runs your daily waking activities, such as making decisions, relating to others, and so on. Your subconscious mind, however, carries memories of all your experiences. It is the storage center for all the information your conscious mind sends it, based on your daily experiences. Your subconscious mind is a computer that is fed the data of your every thought, feeling and experience.

Relating this to the example of weight control: if you get up every morning and worry about what clothes will fit, if you dread getting on your scale, if you dislike being seen in public, if you think about going on a diet but doubt that it will work (they don't—see Chapter 3 on healthy weight), you are programming your subconscious computer in a negative way. Your subconscious mind creates reality according to its programming. If you think of yourself as fat, as having little self-control, as being unable to change, you will see those beliefs reflected in your life—you won't lose a pound.

The same is true for every other area of your life. Your subconscious beliefs and thoughts about yourself, your relationships with others, your money, your material possessions, your job, and so on, will be faithfully re-created in your life. Now you may be thinking, "That isn't true for me. I know that I really want to lose weight and tone up my body (or make more money or have a good relationship) but I'm not experiencing that in my life." The answer is that there is a vast difference between wanting something on a *conscious* level and wanting it on a *subconscious* level.

The conscious mind and subconscious mind are often in conflict. Consciously you may want something, yet subconsciously you create mediocrity or failure. That's why positive thinking as commonly perceived doesn't work. It doesn't do much good to force yourself to think positive thoughts if your subconscious still harbors many negative beliefs. What you need to do is to reprogram your subconscious mind to break the vicious cycle of negative beliefs creating your negative reality. We will examine methods of reprogramming later in this chapter. In addition, you must make some behavior changes on a conscious level that will contribute to new beliefs.

The birth of excellence begins with our awareness that our beliefs are a choice. You can choose beliefs that limit you, or you can choose beliefs that support you. The key, says Anthony Robbins in his motivating book *Unlimited Power*, is to choose beliefs that are conducive to success and to discard the ones that hold you back. It is our belief that determines how much of our potential we'll be able to tap, he says. Beliefs can turn on or shut off the flow of ideas. Virgil agreed. He said, "They can because they think they can."

What You Think About You Bring About

The law of correspondence says, "*As within, so without.*" It says that your outer world tends to be a reflection of your inner (subconscious) world—like a mirror. What you see in the world around you will be consistent over time with the world inside you.

The law of concentration says that "*Whatever you dwell upon grows in your reality.*" Studies reveal that successful, happy people think about successful, happy things most of the time. By the same token, unsuccessful, unhappy people constantly dwell upon people they dislike, the situations they are angry about and the events that they don't wish to occur in their lives. And whatever we think about most of the time, we bring about in our lives. Those two laws in combination explain much of success and most of failure.

So the starting point in making your dreams a reality is to discipline yourself to think and talk about only those things you want, and to refuse to think and talk about anything other than what you want. These can be tangible as well as intangible things. Besides thinking and talking about the new job or house you desire, talk and think about healthy things such as being grateful instead of unappreciative. Be loving instead of angry. Push all negativity, fears, doubts, and self-sabotaging, limiting thoughts and visions aside. You'll discover that all manner of remarkable things happen in your life that bring you closer to your goals when you take your thoughts off your problems and focus instead on your goals. "Speak the affirmative; emphasize your choice by utter ignoring of all that you reject," says Emerson. Don't accept anything less than what you want and focus on that which has your heart.

It's equally important to capture the *feeling* of the goal fulfilled, of whatever it is you desire, whether it's being prosperous, fit and healthy, being in a loving, supportive relationship or being very successful at work. Then you'll start acting that way and finally become it. The key to the process is to capture the feeling, because when you do that you've captured the ability to internalize it. Then it's only a matter of time. Feeling refers to the intensity or amount of emotion you bring to your mental pictures. Emotion is central to all accomplishments. There is a formula, $T \times F = R$: *thought* times *feeling* equals *realization*. This means that the thought or picture multiplied by the feeling or emotion that accompanies it equals the speed at which it occurs in your reality.

If you see your world only according to what surrounds you right now, you are judging by appearances and limiting what you are going to have. Instead of thinking, "I'll believe it when I see it," think "I'll see it when I believe it."

Trust in God and Hang On

Trust in God, the divinity within, regardless of appearances. The very best help for everything in life comes through trusting God and letting God take over, by letting God reveal the highest and best way to us and through us. Trust in divine order to unfold great and wonderful works in your life.

When you plant seedlings, you know that there is a timing and order before a single flower or fruit appears. Your careful cultivation may encourage the buds, but the seedlings follow God's orderly design of growth. The divine plan for you is orderly, too. Favorable conditions for your physical, mental, and emotional needs promote good results, but your spiritual evolvement provides complete fulfillment.

Following nature's clues, realize that neither love, friendship, nor worthwhile accomplishment can be forced. So simply be the best kind of friend or co-worker possible and enjoy watching God's order produce wonderful results. Such results may not happen according to your own or another's plans, but they will happen when you live a life surrendered to God. And they may be even better than expected.

Here's an example of how my surrender to God changed my life for the better. Not long ago I was involved in a committed, monogamous relationship with a man I believed was my life partner. We had lots in common, or so I thought at the time, and were making definite plans for our future together. I had occasional flashes of intuition that all was not well, but I chose not to believe them. One morning after our discussion about planning our engagement, I sat at my altar and talked to God. I turned the relationship over to Him and asked that God's will be done and guide me and us in all our future plans. I was so happy and grateful for the relationship.

Sometimes I feel God's presence as a gentle breeze guiding my way. Other times it's more like a tornado or a cosmic two by four hitting me over the head! That very day I met a messenger from God in the form of a friend of this man who felt I deserved to know facts which, as I later confirmed, were true. The man with whom I was deeply in love was, in actuality, very different than the image he wanted me to believe. He was leading a double life; he was very dishonest, unethical, and not monogamous. He even plagiarized several of my writings. The foundation of any relationship is trust and honesty, but I discovered that our relationship was based on a lie. His word meant nothing. He later admitted to me that I was so trusting of him that he found it very easy to lie to me and get away with anything.

As you can imagine, the news hit me like the above-mentioned tornado! The pain and betrayal I felt was almost too much to bear. Yet I knew that God never gives me more than I can handle. Confucius said, "To be wronged is nothing unless you continue to remember it." My life is now continually and richly filled with blessings. I'm grateful for the experience, which has taught me to be more discerning and to listen more carefully to my intuition. Clearly, that relationship was not for my highest good and it wasn't until I turned it over to God that I realized the truth of our incompatibility.

I believe that trials do not come to destroy you, but to help you appreciate God better. They are the effects of conscious or unconscious action in the past, somewhere, sometime. To overcome your trials you must resurrect your consciousness from the environment of spiritual ignorance. I affirm often: "Heavenly Father, I know that You are coming to my aid, and that I will see Your gift in this challenge bursting forth. My power to overcome is greater than all my trials, because I am your child. Thank you Father for guiding me and blessing me."

It's from the invisible that the visible is made. William James of Harvard University wrote, "Belief creates the actual fact." So believe, feel, and give thanks in advance (which shows faith in the process) that your goal is now your current reality.

As we change our consciousness, we change our lives. Because thoughts create form, the very thing you believe becomes reality for you *because* you believe in it. Richard Bach, in *Jonathan Livingston Seagull*, said, "Don't you believe what your eyes are telling you. All they show is limitation. Look with your understanding, find out what you already know and you'll see the way to fly."

The Power of Feelings

You must also say what it is you desire. Be specific. You must put in mind that which you choose to bring into your life. You must direct the power within to create what you want. The creative principle works according to the seeds that you plant. Therefore it's imperative that you plant the seeds that you desire to grow. When you plant seeds that you don't want to grow, it's out of a lack of understanding. If you plant love, you get back love. If you plant scarcity, disease and disaster, you get back scarcity, disease and disaster. So, say what you want, be specific, and act "as if," that is, act as if what you want were already true.

It's important to understand that belief can be embodied in subconsciousness through "the path of emotions." If an idea excites your interest, your interest will stimulate your emotions, particularly feelings of love, and when the feeling reaches the stage of passion it will then be recorded as a belief in the subconscious mind.

Let's take a closer look at the role of feelings in being the person you want to become. Your feelings are the power that creates. Just to simply visualize something without deep, passionate feelings will do little good. From the extensive research I have done in the field of human potential and manifestation, I have come to appreciate the role of feelings. I like to describe feelings as an electromagnetic force field that is so strong it sends up a vibration that pulls like vibrations to itself. It is a magnet for similar energy entrains. The result: more of those situations that produced the feeling to begin with.

Human behavior specialists know that success begets success and failure begets failure. It is a proven fact that when one makes money, other money comes more easily. A millionaire, for instance, would tell you that after she or he made one million, the second, third or fourth million came more easily and with little additional work. The more money you have, the more money is attracted to you. It works on a law akin to that of magnetism. After interviewing many highly intelligent, successful people with diverse backgrounds and vast experience, the conclusion I came to was that what you think about and how you feel about things are the determining factors in the way your life works out.

Any feelings we want we can have by simply feeling them. It's this powerful force of feeling that acts as a generator to bring into creation that which we desire. Negative feelings bring negative results. Positive feelings bring positive results.

As I lecture around the country and worldwide, I often hear statements such as: "I continually affirm, visualize, meditate, and believe in my highest good, but I rarely see results." Most of the time it's because the receiving channels have not been opened. This can be done by practicing forgiveness toward ourselves and others, and by releasing all fear, anger, guilt and any blockages to the presence of love inside you. (I discuss this more fully in my books *Choose To Live Peacefully* and *Choose To Live Each Day Fully*.)

Positive Actions Bring Positive Results

Let's take a look at some external, conscious changes you can make. For example, if you feel that your beliefs about money are creating negative results in your life, examine the behaviors that support those negative beliefs. Maybe you are frugal in your grocery shopping: you always buy the cheapest of every brand and skip the luxuries. Although frugality might be wise in light of your current financial situation, you should be aware that it also tends to reinforce your belief that you have very little money. One way to attack this belief would be to substitute a new behavior for an old one. In other words, the next time you're in a grocery store, allow yourself to indulge in a little luxury. And while you're doing it, imagine that this is your present reality and *feel it*.

If your problem is loneliness, make it a point to smile at one stranger every day, just as if you had plenty of friends and an abundance of love to share.

If you are overweight, buy yourself something appealing that you would normally have denied yourself because of your present weight.

It's important to remember that living your vision and creating what your heart desires is related to how you feel about yourself. If you feel that you are important enough to ask, and divine enough to receive, receiving will be your reward. If, on the other hand, you feel unworthy, it will be almost impossible for abundance to flow into your life. "Think of how a tree unfolds to all of its magnificent potential, always reaching for the sunshine and growing and flourishing," writes Wayne Dyer in *You'll See It When You Believe It*. "Would you ever suggest to a tree, 'You should be ashamed of yourself for having that disgusting moss on your bark, and for letting you limbs grow crooked'? Of course not. A tree allows the life force to work through it. You have the power within your thoughts to be as natural as the tree." He reminds us that all we need to do is be ourselves.

The more time you spend focusing on your goals and acting "as if"—imagining yourself as already having achieved a goal—the more likely and quickly you will be able to achieve it.

You Get Back Multiplied What You Give Away

Here's another important aspect of changing your subconscious image—the law of circulation which states that *you get back multiplied what you give away.* You must first give away the very thing you desire. If you desire increased prosperity in your life, share what you do have with others. Don't hoard it, because that would be a manifestation of a fear that there might not be enough.

When you have decided what you want, it's important to give a tithe. Tithe gifts can be in monetary form or a giving of yourself in time and/or deposits of love. Tithing traditionally meant to give a tenth of your income to your church. But tithing doesn't necessarily have to go to a church. I tithe money to those individuals or organizations who feed my soul and nourish my spirituality and who are making a positive difference on this planet. I also give money and time to those individuals less fortunate than I. It is futile to say, "Yes, when I get this money I will give a tenth of it as a tithe." You must start helping before that, you must start assisting those in need. If you do that, you will be living the spirit of, "Give that you may receive."

One day, after writing my precise prosperity affirmations and goals on cards, I went to the grocery store. While waiting in the checkout line, I suddenly called out to the harried mother in front of me, "I'll pay for those." Needless to say, she was astonished. Quite honestly, so was I. The words seemed to have just popped out of my mouth. After some hesitancy, and some excellent persuasion on my part, she let me pay her bill. I felt terrific! It is said, "To give is to receive," and it surely rang true for me that day in the market. The pleasure I received made me feel rich inside. But that's not the end of the story. Later that same day I ran into a person whom I had counseled several months before. At that time she had been unable to pay, and so I wrote it off as a loss. But that day she wrote me a check.

To act "as if" takes courage and trust. It's hard to start giving when you don't think you have enough. I realize that some of you will want to get out there and participate and have fun, but are scared. You must go out into the world as if you had the courage— and then you'll find that the courage you wanted is already there. Do the thing and the power is yours. But it begins with a risk. If you don't risk, you don't receive. That's how you generate power.

Your subconscious mind is extraordinarily powerful, but it is a servant, not a master. It coordinates every aspect of your thoughts, feelings, behaviors, words, actions and emotions to fit a pattern consistent with your dominant mental pictures. It guides you to engage in the behaviors that move you ever closer to achieving the goals you visualize and feel most of the time. If you visualize something that you fear, your subconscious mind will accept that as a command as well. It will then use its marvelous powers to bring your fears, instead of your dreams and aspirations, into reality.

Many people feel that their deepest beliefs and feelings are forever a mystery to them. They feel they don't understand the real reasons behind their actions, and as a result they feel powerless to change their actions. You have the power and ability to recognize and change the beliefs you have about yourself. Although your beliefs may seem mysterious and complicated on a conscious level, on a subconscious level they are usually simple. Your beliefs about yourself are based entirely on your past experiences. All of your experiences program your subconscious, and the result is the person you are today.

That is not to say that all you will ever be is the sum of your experiences. However, unless you take conscious control and choose the kind of programming you are feeding into your subconscious computer, you are destined to repeat your past. Have you ever noticed that your life experiences are all very similar—it's just the people who keep changing?

Choose Your Thoughts & Words Wisely

Two other effective ways to reprogram your subconscious mind are creative visualizations and affirmations. The idea is to alter your state of consciousness so you can temporarily set aside the conscious mind and focus your concentration specifically on your subconscious. Suggestions given to your subconscious while in an altered state of consciousness, whether they are images or affirmations, will be at least 20 times as effective as suggestions given in a normal state of consciousness, according to brain researchers. One of the best ways to alter, or slow down, your state of consciousness or brainwave activity is through relaxed deep breathing.

Remember that the subconscious is programmed. It doesn't reason. The subconscious works to create reality according to the programming it has been fed. Although programming is normally accomplished by thoughts and through your life experiences, brain researchers have found that the subconscious is incapable of telling the difference between reality and fantasy, between the real experience and the imagined experience.

So you can have a profound effect on your life by taking time each day to visualize your goals. As George Bernard Shaw said, "Imagination is the beginning of creation. You imagine what you desire, you will what you imagine; and at last you create what you will."

Brian Tracy, friend and human potential expert, host of Nightingale-Conant's *Insight* Tape program (see Resource Directory) and author of the inspiring, motivating book, *Maximum Achievement*, is world renowned for his work on the powers of the mind and visualization. He emphasizes the importance of vividness in mental pictures. The more vividly you can see something that you want in your mind's eye, he says, the more rapidly it will materialize in your reality. Most people have only a vague, fuzzy picture of what they want. They say they want to be rich or healthy or happy. But when you ask them exactly what that means to them, they don't really know.

Tracy says that vividness requires clarity of detail in your mental pictures. The more time you spend examining pictures of your desired goals, or drawing your own pictures of them, or writing out clear descriptions of what your goals and dreams would look like when they came true, the more rapidly the pictures are accepted by your subconscious as a command. Your subconscious mind immediately goes to work to coordinate all of your other resources, internal and external, to bring those desires into your life. "As within, so without." The clearer and more vivid your goal is in your mind's eye, the more rapidly it materializes in the world around you.

Be precise. Be absolutely definite. Know what you want, visualize what you want, and say what you want. It will not do to say you want a lot of money, or that you want a new car or a house. You must state exactly what it is that you want and hold that picture firmly before you.

If you want money, state definitely how much you want. It must be a definite sum. If you are wise, however, you will not bother so much about money. Rather, strive to gain virtues which will be of use to you when you leave this life. No one has ever taken a single coin into the next world. The more money you have, the more you leave for other people. The more you strive for money, the more you make it difficult for yourself to aspire and to attain spiritual values.

On the other hand, the more good you do for others, the more good you take with you. We can never have too much spirituality. We can never have too much purity of thought. And we can never help others too much, for in helping others, we help ourselves. So if prosperity is your goal, make part of your visualization definite plans for how you will help others when you create this prosperity.

Prosperity comes in many ways, shapes and forms, but all are alike in one way—each is a gift from God. A new car, an unexpected check, a smile from a friend or stranger, a breathtaking sunset—these things are among God's wondrous bounty that you can experience every day. When you pray, give thanks to God for answering your prayers. From this day forward, show your appreciation for any future good you will experience by declaring, "Thank You, God, for all the prosperity blessings I have received and will receive." Welcome prosperity graciously and enthusiastically.

Bask in the warmth of God's generosity and give thanks for your blessings every day. *Thank You, God! My needs are met!*

When do you want this goal in your life? Be specific. When do you want this money, car or house? It is not enough to say that you want it sometime in the indefinite future, and of course it is absurd to say that you want it immediately. It is not God's way to drop a gold brick into your waiting hands.

Write down your major goals, in the present tense, on 3 x 5 cards and review them on a regular basis. As you read a goal on a card—for example, "I earn $200,000 per year"— close your eyes for a few seconds, and imagine what it would be like if you were earning that kind of money. Visualize your ideal lifestyle. Get the feeling of success and achievement that goes with that greater income. Then open your eyes, smile, and go about your business, knowing in your mind's eye that you have already succeeded in achieving your goal.

Also, feed your mind a clear mental picture of your desired goals for the coming day, the coming week, and the coming months just before going to sleep at night. I do this every night for about ten minutes. As you drop off to sleep, your brain wave activity naturally slows down (as it naturally speeds up upon awakening), at which time your subconscious mind is the most receptive to the input of new commands. Since your mental pictures are a command, take those last few minutes before you fall off to sleep to daydream and fantasize about exactly the person you want to be and the life you want to have. Your subconscious mind will then take the picture down into its subconscious laboratory and work on it all night long. What often happens is that you wake up in the morning and have ideas and insights to help make those mental pictures a part of your life.

A few years ago one of my goals and dreams was to have a home-away-from-home, somewhere out in nature, where I could go to write and have some quiet and solitude. While I wasn't sure where I wanted this home to be, I was very clear on some of my specific requirements. I wanted the home to be away from a large city and crowds of people, surrounded by trees and nature's sounds. The home itself needed to have lots of wood and windows, a spectacular view, and lend itself to my healthy lifestyle—sun, fresh air, organic garden, great for working out, etc. So for a few months I visualized this home. I wrote down on 3 x 5 cards my vision and gave thanks that it was already a reality.

About six months later, I was invited to give a seven-day workshop in Coos Bay, Oregon located on the southern coast. I had been there a few times before, giving several Sunday services at the Unity-by-the-Bay church and thought it was a beautiful area, but never considered buying a home there. One evening I had a break during my workshop and was invited to visit some dear friends, Wally and Gloria, who live on top of a forested hill overlooking Coos Bay. During our conversation in their home, they mentioned that the house next door was for sale. I acknowledged their comment and didn't give it any more thought—that is until later that night. In the middle of the night, I was hit by another cosmic two by four and immediately realized I was supposed to buy that house next door to my friends. My realization seemed absurd because I hadn't even looked at the inside the house. I just had this knowing that this home was supposed to be mine and would be the perfect place for my personal retreats and to write.

The next morning I called my friends and, upon hearing my news they were delighted, even though they thought I was a little crazy. I called the realtor, Arch Wilkie, and learned that the house was in escrow and about to close. He would be happy to show me other homes, but this one was no longer available. I responded with, "You don't seem to understand. That's my home and I'm not interested in looking at any others." So I left Arch my number and asked him to call when it was available. As it turned out, it did become available, I gave an offer, and it's now our retreat home (God's and mine). It didn't come without roadblocks, I might add. The path of least resistance isn't always the best. The whole process of creating the home presented me with one challenge after another and also taught me numerous lessons—like the importance of belief and faith, not judging by appearances, if it's to be, it's up to me, being thankful for everything seen and unseen, and beholding the divine in everyone and everything. By the way, my home in Coos Bay is on top of a hill, surrounded by trees, overlooking the bay, has lots of light and is filled with angels. I never thought of Coos Bay as a place for my home-away-from-home. Now that I have it, I realize it's the perfect place for me and was made possible because of my partnership with God.

Take a Word Inventory

Be aware of everything you say during the day. Take an inventory of what you actually say. Speak only those words that are positive, loving and uplifting. The words you think and speak have a tremendous influence on your life.

We literally live the words that have become a permanent part of our thinking and speaking patterns. If we say positive, joyful, spiritual, life-enhancing words, we begin to live happier, more joy-filled lives. In Proverbs we find this statement: "Pleasant words are as a honeycomb; sweet to the soul and health to the body." Isn't that a beautiful thought? Just as we need to be careful about the food we put into our bodies, we need to be every bit as careful about our words and thoughts, for they are food for our bodies and souls.

I have found that from time to time I get into bad habits with my words. Not too long ago, I was driving with my close friend Rev. John Strickland. The day was hot and the traffic was heavy. A rude, reckless driver cut me off. I said in a loud voice, "I hate it when somebody does that to me!" John looked very startled to hear that come out of me. He said, "Don't use the 'H' word. That's a terrible thing to put into your consciousness. You should say instead, 'I prefer for drivers not to cut me off in traffic.' And then silently bless the driver."

Well, I was in no mood to listen to a lecture. I felt like saying to him, "I hate it when somebody lectures me!" But I didn't do that because he was absolutely correct. I have thought fairly frequently about that and other careless statements. Have you ever said, "That burns me up?" "They're driving me crazy?" or "This is back-breaking work?" These seemingly harmless expressions program garbage into your subconscious mind. The subconscious does not know that you don't really mean it. It just plays those ideas out into your life, into your experience, as if that's what you really, really want.

So what can you do to help yourself become aware of self-sabotaging words? I asked a couple close friends with whom I spend time to call my attention to every word or expression I say which is not positive. I've learned to pay attention to what I say (most of the time) and to interrupt negative expressions. I usually say or think to myself "cancel" or "erase" and then change the words. I have also imagined in my mind's eye a large screen in which I write any negative expressions I've used and then draw an "X" or a heavy line through the words. I've done this on paper, too, and then burned it. Use any method that is effective for you.

It is important to find positive ways to say exactly what you mean. For instance, replace "I'm sorry" with "I apologize." That is, after all, what you mean. Change "I'm afraid you have the wrong number" to "You have the wrong number." As you find more ways to speak more accurately, you stop feeding your subconscious mind with misinformation about yourself.

Your words communicate more than you intend them to reveal, for they spring from your deepest thoughts. They tell others how you feel about yourself and the world around you. You are as good as your word. In my opinion, when it comes to keeping your word, there is no such thing as a small situation. Perhaps it would be no big deal for you to say you're going to call someone and then not do it; but it can be very important to the other person. It's very important to me that my friends and business associates be accountable and that their words count. In fact, when I learn that someone doesn't follow through on what they say they're going to do, and it's apparent that it's a pattern, I choose not to spend time with that person. I'm inspired by people who make their word count.

To me, a verbal agreement is as important as a written one. In fact, I have verbal agreements, as opposed to written ones, with most of the companies for whom I do consulting. People know my word is good and they can count on me.

Every time my friend, Gary, makes a promise, no matter how small or seemingly insignificant, he keeps his word. If he makes plans with someone and then is offered the opportunity to do something more exciting or interesting, he never hesitates, saying: "Thank you, I'd love to do it, but I already have a commitment." Gary's behavior invariably brings two reactions, both positive. The first friend is pleased because he and Gary stick to their plan, and the second friend is also impressed. While sorry that Gary can't join him, he appreciates the fact that Gary can be counted on. Gary is not only well liked, he is also very successful. I believe that success and accountability go hand-in-hand. His word is his bond, and his friends and business associates all trust him. Gary is as good as his word, friends say of him. To me, there can be no higher praise than that. Make your word count. It's a gift you give to your family, friends, business associates, community and the world.

Fill your consciousness with positive things. There was a study conducted at Sussex University in which 30 subjects were shown a 44-minute television news broadcast in which the topics were either positive, negative or neutral. Not surprisingly, it was shown that negative new broadcasts put the subjects in a bad mood and made most of them edgy. I've noticed the same thing when I watch television news. We always have a choice about what we watch and give attention.

When you choose to be filled with a love of life and of God, you communicate joy through your words and actions. Because you know that God is so much a part of you and all that you do, you just naturally express love. Your words reach out to touch and uplift everyone around you. No matter what the subject is, the inner reality of God's presence stays the same. God's love and peace affect you in a deeply personal way, which is revealed through your words and actions. In Proverbs 15:1 we read, "A soft answer turns away wrath, but a harsh word stirs up anger."

I want to emphasize that your subconscious beliefs create your reality. All that you ever dreamed, desired, or thought consistently is what you have at this very moment. If things aren't just the way you would like them to be and you desire change, you must change your beliefs, thoughts, emotions, feelings and words. The best way to predict the future is to create it. You can choose to be a proactive agent in charge of what happens to you in life. You can make your dreams a reality.

Your Heart's Highest Vision

What's life without dreams? Do some people say you are a dreamer, hinting that you are something less than you should be? They don't know that you are using the tools of imagination and faith and painting a scene that is a real possibility for you. You recognize your dream as it takes shape, alert to the good that is unfolding right before you. Yes, be a dreamer—a dreamer of what God has created for you to have and explore and share in this wondrous world. Never let anyone, including yourself, convince you that your dreams can't come true, not when you know they come from the divine good awaiting your acceptance. You dream the dreams that are inspired by Spirit and follow them in ways that bless you and all those whose lives you touch.

Visualization is a powerful tool that can carry you towards achieving your dreams and goals. Your job is to use the power of visualization consciously and continuously to create the kind of future you want for yourself.

Your imagination is your window to your life's upcoming adventures. Albert Einstein said that he conceived of the theory of relativity by visualizing "what it must look like to be riding on the end of a light beam."

Henry David Thoreau once said, "If one advances confidently in the direction of his dreams, and endeavors to live the life which he has imagined, he will meet with success unexpected in common hours." I love that. It always works, but it takes getting out there and advancing confidently in the direction of your dreams.

What are your dreams? What is your vision? What do you expect to achieve in life? An important part of the process is expectation. Always expect to achieve your highest good, the best life has to offer, and live so that the best may become a part of your experience. Never allow anyone or anything to cause you to doubt your power and ability to live your vision—to manifest your goals and dreams.

I've come to realize that there's an unfathomable, yet recognizable, divine order to this universe. It's ever present and always working in alignment with what we need for our highest good and spiritual unfoldment and growth. I've learned not to analyze or question it anymore. It asks only for our trust, faith and courage.

Courage and the Bear

It takes courage to be the best we can be and to act with faith. Each moment provides an opportunity to behold the spirit of God in all. It takes courage to act in the face of fear and to trust that divine order is at hand. True courage enables us to live in the present moment and make choices rather than be a victim and settle for what life gives us. It's a God-given quality that can be called upon at any time. I definitely called upon it not long ago when my fear almost paralyzed me.

As I regularly do, I went to the Sierra Nevada Mountains alone for a few days of quiet, meditation, fasting and prayer. On this particular trip, I had a very small cabin next to a placid, beautiful lake. The day before I came home, I decided to take an all-day hike in the mountains. I left at around dawn and hiked uphill for most of the morning. Around two in the afternoon, I decided to sit down, relax and meditate by a tree. It was unusually quiet that day; I passed only five people on the trails. Sitting crossed-legged with my eyes still open, I could see paradise—several lakes and most of the Sierra. With each breath, I felt more peaceful, relaxed and connected with the spirit of life. I closed my eyes and began to concentrate on my breath, slowly inhaling and slowly exhaling. It felt wonderful. In a few more moments, I was totally absorbed in my inner world, not at all distracted by my surroundings, except for one minor thing. I thought I could hear some leaves moving. Often, when I'm meditating outdoors, I'm extra sensitive to nature's sounds. I figured I was in tune with the leaves and their musical dance. After a few more minutes, however, the sound of the leaves moving got louder. Slightly curious, I opened one eye. What I saw made my heart jump. No more than ten feet in front of me was a huge bear.

My first reaction was unbridled fear. The bear just stood there and stared at me. My second reaction was to ask God what to do. The answer was instant and, as I look back on the situation, somewhat off the wall. I was told to breathe slowly and deeply—as best I could. I was also told to smile at the bear and say some kind words from my heart. I gave it my best shot. I told the bear (in a voice about three octaves higher than usual!) that he was beautiful, his fur looked shiny and soft in the afternoon sun, and that I didn't intend on being his lunch. By talking to him, I actually began to feel relaxed. As I acted with courage, the fear slowly began to disappear. For about five minutes, I spoke to the bear while he just looked at me.

Then something really amazing occurred. I sensed that the bear was talking with me and responding to my comments. He even seemed to smile. Yes, part of me was still a little scared, but not paralyzed or mentally frozen. I paid attention, felt all my emotions fully and actually enjoyed the experience.

Then the bear started to move in my direction. I wasn't quite ready to hold out my hand to pet him. Before he got to me, he turned around and left. As I watched him shuffle away, I reflected on my extraordinary experience, one in which I learned that courage is inside of us all just waiting to rear its beautiful head.

We develop and strengthen our courage by using it. Don't let it go to waste. Trust in who you are. Be all you were created to be by living more from inner guidance. Each day, each moment, provides an opportunity to behold the spirit of God in all people and all creatures. We can all be centers of harmony just as we are, right where we are. Regardless of age or physical or material status, we can feel the joyful, radiating harmony of God moving through us and among us. With God as our partner, every day is a glorious, new adventure.

Patient Persistence in the Good

I continue to live in awe of the magnificent adventure life continually is. I'm convinced that it's extremely important to always imagine and think about your heart's desires, while at the same time letting go of thoughts of what you don't want. In other words, let your imagination work for you and not against you. Make friends with your thoughts. Know that you are exactly where you need to be in life and, at any moment, you can choose to experience something else simply by taking responsibility and consciously choosing to think differently. This reminds me of the fantastic line by writer Nikos Kazantzakis: "You have your paintbrush and colors. Paint paradise, and in you go."

There is power in what you think and say. But I'm not saying that all you have to do is put different pictures in your head and say a few positive words and immediately your life will turn around. I am saying that in order to change, you must start with your images, thoughts and words. They will then get stored in your subconscious as reality. Then you will start acting on that new reality. I use visualization for everything from creating or healing relationships, to increasing my prosperity and fitness level, to finding parking spots, to tapping into higher levels of creativity and peacefulness.

When we see evidence of adverse conditions in the world or our personal lives, we may find it difficult to believe that God's power is at work. Yet even in the midst of circumstances that we cannot personally understand, we can affirm that God's love is healing, strengthening, and preparing the way for good. Regardless of appearances, we can always trust God to bring order to chaos and peace where there seems to be disharmony. We accept our own part in the overall scheme by holding firmly to the truth about ourselves and others. Instead of focusing our attention on negative conditions, we let our thoughts be loving and reflective of our true nature. The good thoughts we sow will help us remain patient as we wait for God's good to unfold.

These days most of my visualizations and affirmations have to do with being in perfect harmony with the superconscious mind—the divine within—and staying open to this guidance. I want to be an open vessel through which God's will is manifest in my life. My human mind is not usually aware of what God's will for me is, but the divinity within me is. Every day, through prayer and meditation, I consciously surrender all to God, holding nothing back; and I ask for awareness, strength and courage to act on the guidance I receive. In adopting this way of thinking, I have seen more changes and far greater fulfillment in my life than I could have imagined possible.

The indwelling Spirit makes all things new. This divine power completely regenerates, renews, restores and rebuilds your life and world according to divine reality. I realize that Spirit can do for me only what it can do through me. "When you unlock the human door you are caught up in the life of the universe where your speech is thunder, your thought is law, and your words are universally intelligible," said Ralph Waldo Emerson. In quiet and stillness, that which is for your highest good is waiting for you to claim it. You will never have to search for it.

In All Things, Be Grateful

I once read a story of a small boy, about ten years old, who came into a restaurant and sat at the counter. The waitress came over and put a glass of water in front of him. "How much is an ice cream sundae?" he asked.

"Fifty cents," replied the waitress.

The little fellow pulled his hand out of his pocket and studied a number of coins clutched in it. "How much is a dish of plain ice cream?" he asked. There were many people waiting at the counter and the waitress was slightly impatient.

"Thirty-five cents," she said brusquely.

Again he counted the coins. "I'll have the plain ice cream," he said.

The waitress took his money, brought the ice cream, put it in front of him and walked away. When she came back a few minutes later, the boy was gone. She stared at the empty dish and then swallowed hard at what she saw: there, placed beside the empty dish, were two nickels and five pennies, 15 cents—her tip. That was some time ago, but she still keeps those seven coins as a gentle reminder that little people are just as important as big ones—especially to themselves.

It's so easy to be grateful when all is going our way. But what about when life challenges us? I recall Helen Keller's remark: "I thank God for my handicap, for through that, I have found myself, my work, and my God."

We don't have to have problems to grow. We can grow in spiritual maturity as we turn to God. But it seems to me that only a faith and belief in God and His goodness can give us the understanding and strength to be grateful in the midst of challenge, and the courage to live more from our ever-present inner guidance.

Let go and let God's spirit of love and light direct you. It's in surrender that we find everything we are seeking. Begin each day with an expectant attitude. Look for the special blessing each person and situation has for you. Be open to new good, and give thanks that God is always with us on each new adventure.

First thing in the morning, and anytime during the day, pause and invite God's spirit of love and light to guide you along your way. At home, in your car, at work, let go of anxious thoughts and let God's spirit of light and love fill your heart and mind. Moment by moment, realize the presence of peace and harmony within you. As you let go of worry and fear, invite God's spirit to fill your mind. Become one with God. You are a beacon of love and light shining forth into the world.

When you know your heart's desire, and turn everything over to God, the perfect plan is set in motion as you let God direct you in all matters. You must take action and have complete trust in that action, knowing that God's love is directing you. The more we trust God, the more our minds and hearts and lives will be filled with divine power, love and success. When you understand this concept and integrate this knowledge into your life, you will be able to turn your dreams into reality and create a healthier, happier life than you ever imagined possible.

*"You are never given a wish without also being given the power to make it true." —**Richard Bach***

SEVENTEEN

Serenity & Solitude
Essential Ingredients for Quality of Life

S*eek time to be alone; and in the cave of inner silence, you shall find the wellspring of wisdom.* —**Paramhansa Yogananda**

One of the true masters of the art of serenity was Thomas Edison. It seems that when his factory burned down years ago, he did not bemoan his fate. When newspaper editors went to interview him immediately following the disaster, they found him calmly at work on plans for a new building.

Another master of this art was Ralph Waldo Emerson. As his library of precious books was on fire, writer Louisa May Alcott tried to console him. The great philosopher said to her, "Yes, yes, Louisa, they're all gone, but let's enjoy the blaze now."

Men such as Edison and Emerson mastered the art of serenity. According to Webster, serenity has to do with the quality or state of being serene—calm, tranquil, peaceful, quiet, noiseless. But to master this art of serenity, we need also to master another art, that of being alone.

Solitude & Silence

Everyone needs time for solitude and silence. During those precious times can be found the peace of your own company. While few of us would choose lifelong solitude, all of us need at least some time to ourselves. We may differ from friends, colleagues, and partners in the amount, frequency, and urgency of our need, as well as in the way we spend our personal time. We may have trouble carving out periods of privacy, or even feel guilty claiming them. But when we're deprived for too long, we experience distress and lack of balance.

Paramhansa Yogananda, in *Man's Eternal Quest,* says this about solitude: "Be alone within. Don't lead the aimless life that so many persons follow. Meditate and read good books more. . . . Once in a while it is all right to go to the movies and have a little social life, but mostly remain apart and live within yourself. . . . Enjoy solitude; but when you want to mix with others, do so with all your love and friendship, so that those persons cannot forget you, but remember always that they met someone who inspired them and turned their minds toward God."

It's hard to practice solitude and silence when we are constantly bombarded with a barrage of noises that seem to be part of living in our technological society. When we think we've carved out some quiet time, we become more sensitive to subtle sounds such as the refrigerator motor, air conditioner, heater, distant traffic or the dripping faucet.

It's not easy to find absolute silence in the outer world, but you can find silence inwardly. Within each of us there is a peaceful silence waiting to be embraced. It's the harbor of the heart, and when rediscovered, your life will never be the same. In the Bible we read, "For God alone my soul waits in silence" (Psalms 62:1). And Yogananda said, "Calmness is the living breath of God's immortality in you." He also said the following, which I have written and posted on my bathroom mirror: "Always remember that seclusion is the price of greatness. In this tremendously busy life, unless you are more by yourself, you can never succeed. Never, never, never. Walk in silence. Go quietly; develop spiritually. We should not allow noise and sensory activities to ruin the antennae of our attention, because we are listening for the footsteps of God to come into our temples."

Mystics, saints, and spiritual leaders of the past and present have all advocated periods of silence for spiritual growth as a practical way to find balance and to be made whole again.

Concomitant with silence is spending time in solitude. Ah-h-h solitude! Even the word evokes peace within me, perhaps because it's such an important and vital part of my life. On solitude, Henry David Thoreau wrote in his *Journal,* March 20, 1841, "It is a great relief when for a few moments in the day we can retire to our chamber to be completely true to ourselves. It leavens the rest of our hours." In *Walden,* he added these two wonderful thoughts on solitude.

> *"I have a great deal of company in my house;*
> *especially in the morning, when nobody calls."*

> *"I love to be alone.*
> *I never found the companion*
> *that was so companionable as solitude."*

How do you feel about being alone? There is, indeed, a difference between aloneness and loneliness, the two sides of solitude. Loneliness expresses the pain of being alone; solitude expresses the joy of being alone.

Sometimes finding time to be alone is a difficult thing. In *Gift from the Sea*, Anne Morrow Lindbergh says, "The world today does not understand, in either man or woman, the need to be alone. Anything else will be accepted as a better excuse. If one sets aside time for a business appointment, a trip to the hairdresser, a social engagement, or a shopping expedition, that time is accepted as inviolable. But if one says: 'I cannot come because that is my hour to be alone,' one is considered rude, egotistical, or strange. What a commentary on our civilization, when being alone is considered suspect; when one has to make excuses, hide the fact that one practices it—like some secret vice."

One of my friends has three children. She rarely has time to herself. She is very busy working and raising the children. She often finds herself rushing between the children's dance lessons, doctor appointments, grocery shopping, and other household errands. When she told me how she spent her days, I became exhausted just listening. I suggested she give herself permission to call some time her own. Now, after she drops off a child at dance lessons, she either pulls out a favorite book and reads in her car or she spends the time in meditation. There are no phones, no people, no distractions. She has an hour of quiet and solitude to do or think as she pleases.

When I'm conducting a workshop, I often ask the participants to go outside for fifteen minutes and stroll the grounds, alone, in silence. I have them experience and practice being totally involved and absorbed in what they see, smell, feel, touch, or hear. I want them to let nature's beauty into their awareness. No matter what part of the world we are in, I always have participants come to me afterwards and say that this was their first experience of being truly alone and finding peace in their own company.

What I have discovered in taking this kind of walk is that I feel a subtle, gentle communion with nature. I build a garden of the soul. The flowers, trees, birds, clouds, and even insects seem to be in harmony with me. It rejuvenates my entire being and allows me to be more fully aware of my environment, sensitive to nature and connected to feeling my oneness with all life.

I devote a few hours a week to private counseling. With many clients, the session may first begin with an invigorating hike in the beautiful Santa Monica Mountains. I find this to be a wonderful way to let go and surrender to the spirit of life. Listening to the silence and sounds of nature is a great way to feel serene and in touch with your feelings, hence making it easier to express yourself. By the time our session is over, we both feel rejuvenated physically, mentally, and spiritually.

Several years ago, I spent time in a monastery in which disciplined silence was required 24 hours a day. At first, it was difficult. There was so much I was feeling, experiencing, and seeing that I wanted to share with the others. And then, slowly and subtly, I discovered that the silence was overwhelmingly blissful. It was almost as though a gentle wave of peace rolled over me. There was nothing but silence—all around me, through me, and everywhere expanding and reaching out to touch all creation. Things that touch the heart are often difficult to put into words, and this was one of those experiences. I just knew that I loved the silence, reveled in it, and wanted to have it with me always.

Since that time at the monastery, I carry this silence with me. Even in conversation, I am aware of this quietness beneath the sounds of people's voices. And although I sometimes lose awareness of it, I can recall it and let it once again be a source of great peace and joy, like the awareness of a close and loving friend.

Since my experience at the monastery, I now find time for regular periods of solitude and silence. I recognize that I choose more solitude than most. Not only do I meditate at least twice a day, but I also take off several hours once a week, one weekend a month, and a few days with each change of season to simply be alone and embrace silence. In fact, as I write this chapter I'm celebrating a new glorious season and am spending a few days in Coos Bay, Oregon away from most activity of my usual world. This regular supplement of solitude and silence greatly enhances all areas of my life. It nourishes my soul.

"The most important time for me to have to myself is the half hour when I get home after a hectic day of work and doing errands," says Dejla Asli, a dear friend and cosmetician at Georgette Klinger Salon on Rodeo Drive in Beverly Hills, California. "My family and friends sometimes don't understand why I still want that after being alone some of the day. But at home, that half hour is really for myself, for relaxing and meditating. And if I have it, I'm refreshed and can go out socially and enjoy myself, or even go back to work."

Constant activity and noise enervate the body and leave us feeling drained mentally, emotionally and physically. Quality time alone is renewing. I enjoy exercising alone at dawn. I feel great not only because I am alone, but also because I'm working out and find pleasure in my own company. There's also serenity in being self-sufficient—feeling complete, whole, and satisfied with myself and what I'm doing—whether I'm working or enjoying a respite of relaxation and solitude.

"Silence will help you see clearly exactly what is out of balance in your life," says Barbara De Angelis, Ph.D., in her wonderful book, *Real Moments.* "It creates an opening through which you can receive truth, perspective, strength, healing, revelation."

When was the last time you were *alone*—I mean really alone—and in silence without radio, video, or tapes, listening to the silence of your heart, being at peace with your own company?

Here are some simple ways De Angelis suggests to create and experience more silence in your life:

Carving Out Time to Be Alone

- Drive with your radio turned off. Cars are great moving awareness centers. I consider them "sacred spaces."
- Don't turn on your TV if you're not really watching. Background noise keeps your mind restless and suggestible to unwanted influences.
- Keep your telephone from becoming a disruptive force. Turn the ringer off and the volume down on your answering machine a few days each week. Sometimes I gather my messages at the end of the day and return the calls in one sitting.
- Exercise without your personal stereo. If outdoors, listen to nature. It can be more meditative. Move to the rhythm of your thoughts.
- Sit in silence by firelight or candlelight. "Watch the flames. Listen to logs crackle, or watch the wax drip down the side of the candle," says De Angelis. "Imagine the light illuminating all of the dark or hidden places inside of you. Enjoy the simplicity of the moment."

There's an old saying that God gave us two ears and one mouth so we may hear more and talk less. How well we use our ears will play an important part in determining what we learn as we go through life. The more I spend time in silence, the more I appreciate the power of brevity and silence when conversing with others. One of my college exercise physiology professors was short and thin. But to me he was a living example of the power of silence. In his quiet manner, that professor conveyed firmness and fairness—but not fear. He deserved and received wholesome respect from everyone.

President Abraham Lincoln could have rambled on at Gettysburg, but if he had done so I'm sure nobody would have remembered it. He chose to be brief, and with it came power, eloquence, and fame. Shakespeare observed, "Where words are scarce, they are seldom spent in vain."

Silence is golden. It can persuade, dissuade, heal, inspire, command, console, win elections, promote good health, and bring about greater happiness and harmony in your life. Even when you are with other people, silence can help you communicate ideas, feelings, beauty, strength, or understanding without uttering a sound.

Understanding and accepting another's need for private time is more difficult for those who don't want to be by themselves. Some of us are apt to feel rejected when our company is turned down in favor of "nothing"—that is, the other person's being alone. It is not a rejection, although it may be misunderstood that way.

Often the issue is finding time. You must choose to *make* the time. Make privacy a priority in your life. Privacy is a universal need. There will always be others who want some of your time. In order to get quiet time to yourself, reserve a regular period in your daily schedule when your family and friends around you know that, barring emergencies, you expect to be left alone. It helps to explain your needs clearly and specifically to others.

Find a way to fit this privacy into your life. For some, solitary exercise may be all that is needed to maintain that balance throughout the day.

Others spend several minutes alone one or more times a day in some type of meditation. This spiritual exercise acts like a shock absorber to life, allowing life's experiences to touch us more gently. Still others embark on longer silent retreats to go more deeply into their own consciousness and clear all channels. Whether for short or extended periods of time, retreating from the outside world will enhance and enrich all areas of your life.

I believe that all the other good things we endeavor to provide for ourselves—sound nutrition, daily exercise, vitamin supplements, material wealth, and so on—will be of limited value unless we learn to live in harmony with ourselves, which means knowing ourselves and finding peace in our own company. Peace is a natural consequence of time spent alone. In time spent alone we realize we are never really alone and that we can live more fully by focusing on inner guidance rather than on externalities. Too often we look outside ourselves for our worth and forget that nothing will ever be enough until *we* are enough. When we recognize that we are already enough, everything else will be enough. It all starts on the inside. "Perception is a mirror, and what I look on is my state of mind reflected outward," it says in *A Course in Miracles*.

"Privacy," stated former Supreme Court Justice Louis D. Brandeis, "is the right to be alone—the most comprehensive of rights, and the right most valued by civilized man." And woman!

As we open our hearts to silence, we access the most powerful healer of all—the healing power of love, of God. In silence, deep within our hearts, each of us knows the truth.

Wisdom According to FedEx

Have you ever wanted to reveal to the world the deep inner truths that you receive from your times of silence? What if someone said that you knew the secret of happiness and put you on a stage to tell it? The "Totally Hidden Video" television show set up a convincing prank on precisely this theme which was revealed in the delightful book, *I Had It All the Time*, by Alan Cohen.

For the gag, a Federal Express driver was asked to deliver a package to a religious temple (fabricated by the television show). Unknown to the driver, the pranksters had taken a photo of him and replicated it as a painted portrait, depicting the young man dressed in the royal regalia of the fictitious sect.

When the delivery man arrived, the disciples (actors hired by the program) took one look at him and began buzzing excitedly. They ushered him to the front of the sanctuary and invited him to sit on a plush cushion of honor. Then they revealed to him that he was the chosen one, the long-awaited prophet foretold in their scriptures. To allay any doubts, a servant parted the altar curtain where, lo and behold, hung the majestic portrait of the deliverer, painted by a visionary centuries ago.

"Please," begged a disciple, "give us some words of wisdom."

The driver surveyed the portrait and looked over the throng of expectant devotees. A hush fell over the assembly. He sat down on the pillow, took a deep breath, and spoke: "Life," the sage explained, "is like a river."

The disciples "oohed" and "aahed" on the heels of his utterance, hanging fervently on every sacred word.

"Sometimes life flows easily, and sometimes you encounter rocks and rapids," the guru illustrated, "but if you hang in there and have faith, you will arrive at the ocean of your dreams."

Again the students swooned with ecstasy. More "oohs" and "aahs." This was indeed the day they had been waiting for!

"Well, that is about it," Swami FedEx curtly concluded. "I have to go now and make some more deliveries."

Reluctantly the devotees rose, bowed reverently, and sheepishly cleared the way for the anointed one. Amid profuse veneration he made his way to the door.

Now here is the amazing postscript to the story: the program played the same trick on several FedEx drivers, each of whom found profound words the moment he sat on the cushion. The invitation to wax profound brought forth the inner wisdom in these unassuming fellows.

Deep within our heart, we all know the truth. The answers we seek, the power we strive for, the happiness and health that we want, and the acknowledgment we attempt to gain, abide inside us. Given the opportunity (being placed on the cushion), or the challenge (being pushed up the rapids), we know what we need to know and do.

Simplify, Simplify!

"Live simply so that others may simply live." —**Gandhi**

A natural outgrowth of the practice of solitude is the desire to slow down and forego the hurry habit. There's an American sickness I've seen growing over the past years: the *hurry* sickness, the *busyness* sickness. We see it everywhere—instant breakfasts, fast foods, in-and-out cleaners and burgers, one-minute managers and twelve minute fitness programs. I wouldn't be surprised to see a new book about "one-minute sex." I hope not.

To let go of the busyness of life requires simplifying our lives. Simplify! What a wonderful word and a powerful process it represents. I have discovered great joy in simplifying all areas of my life. This includes my thoughts, what I say, how I choose to spend my time, how I arrange my closets, cupboards and garage—everything.

To simplify is so freeing and feels so good. For example, look at the foods you eat in one meal. It's hard to appreciate any one of them fully when so many are mixed together. Similarly, you can have a fantastic collection of art objects in your home, but if you have too many—if it's cluttered—then appreciating each piece fully is difficult.

In his delightful little book, *How You Can Talk With God,* Yogananda said, "Why do you consider nonessentials so important? Most people concentrate on breakfast, lunch, and dinner, work, social activities, and so on. Make your life more simple and put your whole mind on the Lord." What great advice!

When your life gets too complicated and out of balance, you become less sensitive to your own needs and the needs of your family and friends around you. When you consciously choose to simplify, your life slows down and you are better able to live in the present moment, with a sagacious awareness of your own inner guidance and divinity. Often we live so harriedly and hurriedly that we don't pay attention to what's really important. Our lives are cluttered with superfluousness.

In the play *Our Town*, there is a most poignant scene when little Emily dies and goes to the graveyard. She is missing life at Grover's Corners and asks if she might have the opportunity to go back in time just for one day. Her request is granted and she selects her 12th birthday for a "rerun" visit. She sees this event from a new perspective. She learns something about loving life that she never realized while she was alive.

Emily comes down the stairs in her birthday dress, her curls bouncing, so happy because she is the birthday girl. Mama is so busy making a cake *for* her that she doesn't look up to see her. Papa comes in and is so busy with his books and papers and making money that he walks right by. He doesn't even see her. Her brother is in his own scene, and he's not bothering to look either.

Finally, Emily ends up on center stage alone, in her little birthday dress.

EMILY, in a voice that her family cannot hear:

Please, somebody, look at me. *Going to her mother once again:* Mama, please, just for a minute, look at me. *Nobody does. She turns to the gods.* I can't go on. It goes so fast. We don't have time to look at one another. I didn't realize that so much was going on and we never noticed. Take me back . . . up the hill . . . to my grave. But first. Wait! One more look. Good-bye world. Good-bye Grover's Corners . . . Mama and Papa. Good-bye to clocks ticking . . . and Mama's sunflowers . . . and food and new ironed dresses . . . and hot baths . . . and sleeping and waking up. Oh earth, you're too wonderful for anybody to realize you. . . . Do any human beings ever realize life while they live it— every, every minute? *Again looking to the gods.* Take me away. I forgot how difficult it was to be a human being. Nobody looks at anybody anymore.

Truly there are no ordinary moments. Every moment is a miracle waiting to be recognized. Simplify. Pay attention to what is really important and essential in life. Be a miracle finder.

Unclutter Your Life

What can you do to simplify your life right now, today? One surprisingly effective place to start is by cleaning out and simplifying one of your closets, some cupboards, or your garage. Keep that up for fifteen minutes each day until you have finished with your entire home. As a result of this disciplined exercise, you will find yourself easily and naturally beginning to simplify other areas of your life—how you spend your time, what you think, and what you say. This technique is not only freeing and refreshing, it also supports you in feeling more serene, peaceful, and in seeing your life from a higher perspective. The technique works because outside and inside always reflect each other; change one and you influence the other.

Living Fully and Living Simply Go Hand-In-Hand

There is a trend toward simplicity, claims Stanford Research Institute social scientist Duana Elgin in his book, *Voluntary Simplicity*. He states, "To live with simplicity is to unburden our lives—to live a more direct, unpretentious, and unencumbered relationship with all aspects of our lives; consuming, working, learning, relating and so on. Simplicity of living means meeting life face to face. It means confronting life clearly, without unnecessary distractions, without trying to soften the awesomeness of our existence or masking the deeper manifestations of life with pretensions, distractions and unnecessary accumulation. It means being direct and honest in relationships of all kinds. It means taking life as it is— straight and unadulterated." That rings true for me.

Letting go of clutter, living honestly, simply and freely, without pretensions, encumbrances and superfluity is what living fully and joyfully is all about. Perhaps we can head in that direction by having fewer desires and being more selfless. The venerable Lao-Tzu said:

> *"Manifest plainness*
> *Embrace simplicity*
> *Reduce selfishness*
> *Have few desires"*

At one time in my life, I found great pleasure in collecting material things. My income was generous and I would delight in buying lots of clothes, appliances, electronics, gadgets, cars, etc., until I got to the point that I was seeking fulfillment from what I collected rather than from the divinity within. In pursuit of many material goals, I began to lose sight of my spiritual goals, through which all fulfillment, happiness and peace come. I was looking outward to my collection of stuff rather than within, to my true nature, for my value and worthiness as a human being.

Fortunately, I discovered that what the world holds for me is not as important as what I bring to the world. When I realized that, it became clear to me that I wanted to live more simply—in every aspect of my life. I have found that I can live well and still live simply. I still buy clothes and other items these days, but more often I'm giving away things and finding ways to make my life more simple, less complicated.

Here's an inspiring passage from the wonderful book, *The Simple Life,* by Joan Atwater.

> Our lives are overburdened, and living often seems to us a terribly complicated affair. The problems of the world are so incredibly complex and we see that there are no simple answers. The complexity always leaves us with a feeling of helplessness and powerlessness. And still, amazingly enough, we go on, day by day, always half subconsciously yearning for something simpler, something more meaningful.
>
> So how we look at our lives and living becomes tremendously important. It's up to us to bring this authenticity, this simplicity, this directness, this unburdened clarity into our looking. If such a thing as living life fully interests you, then it's up to you to learn about it and live it.

Isn't that fantastic? If living fully interests you, then do it fully! How can you simplify your life in order to fulfill your purpose more easily and live more fully? We can assist each other on our journey through this miracle called life, but no one can live your life for you. In the end, it comes down to choice. Once you become aware that you are choosing everything, you can take over your own life and live it the way your Higher Self knows how to live it. You can choose to let go of clutter and complexity in favor of serenity, peace and happiness—a more spiritual life.

To Find Happiness, Serve

When your life is less cluttered, you have more time to focus on what's really important, like being of service and letting God's will navigate your thoughts, words and actions. It was Albert Schweitzer who said, "I don't know what your destiny will be, but one thing I do know: the only ones among you who will be really happy are

278 • MAIN INGREDIENTS

those who have sought and found how to serve." I believe that service is the key to a happy life, to a spiritualized life—and it is also the key to spiritualizing business.

Whether or not we belong to a church or service organization, or have a job that provides meaningful service opportunities, not a day goes by that we can't at least serve one other human being by making deposits of unconditional love. It's not the deed that is essential, rather the important thing is the loving serviceful attitude—because success and saintliness are more a product of inner consciousness and attitude than efficiently improving the world's outer condition.

Yogananda said: "Instead of making money and greater profits your goal in business, make service your goal, and you will see the entire plan of your life change. Business for private profiteering is wrong." Now that doesn't mean that we shouldn't make a legitimate profit. It just means that service, not money, should be our goal; then profit follows automatically. Profit is the natural result of service. Values can be profitable, as the best entrepreneurs know. One such businessman is Tom Chappell, president of Tom's of Maine and author of the excellent book, *The Soul of a Business,* which is subtitled, *Managing for Profit and the Common Good.*

There is intrinsic security that comes from service, from helping other people in a meaningful way. One important source is your work, when you see yourself in a contributive and creative mode, really making a difference. Another source is anonymous service— where no one knows it, no one necessarily ever will, and that's not your concern, but rather your concern is blessing the lives of other people. "It is high time the ideal of success should be replaced with the idea of service," said Albert Einstein.

Victor Frankl, author of *Man's Search for Meaning,* focused on the need for meaning and purpose in our lives, something that transcends our own lives and taps the best energies within us. The late Dr. Hans Selye, in his monumental research on stress, basically said that a long, healthy, and happy life is the result of making contributions, or having meaningful projects that are personally exciting, which contribute to and bless the lives of others. His ethic was "earn thy neighbor's love."

In the words of George Bernard Shaw:

"This is the true joy of life: being used for a purpose recognized by yourself as a mighty one, and being a force of nature instead of a feverish, selfish little clod of ailments and grievances, complaining that the world will not devote itself to making you happy. I am of the opinion that my life belongs to the whole community, and as long as I live it is my privilege to do for it whatever I can. I want to be thoroughly used up when I die. For the harder I work the more I live. I rejoice in life for its own sake. Life is no brief candle to me. It's a sort of splendid torch which I've got to hold up for the moment and I want to make it burn as brightly as possible before handing it on to future generations."

Yogananda suggests that each day we find ways to do some good. Perhaps give to a worthy cause or help some individual. Sometimes all a person needs is some understanding, attention or compassion. See God in everyone, no matter how erring the person may be. When you mentally put yourself in the position of others, it is easier to understand them, to act with kindness, and to help. "The one thing that will help to eliminate world suffering—more than money, houses, or any other material aid—is to meditate and transmit to others the divine consciousness of God that we feel. Everyday radiate His consciousness to others," explains Yogananda.

Someone once said, "Service is the rent we pay for the privilege of living on this earth." And there are so many ways to serve.

EIGHTEEN

Acts of Kindness
The Joy Factor

O f course I love everyone I meet. How could I fail to? Within everyone is the spark of God. I am not concerned with racial or ethnic background or the color of one's skin; all people look to me like shining lights! —**Peace Pilgrim**

I could hear the frustration in her voice the moment I picked up the telephone. When you've known someone for years, it's often easy to ascertain when something is bothering them even before words are spoken. Have you noticed that with your close friends or family members? My friend Rose called me because she was on the verge of quitting her job, even though she loved her work. She needed some guidance.

Rose is a very talented window dresser for a popular store on Rodeo Drive in Beverly Hills. Every couple of weeks she is in charge of changing the window. Rose's talents are so well-known that people come from miles around just to see what she has created in the window. She loves what she does, but she had been having a very difficult time with her boss. During our telephone conversation, she described how she was convinced that she was unjustly criticized by her supervisor and felt that some of her best work was rejected and unappreciated. She also felt he was deliberately rude and unfair to her.

Because I believe that we always attract to ourselves the equivalent of what we think, feel, believe, and put our faith in, I lovingly suggested to my friend that maybe she, rather than her boss, was the one in need of a new attitude. I asked her how she felt about him.

Rose confessed to me that her mind was filled with criticism and unkindness toward this man and that she rarely felt positive in his presence because of the way he treated her. She even revealed to me that every morning as she walked to work, she visualized the entire scenario of how she knew she would be treated by him that day. Rose confirmed my observation about the law of correspondence. I explained that he was merely bearing witness to her concept of him.

When Rose realized what she had been doing, she agreed to change her attitude and only think of him in a loving, kind way. I recommended to her that, before drifting off to sleep at night, she visualize her boss congratulating her on her fine designs and creativity and that she, in turn, see herself thanking him for his praise and kindness.

To her delight, after only seven days of practicing her visualizations, the behavior of her employer miraculously reversed itself. Rose soon discovered for herself that her own attitude toward him was the cause of all that irritated her. She proved the power of imagination and kindness. Rose's persistent desire to replace love and tenderheartedness for unkindness influenced his behavior and determined his attitude toward her. It is always the same—as within, so without.

Humans are powerful spiritual beings meant to create good on the earth. This good isn't usually accomplished in bold actions, but in singular acts of love and kindness between people. It's the little things that count, because they are more spontaneous and show who you truly are. The amount of love and good feelings you have at the end of your life is equal to the love and good feelings you put out during your life. It's that simple. "What a splendid way to move through the world," writes Jack Kornfield in *A Path with Heart*, "to bring our blessings to all that we touch. To honor, to bless, to welcome with the heart is never done in grand or monumental ways but in this moment, in the most immediate and intimate way."

The Religion of Kindness

It was the Dalai Lama who said, "My religion is very simple—my religion is kindness." Gentleness and kindness go hand in hand. Gentle means kindly, mild, amiable, not violent or severe. Gentle also implies compassionate, considerate, tolerant, calm, mild-tempered, courteous, and peaceful. But I think the best synonym for gentle is tenderhearted. I love that word! And I also love being around people who are tenderhearted. What about you? Think about those people you love to be around the most, with whom you feel the most enthusiastic, positive and can be yourself. You'll probably say they're loving, supportive, kind and maybe even tenderhearted.

To be treated with tenderheartedness and kindness, we must first offer that quality to the other person. Respond to others exactly as you would want to be treated. No one likes to be belittled, ignored, or unappreciated. Everyone likes kindness, patience, and respect. In Ephesians 4:32, we read, "Be kind to one another, tenderhearted, forgiving one another, as God in Christ forgave you."

"Random acts of kindness" is a slogan that's been catching on around the country. Oprah Winfrey has even devoted a few of her programs to people offering unsolicited acts of kindness to others. Acts of kindness are those lovely things we do for no reason except that, for a moment, the best of our humanity and heart comes forward. Every day we are presented with hundreds of opportunities to practice kindness towards our fellow humans. These gestures aren't expected or anticipated. Don't ever underestimate the power of kindness. In the process, we are transformed. We become, in a sense, an angel for a moment and touch the divine when we give to another pure love and joy without expecting something in return. We become twice blessed, for in blessing another we bless ourselves. In showing love and kindness to another, we also increase our self-esteem. Acts of kindness connect our heart with the heart of another person and create pathways through which our love can flow.

Sometimes these acts of kindness are made anonymously and sometimes not. But in the process, we can't help but be changed ourselves. In giving of our highest selves, purely out of love, our body, our heart and our environment change, and for an instant we realize that loving and being loved is the one true human vocation. We feel connected to the love in ourselves and the love in others.

I'll never forget the morning of January 17, 1994. It was 4:31 a.m. and I was meditating on the floor in front of my altar. My first reaction was that God was speaking to me! A couple of seconds later, I knew it was the biggest earthquake I had ever felt. I will never forget the terrifying sensation of holding on to the corner of my bed and listening to everything in the house crashing. It felt and sounded like the end of the world had arrived. I felt certain that I was going to die. Most everyone who went through this experience felt like the epicenter was under their own home, and that it was more like four minutes than forty seconds. I can honestly say that for those moments and for the hours that followed, I was living totally in the present moment.

But what's germane here is the response from the community. Adversity always brings gifts and powerful lessons. Families, friends and even strangers reached out to one another with true compassion and kindness. Sharing the same experience brought people together on common (if shaky) ground, opened hearts and woke up our spirits. Southern California, in a sense, was invigorated with a newfound compassion and kindness.

It permeated everywhere and lifted the hearts of all. Statistics revealed that in the days following the earthquake the crime rate was the lowest it's been in years. We were all forced to slow down and to see more clearly what's truly important and essential in life: not the things you possess, not even the work that you do, but the people in your life, the heart-to-heart connection you have with others and the love you give.

What's truly essential is invisible to the eye; it can only be seen and felt with the heart. "When strangers start acting like neighbors, communities are reinvigorated," says Ralph Nader. Acts of kindness send out a positive ripple into the world that is magnified by everything it encounters. Acts of kindness help bring us back to the feeling that people are basically good and kind. The love you have to give never runs out, for the more you give, the more you have to give. Ralph Waldo Emerson said, "It is one of the most beautiful compensations of life that no man can sincerely try to help another without helping himself."

Sometimes, however, we get so caught up in our responsibilities and commitments to family, friends, work, and doing what's expected of us that there's little left to give to others, let alone ourselves. That's when we need to step outside the ordinary and enter into the realm of the extraordinary and magnificent. With willingness and a little effort, you can create miracles in your life and the lives of others. You can become an angel, transforming the lives of others simply by giving with love. On my refrigerator is this quotation from *A Course in Miracles:* "Miracles occur naturally as expressions of love. The real miracle is the love that inspires them. In this sense everything that comes from love is a miracle."

For random acts of kindness to flourish we need to begin in perhaps the most difficult place of all, our own hearts, with simple acts of kindness toward *ourselves.* It is essential that we refuel our own spirits so that we will want to be compassionate to others. Then we can truly give to others from a heart overflowing with loving kindness. "Let us not be satisfied with just giving money," says Mother Teresa. "Money is not enough, money can be got, but they need your hearts to love them. So, spread your love everywhere you go."

Kindness at the Airport

Last month I was moved by a gesture of love at the airport. I was leaving Portland, Oregon to fly to Los Angeles. Because of stormy weather, most flights were delayed and some were canceled. The airport was crowded yet, fortunately, my flight was scheduled to leave on time. As they announced the final boarding, I noticed a harried man run up to the counter with his briefcase in one hand and ticket in another. He was told by the ticket agent that his reservation had been cleared and his seat given away. She told him that she would do everything she could to get him a seat on a later flight.

Well, he went meteoric. Everyone in the terminal could hear his frustration. He had an important meeting in Los Angeles that he couldn't miss. I felt for him because I've been in similar situations where I couldn't afford to miss a flight. In his tirade he yelled out that he wanted to see a supervisor.

All of a sudden a woman who looked to be in her 70s walked up to this man and said that she wasn't in a hurry and would be happy to give him her seat. As you can imagine, this man stopped right in his tracks. It almost looked like he was going to cry. He apologized to her, to the ticket agent and to everyone around for his behavior and thanked the woman for being an angel in his life. He boarded the flight smiling, relieved and much wiser. What a blessing for this lovely woman, too. The man wasn't aware of this, but the airline got the woman on another flight just three hours later, and also gave her a free round-trip ticket to any destination served by Alaska Airlines. So she was truly twice blessed.

Let Your Heart-Light Shine

Reaching out with a kind act or word of praise or appreciation can be so simple. Yet sometimes we assume that others "have it together" and don't need our kindness. Wouldn't it be better to move beyond our assumptions and to offer the kind of thoughtful-ness we would appreciate receiving—a compliment, a smile, a hug, a pat on the shoulder, a note of thanks or just a question that shows concern? If your kind gesture goes unnoticed or is refused, it doesn't matter, because in giving to another, you give to yourself.

Take smiling, for example. Everyone can do it. If you're not used to smiling, practice in the mirror by pulling up on the corners of your mouth! It's so simple, and yet so effective. Learn to smile sincerely, from your heart. Did you know that it takes more muscular effort to frown than it does to smile?

Smile at family and friends, at strangers, everyone you meet or pass during the day today. Do you realize how many lives you can touch simply by smiling? You smile at one person and he or she catches the good feeling and smiles at another person, and so on until your smile has indirectly affected the lives of several thousand people in one day.

A few years ago I had an illuminating experience as I was flying across country, coming home after a two-week lecture/TV tour. I was tired and needed to get some work done. I was hoping the seat next to me would be vacant, because I felt like being alone and not talking to anyone. No such luck. An elderly man sat down next to me and started talking a mile a minute. My inclination was to let him know I didn't feel like talking, yet my heart told me to simply listen and wait. With some resistance and initial resentment, I quietly listened and learned a wonderful lesson that day. Brief encounters can be fantastic. Regardless of whether a friendship lasts a few minutes or a lifetime, each relationship has value. I learned this man was a retired pilot and had flown everything from biplanes to supersonic stunt jets to ultralights. Because I love to fly, I delighted in five hours of stories and adventures. Although I never saw him again, I'll always be grateful for our brief exchange and for my lesson in openness.

Next time you meet a new person, be aware of your reactions. Are you being cool, standoffish, keeping the person at arm's length with small talk, wondering what they're after? Are you feeling a little uncomfortable, uncertain about where this new encounter is headed? If you are concerned about getting too involved, remember that your involvement need extend no further than this one meeting if you don't want it to. Take your cue from kids, who often can have a great time together even if they know they may never see each other again. They are not averse to gaining something for fear of losing it. Set out to find this new person's funnybone, or find some other way to put him or her at ease. When you show that you trust and respect someone, barriers immediately begin to drop. If you let your childlike trust take over, and you feel positive about being able to handle anything that comes along, your very attitude of certainty will see you through. Every chance you get, put a smile on your face as a gift you give yourself and others.

Or how about writing a note of thanks or appreciation? You don't need a special occasion to send a card or note to someone. You think you're too busy to send a card or note? It doesn't take much time. I love to write letters and am very faithful, as most of my close friends will attest. Sometimes I'll go to a card store and purchase several dozen cards to have on hand. Isn't it fun to receive a card from a friend for no reason at all? It may even be quicker than the telephone.

Last week a friend and I were having dinner at a local restaurant. It was early evening and the restaurant wasn't very busy, and my friend and I had the opportunity to visit with our waitress. We found out that she was in her early twenties, had two children, was a single mom, was putting herself through college and was working two jobs just to make ends meet. In spite of all her challenges, she was cheerful, enthusiastic and a joy to be around. When we got our bill, my friend and I decided to do something special. Even though the bill was under $30, we left a $100 tip. What a great feeling!

You can't speak or think negatively about another without that criticism becoming a part of your own reality. Your subconscious mind is simplistic and believes that what you're saying about someone else is what you believe about yourself. Similarly, being kind towards another really is being kind to yourself.

In Romans 12:21, Paul admonished, "Do not be overcome by evil, but overcome evil with good." This rang true for me not long ago when I visited a friend in the hospital. When I walked into her room, she began complaining that her nurse was forgetful, rude, short with her, and altogether not very pleasant.

When my friend left the room for therapy, this nurse came in to change the sheets. I could see and feel pain and anguish on his face and in his heart. I offered a few kind words about how much I appreciated his hard work and dedication. That opened the way for him to reveal the incredible hardship in his life. His wife still lived in South Africa, his two children had recently died from medical complications, and he was working a double shift just to make ends meet. Before he left the room, I gave him a big hug. He started to cry. Sometimes all it takes is a hug or a kind word and the emotional floodgates open. During the following couple of weeks, whenever I visited my friend, I took the nurse some of my homemade bread, which he loved and appreciated. Both my friend and I learned a valuable lesson during those two weeks about how important it is to reach out to others with kindness, even though you have no guarantees of what you'll get in return. Always let your heart-light shine in dealing with others.

Sometimes the kindest gestures may go unnoticed. I love to put coins in parking meters when I walk down the street if I find some that have expired. The drivers of the cars may never know, but it makes me feel good. Sometimes I send a note anonymously with a kind word or a few dollars when I know the recipient is in need. It takes so little to do so much.

Sometimes gestures are absolutely noticed. Not long ago when I was in Coos Bay, Oregon, my wonderful friend Helen Guppy accompanied me to a radio station where I was scheduled to do an interview from 11 p.m. to midnight. When the interview was over, the radio station closed and everyone left. Helen and I walked to my car only to discover that it wouldn't start. I lifted the hood to see if anything looked out of the ordinary. Helen reminded me that we were not in the best area of town, blocks from a telephone, and that it was cold and beginning to rain. I told Helen that we needed to imagine and affirm that an angel would help us out of this dilemma.

As we were getting back in the car to see if an angel would start the engine, a cab drove by. The driver stopped and asked if we needed any help. Helen whispered to me to have faith even though he didn't look like the angel she imagined. I agreed. He looked under the hood and instantly checked the battery. It was out of water. He happened to have some water in his cab and he filled the battery reservoirs. He also told us an interesting story. He had just dropped off a passenger several blocks away and was heading home since his shift was over. Something inside him guided him to take a totally different route home that evening, one he had never taken before. He thought it was odd but did it anyway. That's when he saw Helen and me looking under the hood and wondered if we need help. We told him that he was our imagined angel. He smiled. Then he followed us back to my home to make sure the car didn't stall, then said good-bye.

That's not the end of the story. The next day I found a book on angels "anonymously" left at my door, but Helen and I both know who left it. William Penn described well the act of kindness from the cab driver when he wrote, "If there is any kindness I can show, or any good thing I can do to any fellow being, let me do it now, and not deter or neglect it, as I shall not pass this way again."

Reach Out and Touch Someone

Each of us can make a difference in the world. By our intentions and through our attitudes, we can choose to see heaven or hell. Alan Cohen writes in his delightful book, *Joy Is My Compass,* that "the difference between a saint and a sourpuss is that the sourpuss sees his daily interactions as a nuisance, while the saint finds a continuous stream of opportunities to celebrate. One finds intruders, the other angels. At any given moment we have the power to choose what we will be and what we will see. Each of us has the capacity to find holiness or attack all about us." Make a difference in your world by giving deposits of love and kindness every chance you get. You never know how profound your gesture can be in someone else's life.

A few years ago a friend and I went to see a play in Los Angeles. After it was over, we decided to get something to eat at a coffee shop down the street. It was late and few people were in the restaurant. After awhile I noticed a ragged woman who obviously didn't feel good about herself. The waitress told us that this woman came in every Saturday evening at the same time. As I was talking with my friend, I couldn't help but notice the woman's appearance. In her mid-fifties, she had dirty clothes and matted, greasy hair, and carried a backpack as her purse. I could sense her sadness and loneliness. I was keenly aware of my desire to reach out to her, but I didn't really know what to do.

My friend had to leave, but I decided to stay. I went over to the woman's table, touched her hand, and asked her to keep me company while I finished my meal. At that point she started to cry, and I thought to myself, "Susan, you certainly misread your inner signals this time." As I sat down to try and mend the situation, this woman, Gloria, told me I was the first person to approach her with genuine warmth and caring in years!

Well, Gloria and I talked for an hour and she invited me to her apartment a couple blocks away. In her cramped and disheveled one-room apartment I listened through the night to her life story.

I found out that Gloria hadn't worked for months and that she had no family and rarely had visitors. As she spoke of her love for children, I remembered a telephone call I had received two weeks before. A friend who owns a day care center had called, asking me if I could recommend someone for an opening as a teacher's aide. I will never forget the sparkle in Gloria's eyes as I told her the details of this possible job.

Amazingly, it was now eight o'clock in the morning. I suggested she take a shower and then we could return to the coffee shop for breakfast. We also called the day care center owner. The position was still open, and I arranged for Gloria to have an interview later that day.

In the meantime, I helped Gloria curl her hair, showed her how to apply some makeup, and helped her to pick out a clean dress to wear for the interview. It was wonderful to see her transform before my eyes. As it turned out, Gloria got the job and began work the next week. After several weeks, I paid a surprise visit to Gloria at the center. I could hardly believe my eyes. She looked ten years younger and was aglow with enthusiasm. The children all loved her and so did the center's owner. She invited me to her apartment for dinner that evening. I didn't recognize her home either. She had cleaned and painted every inch and even had a couple of plants on her dresser. I was so touched. Gloria was radiantly alive and happy, as she was meant to be.

From this experience I truly learned the value of reaching out to someone even though you have no guarantee of the outcome. I believe that's what living is all about—person to person, heart to heart. Life is not a spectator sport. Participate in the adventure of life. You cannot induce permanent change in someone by doing for them what they can and should do for themselves, but you can be a catalyst for change. With love in your heart and a willingness to risk and be vulnerable, all will be right. As the great teacher Jesus said two thousand years ago, "Love thy neighbor as thyself."

This week go out and meet someone new. Introduce yourself to people, even if it feels funny at first. This will help shake off your inhibitions about talking to strangers. Trust new friends and yourself to make the best of the situation. Find out what it is you have in common. The more you do this, the more you'll discover, as I have, that what we have in common with each other far outweighs the differences, and further, that it's the differences that make friendships stimulating and exciting. "You will find as you look back upon your life," says Henry Drummond, "that the moments when you have really lived are the moments when you have done things in a spirit of love."

It takes a strong person to be gentle and kind. "Tenderness and kindness are not signs of weakness and despair," writes Kahlil Gibran, "but manifestations of strength and resolution." We always feel at peace with such a person, don't we? When we relax and get centered in the divine flow, we can feel God's gentle presence within us and express that gentle kindness toward ourselves and others.

Richard Bucke was a physician who studied the personality traits of those he felt had "cosmic consciousness." His book, *Cosmic Consciousness,* is one of classics of mystical experience. Of Walt Whitman, someone with a supremely well-developed mystic sense, Bucke wrote the following which, for me, shows Whitman's kindness and compassion and his ability to let his heart-light shine.

> When I first knew Walt Whitman I used to think that he watched himself, and did not allow his tongue to give expression to feelings of fretfulness, antipathy, complaint and remonstrance. . . . After long observation . . . I satisfied myself that such absence or unconsciousness was entirely real. . . . He never spoke deprecatingly of any nationality or class of men, or time in the world's history . . . or against any trades or occupations—not even against any animals, insects, plants or inanimate things, nor any of the laws of nature, or any of the results of those laws, such as illness, deformity or death. He never complained or grumbled either at the weather, pain, illness or anything else. He never in conversation . . . used language that could be thought indelicate. . . . He never spoke in anger. . . . Never exhibited fear, and I do not believe he ever felt it.

There have been many teachers in my life who have taught me about kindness and have shown me, by example, that angels walk among us. My mom, June B. Smith, is one such person. She lives her life doing kindnesses for others and has been my greatest inspiration. I'm always telling Mom that when I grow up, I want to be just like her.

Another angel is my dear friend Helen. Although her wings are invisible, they are quite obvious to me. Her greatest joy comes from helping others, whether she knows them or not. Her life is about blessing the lives of others and, in return, she is filled with joy and happiness. Along with my mother, Helen has taught me the true meaning of unconditional love and kindness.

The Health Benefits of Small Pleasures

As Jack Kornfield said, "Even the most exalted states and the most exceptional spiritual accomplishments are unimportant if we cannot be happy in the most basic and ordinary ways, if we cannot touch one another and the life we have been given with our hearts."

To be gentle and kind to others, we must first be gentle and kind with ourselves. There's no need to be hard on yourself, to beat yourself up when you make a mistake, choose incorrectly, or repeat the past. Be kind and understanding of yourself. Be especially kind to yourself if you behave in a way that you dislike. Always talk kindly to yourself, and be patient when you find it difficult to be a "holy" person. Forgive yourself, and then when you do not act as you want, use your actions as a reminder of where you are and where you are not. Be your own best friend.

A study has uncovered a surprising benefit to working small joys into your day-to-day schedule. It can help give your immune system a boost. Researchers in the Department of Psychiatry at State University of New York at Stony Brook asked 100 volunteers to fill out an evaluation of daily ups and downs; they compared this information with antibody activity in the participants' saliva, which indicates immune system fluctuations. Their finding: The stress of a negative event weakens the immune system on the day it occurs—

but a *positive event can strengthen the immune system for two days or more.*

"In other words, positive daily events help immune function more than upsetting events hurt it," says Arthur Stone, Ph.D., the psychologist who conducted the study. Among the everyday events that boosted subjects' immune systems: pursuing leisure activities (such as jogging) and spending time on a favorite hobby or special interest. Take time to be kind to yourself with life-affirming pleasures and activities.

The Health Benefits of Love and Kindness

Also, just as God forgives us, we must continually forgive ourselves. Forgiveness is an act of self-love, rather than some altruistic saintly behavior. In working with countless people over the years, I have come to the conclusion that an absence of forgiveness is tantamount to staying imprisoned in an unawakened life. Forgiveness is as important to learn and practice as are all of the other principles discussed in this book.

The more you extend kindness to yourself, the more it will become your automatic response toward others. Fill yourself with love even toward those who would do you harm—which is what all spiritual leaders of all times have said—and see if you still feel anger and revenge. One of my favorite Bible verses is "Love one another" (John 13:34), which is a crucial part of learning to forgive. True forgiveness begins with love. When we learn to love others as God loves us—unconditionally, and without thought for what has happened in the past—we will not have any trouble forgiving them. We will be led out of the darkness of doubt and confusion and into the light of understanding. We will release the painful experiences of the past and invite more positive ones into our lives.

Love and kindness are intimately related with health. This is not simply a sentimental exaggeration. One survey of 10,000 men with heart disease found a 50 percent reduction in frequency of chest pain (angina) in men who perceived their wives as supportive and loving.

Tender loving care is a valuable element in healing. In the insightful book, *Healing Words: The Power of Prayer and the Practice of Medicine,* by Dr. Larry Dossey, I read about a fascinating study by David McClelland, Ph.D., of Harvard Medical School. He demonstrated the power of love to make the body healthier through what he calls the "Mother Teresa effect." He showed a group of Harvard students a documentary of Mother Teresa ministering lovingly to the sick, and measured the levels of immunoglobulin A (IgA) in their saliva before and after seeing the film. IgA is an antibody active against viral infections such as colds. IgA levels rose significantly in the students, even in many of those who considered Mother Teresa "too religious" or a fake. In order to achieve this effect in another way, McClelland later asked his graduate students simply to think about two things: past moments when they felt deeply loved and cared for by someone else, and a time when they loved another person. In both cases there was an increase in IgA levels in the students.

The Health Benefits of Friendship

I don't need scientific documentation to know that my close friendships have a positive effect on my immune system. I highly value and feel a great sense of gratitude for the love and support I receive from my friends, and for the opportunity to care deeply for others. The only way to have a friend is to be one. Friends help sustain us when we're down, comfort us when we're sad, and offer counsel when we're confused. Friends are truly the best kind of wealth we can have—a wealth not calculated in numbers, but in the priceless value of a true friend. Show love and appreciation for your friends. Practice forgiveness and seeing your friends as beloved children of God. Never take your friends for granted. Friendship is as sacred a commitment as any other; our friends are sent by God, for us to help them and for them to help us.

Often in today's society we put our selfish interests first, before loyalty or integrity or commitment to higher values. Since what emanates from us will come back to us at some point, this is ultimately not a winning attitude. We must do what is right for the sake of doing what is right. To have a true friend you must be a true friend. "Some friends play at friendship but a true friend sticks closer than one's nearest kin." Proverbs 18:24. The love shared between two people is the most precious gift we have. I love what Sir Hugh Walpole said about this: "The most wonderful of all things in life, I believe, is the discovery of another human being with whom one's relationship has a glowing depth, beauty, and joy as the years increase. This inner progressiveness of love between two human beings is a most marvelous thing, it cannot be found by looking for it or by passionately wishing for it. It is a sort of divine accident."

I am reminded of a beautiful friend, Molly, who was all of 4'10" tall, but a giant of a woman. Well into her seventies when I met her, she knew how to celebrate life and the importance of being kind and loving to everyone. That was evident in her many friendships. The times we spent visiting together will always be special to me. A vibrant, alive, positive woman, Molly spent her days swimming, walking, doing yoga, or volunteering at the UCLA hospital.

About six months before she died, she found out she had cancer. The shocking news darkened her sunny disposition for the first three days. Then she adjusted to it and decided to make the most of her remaining days. She continued her routine, and seemed as radiantly alive and cheerful as ever.

The last month of her life she spent in the hospital. I was away on a lengthy tour, and when I returned I immediately visited Molly in the hospital. I wasn't prepared for what I saw. During my absence she had lost nearly half her body weight, all her teeth, most of her color but, astonishingly, not her cheerful attitude. Although she was physically unrecognizable, her spirit shone through when she said, "Sunny, I know I've looked better. Let's see if you can perform your magic and fix me up." I asked the nurse to leave Molly and me alone for awhile. I dropped the sidebars on her bed, and we celebrated being together. I brushed her hair, washed her face, and applied a drop of her favorite perfume. Although she could barely move, and she had a difficult time speaking, she still told me a couple of jokes. She also spoke with great appreciation about the flowers in her room and the birds singing to her from the tree outside her window.

She then asked me to lie down next to her, because she needed to talk and she didn't think she had much time left. That final hour she spoke to me about the light and colors she saw and about the peace and joy she felt. She was ready to go to the other side and was actually eager to make her transition. Just before she died she said to me, "Life is meant to be joyful. Don't ever get too serious about life. Laugh every day and live each day as though it were your last. Continue to find ways to give love to others like you have always done with me. Follow your heart and let the beauty of life into your spirit." And then she passed on.

Molly reminded me that we must embrace all of life and live every day as though we were born anew. Erich Fromm said, "Living is the process of continuous rebirth. The tragedy in the life of most of us is that we die before we are fully born." My experiences with Molly also make me think of something Elisabeth Kubler-Ross said in her book, *Death: The Final Stage of Growth.* "What is important is to realize that whether we understand fully who we are or what will happen when we die, it's our purpose to grow as human beings, to look within ourselves, to find and build upon that source of peace and understanding and strength that is our individual self. And then to reach out to others with love and acceptance and patient guidance in the hope of what we may become together."

This is what Molly did with me.

And then there was Isabelle. I met her when she was ninety-three, in the last year of her life. We were both at a photocopy store, where she was making copies of her latest poetry manuscript. I overheard her asking for a telephone to call a taxi to take her home. So I introduced myself and offered a ride. You can imagine my surprise when I found out she lived three doors away from me, having recently moved in. I'll always treasure the year I spent getting to know Isabelle. She showed me the insignificance of chronological age. Young in spirit, Isabelle loved to laugh, most especially at herself. She valued life's simple beauty—clouds, flowers, leaves, rain.

She loved to take a "blind trust walk" with me. Either in our homes, at the beach or at the park, we would walk arm in arm. One of us would have our eyes closed as we walked and explored together. When I was the blind partner she would lead me around for about fifteen minutes, introducing me to all kinds of sensory experiences—the sound of birds or waves, the smell of herbs, the touch of leaves or flowers. It's a fantastic way to practice living in the moment, to heighten awareness, and to learn about trust—letting go and embracing the unfamiliar.

A few weeks before her transition, we were visiting, drinking tea and sharing ideas on world peace. Unexpectedly, it started to rain and Isabelle decided we should take off our shoes and walk outside and celebrate the rain and wet grass. I wish you could have seen her. Ageless and shining, she frolicked barefoot on the freshly cut grass, laughing, singing, and catching raindrops in her mouth. Isabelle, my precious friend, knew how to let her child out to play.

Molly and Isabelle knew that real life was not all work and no play. In fact, they made their work their play. They retained a childlike innocence and curiosity about being alive. Although they knew how to be adult, they allowed their child within to be integrated into their days. Do you know people like this? If so, compare how you feel when you are around them with being around people who have not gotten in touch with their inner child. Mencius, an ancient Chinese philosopher, said, "The great man is he who does not lose his child's heart."

Sometimes the greatest act of kindness is simply to listen to your friend. During a television interview, the "hug doctor" Leo Buscaglia talked about children who have made a difference in someone's life. He told the story of a neighbor whose wife had just died. One of the neighborhood children paid the man a visit and was there for some time. When he returned home, the little boy's mother, believing her son had been bothering the man, asked, "What did you say to Mr. Johnson?" The little boy answered, "I didn't say anything. I just helped him cry." Children instinctively seem to know simply how to *be* with another person and not *do* anything. Take time to understand others' feelings. *The deepest hunger of the human heart is to feel understood.*

Through love and forgiveness, we can live from the heart and in the heart of God. My unshakable belief in the ever-present goodness and availability of God underlies everything in my life. I've come to know that, with God as my source of inspiration, I have a well that will never run dry. Each day is a fresh new possibility to be kind to ourselves and others. And when we live in the heart of God we can let our kindness shine in everything we think, feel, say, and do.

Showing Kindness Day to Day

Every day you have countless opportunities to practice kindness towards yourself and others. Here are some ideas to add to your list.

1. Go to your local shelter and adopt a pet.
2. Offer a ride to a friend who can't get around.
3. Volunteer time at your local library.
4. Pick up some trash as you walk down the sidewalk.
5. Ask your friends and co-workers to tell you their stories of random acts of kindness. In fact, have a party for telling such stories. Emphasis on the pleasure of giving with no strings attached inspires us to do more.
6. Give another person your parking spot.
7. Let another driver get in front of you if they want. Wave and smile at them too.
8. Surprise a forgotten friend or relative with a phone call.
9. Give a present to an underprivileged boy or girl, or to someone for no reason at all.
10. Take all of the clothes you haven't worn in a year to a homeless shelter. Organize neighbors on your block to do the same.
11. Wave hello to pedestrians, even if you don't know them, when you're in your car. It will lift their spirits as well as yours.
12. Let the person behind you in line at the grocery store or hardware store go in front of you.

13. Pay for the groceries of the person in front of you. If they are hesitant, just tell them it will make you feel terrific.

14. When you're in line for a movie, anonymously pay for the ticket of someone behind you in line. Then watch their face as they receive the news. I do this often because I receive such joy watching the expression on the person's face, and he or she has no clue that I'm the one who did it.

15. Order a mail-order gift anonymously for a friend or someone you know who needs to be cheered up.

16. Slip a $20 bill into the pocket or purse of a needy friend or stranger.

17. If you drive on a toll bridge, pay for the next few cars after yours.

18. Laugh out loud and smile often. Even when you're not in the mood to smile, do it. It will lift your spirits. Don't take your life so seriously. Play the game of life and show kindness.

19. If you know someone who's having a difficult day, do something special and wonderful for that friend without telling them you did it.

20. Tell your family and friends often how much you appreciate them and how blessed you are to have their presence in your life.

21. Tell your boss or employees the same things. Everyone wants and needs to feel appreciated.

22. Get your children to go through their toys and select some to give to those less fortunate. Let the children go with you to take the toys someplace they are needed and will be appreciated.

23. Plant a tree or flowers in your neighbor's yard where it's needed—with their permission, of course.

24. Take some beautiful plants to your local nursing home, fire station, hospital, police station, doctor's office or other place of business.

25. Make sandwiches, drive by a city park, and give them out to the homeless people.

26. Leave a flower anonymously on someone's windshield.

27. Look in the mirror every day and tell yourself how beautiful and wonderful you are.
28. Compliment others throughout the day.
29. If you see someone who appears stressed or unhappy, visualize them surrounded by light and love.
30. Be loving and kind to yourself every day, knowing you are a child of God and deserve to live a joy-filled wonderful life.

"If each of you reading this practiced just one random act of kindness a day, starting tomorrow, our world would be transformed."
—Barbara De Angelis, Ph.D.

At the end of most of my workshops we sing the following song by Jai Michael Josefs. The words express beautifully the importance of being kind and loving towards ourselves so that we can offer that love and kindness to others. To change the world, we must first change ourselves.

I Love Myself
The Way I Am

by Jai Michael Josefs

*I love myself the way I am.
there's nothing I need to change.
I'll always be the perfect me.
there's nothing to rearrange.
I'm beautiful and capable
of being the best me I can.
And I love myself just the way I am.*

*I love you just the way you are.
there's nothing you need to do.
When I feel the love inside myself,
It's easy to love you.
Behind your fears, your rage and tears,
I see your shining star.
And I love you just the way you are.*

*I love the world just the way it is,
'cause I can clearly see
That all the things I judge are done
by people just like me.
So 'til the birth of peace on earth
that only love can bring,
I'll help it grow by loving everything.*

*I love myself the way I am
and still I want to grow.
But change outside can only come
when deep inside I know.
I'm beautiful and capable
of being the best me I can.
And I love myself just the way I am.
I love myself just the way I am.*

NINETEEN

Meditation & Prayer
The Key to Transforming Your Life

T he purpose of spiritual work is not really to do things for God, but rather to do the most important thing of all for ourselves: to purify our own hearts. No work for God is more or less important than any other. The Bhagavad Gita states that He accepts even a flower or a leaf as an offering, if it is tendered with devotion. The important thing is to reach the point where all our love, all our energy flows naturally toward Him. —J. Donald Walters

Meditation is an ancient art going back to times long before historical records were kept. John Novak, in his practical book *How to Meditate*, reports that stone seals have been found in the Indus Valley of India dating back to at least 5,000 B.C. showing people seated in various yoga postures. For all these millenia, meditation has survived as a vital science of living.

Only during the past three decades has scientific study focused on the clinical effects of meditation on health. Meditation is so thoroughly effective in reducing stress and tension that, in 1984, the National Institutes of Health recommended meditation over prescription drugs as the first treatment for mild hypertension.

The first research on the physiology of meditation was conducted by Dr. R. Keith Wallace at UCLA. Studying Transcendental Meditation, Wallace found that during meditation the body gains a state of profound rest and the brain and mind become more alert, indicating a state of "restful alertness." Studies show that after meditation reactions are faster, creativity greater, and comprehension broader.

Health Benefits of Meditation

Dr. Herbert Benson, of the Mind-Body Institute at Harvard University, determined that meditation practice can bring about a healthy state of relaxation by causing a generalized reduction in multiple physiological and biochemical stress indicators, such as decreased heart rate, decreased respiration rate, decreased plasma cortisol (a stress hormone), decreased pulse rate, increased alpha (a brain wave associated with relaxation), and increased oxygen consumption.

Scientists are finding that meditation also helps keep us wrinkle-free and healthy. One study showed that people who had been meditating for more than five years were biologically 12 to 15 years younger than non-meditators. A comparison of hospital records of 2,000 meditators and 2,000 non-meditators revealed that the meditators required only half as much medical care. They have 87 percent less heart disease, 55 percent fewer tumors and 87 percent fewer nervous disorders.

The late Dr. Hans Selye, a pioneering Canadian stress researcher, described two type of stress—negative stress and positive stress. The difference between the two, he said, depends upon whether or not you feel in control of the stress. By becoming more aware of your reactions to stress, meditation can assist in providing an increased internal sense of control.

Another medical expert who advocates meditation is Dr. Dean Ornish, a well-known physician from Palo Alto, California and author of the groundbreaking book, *Dr. Dean Ornish's Program for Reversing Heart Disease*. This book has easy-to-follow instructions for a calming routine that includes meditation, yoga, and progressive relaxation.

Dr. Jon Kabat-Zinn at the University of Massachusetts Medical School, author of the marvelous book, *Wherever You Go There You Are*, founded the Stress Reduction Clinic in 1979 to help people suffering from chronic pain and chronic diseases such as cancer, heart disease and AIDS, as well as stress-related disorders such as abdominal pain, chronic diarrhea, and ulcers. According to Dr. Kabat-Zinn, these conditions are often the most difficult to treat, and the patients have frequently tried other, more conventional forms of medicine without complete success.

Dr. Kabat-Zinn designed a stress-reduction program to test the value of using mindfulness meditation to help patients develop effective coping strategies for stress, and to see whether meditation would have any effect on their chronic medical condition. As it turned out, the majority of people improved in a number of different ways.

Kabat-Zinn's stress-reduction program patients also make a commitment to practice on their own each day. Results:

- Virtually all patients, whatever their diagnoses, show dramatic reduction in physical symptoms over the eight-week period.
- Psychological problems—anxiety, depression, hostility—also drop over the eight weeks. Follow-up studies four years after completion of the course show that both physical and psychological improvements are consistent over time.
- Symptom reductions are greater than with other techniques, such as drug intervention, indicating that results don't come from a placebo effect. Somehow, the patient's inner resources for healing are being tapped.
- Patients' self-perceptions change. They view themselves as healthier and better able to handle stressful situations without suffering destructive effects. They feel more in control of their lives, view life as a challenge rather than a series of obstacles, and feel they are living more fully.

In general, Kabat-Zinn concludes that meditation is effective in:

- Decreasing pain.
- Reducing secretion of stress hormones, including adrenaline and noradrenaline.
- Decreasing the amount to excess stomach acid in people with gastrointestinal problems.
- Lowering blood pressure.
- Increasing relaxation.

Meditation and the Breath

Although meditation can take many forms, most techniques can be grouped into two basic approaches: concentrative meditation and mindfulness meditation. Both gradually train you to focus your attention and strengthen your concentration with the result of eventually quieting the mind.

Concentrative meditation focuses the attention on the breath, an image, or a sound (mantra), in order to still the mind and allow a greater awareness and clarity to emerge. To sit quietly and focus on your breath is the simplest form of concentrative meditation. This form of meditation can be compared to the zoom lens of a camera that narrows its focus to a selected field.

Concentration is the ability to tell yourself to pay attention to something and then do exactly that! Our minds tend to drift. We have continuous mental conversations. Most people talk to themselves nearly every minute of the day. Through meditation we control, limit and finally eliminate this internal chit-chat. An effective way to control and master your mind is through breath awareness.

The connection between the breath and one's state of mind is a basic principle of yoga and meditation. Think back to a time when you were frightened, agitated, distracted or anxious. Whether or not you noticed it, your breath was probably shallow, rapid and uneven. On the other hand, when the mind is calm, focused, and composed, the breath will tend to be slow, deep, and regular. It also works in reverse. By consciously taking slow, deep, and regular breaths, the mind will become calm. Focusing the mind on the continuous rhythm of inhalation and exhalation provides a natural object of meditation.

Breath control is the tool that allows you to alter your existing mental state. Inhale slowly and rhythmically through your nose, breathing quietly and deliberately. The incoming breath fills (in sequence): the abdomen, the ribcage and the upper chest. After you draw a full, comfortable breath, hold it for a count of one to three, then release it slowly at the same rate and rhythm as you drew it in. The exhalation procedure is the exact opposite of inhalation: First expel the air from your upper chest, next the ribcage and finally the abdomen. Allow the abdomen to power the breathing process. Try to breathe silently.

Breathe with concentration for a few minutes. Do it now. Settle into your posture and relax (don't slump). Sit on a bench, in a chair or cross-legged on a cushion, folded towels or pillow. (I sit on a quarter moon-shaped pillow.) The crossed-leg position (with elevated buttocks) is great for smooth breathing and proper posture. Place your hands in either of these two positions: The Zen mudra position is right hand palm up on lap, left hand on top of right hand, also palm up, the balls of the thumbs touching lightly. Another hand position is to place left hand on left thigh, right hand on right thigh, both palms up, gently touching your thumb to your index finger. By monitoring the breathing, maintaining proper posture and using one of the hand positions, you stay alert and focused. You are meditating. Notice as you do this that your mind becomes more tranquil and aware.

I use a meditation technique called *Kriya Yoga* which I learned in the inspiring Self-Realization Fellowship *Lessons* of Paramhansa Yogananda (see Resource Directory). This is a very effective way to increase our inner receptivity to God's guidance.

Mindfulness Meditation

The other type of meditation is *mindfulness meditation*. According to Dr. Joan Borysenko, "Mindfulness meditation involves opening the attention to become aware of the continuously passing parade of sensations and feelings, images, thoughts, sounds, smells, and so forth without becoming involved in thinking about them." The meditator sits quietly and simply witnesses whatever goes through the mind, not reacting or becoming emotionally involved with thoughts, memories, worries, or images. This helps the meditator gain a more calm, clear, and nonreactive state of mind. Mindfulness meditation can be likened to a wide-angle lens—a broad, sweeping awareness that takes in the entire field of perception.

Mindfulness is an ancient Buddhist practice which has profound relevance for today, says Kabat-Zinn in his book, *Wherever*

You Go There You Are. Mindfulness has nothing to do with becoming a Buddhist, he explains, but is a way of "waking up and living in harmony with oneself and with the world." Mindfulness is paying complete attention to whatever we're doing, allowing the "mind to be full" of the experience. The opposite of mindfulness is mindlessness, to do things without thinking, without much feeling, automatically and unconsciously like a robot. In mindfulness, we examine who we are, question our view of the world and our place in it, and cultivate some appreciation for the fullness of each moment we are alive. Most of all, it has to do with being in touch with yourself and your world.

We are often more asleep than awake to the unique beauty and possibilities of each present moment as it unfolds. We're usually absorbed in anticipating the future—planning strategies to ward off things we don't want to happen and to force outcomes that we do want—or in remembering who did what to whom and why. Most of us spend very little time aware of the present moment. Such mental manipulation leaves one enormously agitated.

While it is the tendency of our mind to go on automatic pilot, our mind also holds the deep innate capacity to help us awaken to our present, mindful moments and use them to advantage. Those moments are really the only moments we have to live, to grow, to feel, to love, to learn, to give shape to things and to heal. The essence of mindfulness is paying full attention. We come out of automatic pilot and observe more deeply. This allows us to feel more connected to what's going on around us and to develop a greater understanding of the order of things. Just as a garden requires attending if we hope to cultivate flowers and not weeds, mindfulness also requires regular cultivation. The beauty of it is that we carry this garden with us, wherever we go, wherever we are, whenever we remember. It is outside of time as well as in it. Kabat-Zinn calls mind cultivation *wakefulness meditation.* In his book he maps out a simple path for cultivating mindfulness.

The meditative disciplines, whether concentrative or mindfulness, reintroduce calmness and stability into our lives.

Where to Meditate

You don't have to travel to the Holy Land or the Himalayas to find sacred space. Dr. Ornish began reserving a space at home for his meditations when he was an undergraduate in college. "I was living in a one-bedroom apartment, and I didn't have a room I could use for that purpose," he says. "I didn't even have a corner of a room. But I had two closets. One I used for clothing; the other was for meditation," which he did sitting on the floor. He suggests dedicating some space exclusively to prayer or meditation. Doing so enhances your meditation, and makes your room and your home more sacred.

It's easy to dedicate a personal sacred space. For example, Ornish suggests, "you can put up a picture of a religious or holy person, or someone whose image evokes a sense of calmness or peace and love, or just set up a candle—whatever has the meaning for you of being sacred or inspiring."

"Sacred space and sacred time and something joyous to do is all we need. Almost anything then becomes a continuous and increasing joy."
—Joseph Campbell

A sacred place is where you find tranquillity, where you will relish moments of rich solitude. "In your sacred space, things are working in terms of your dynamic," explains Joseph Campbell, "and not anybody else's. Your sacred space is where you can find yourself again and again."

How to Begin

First, decide where you are going to meditate. For more than twenty years I have devoted a corner of my bedroom to my place of meditation. Create some type of altar with inspiring books, pictures or objects like statues, candles, or flowers. Keep it simple and clean. On my altar (which is really a wicker basket) I have placed a natural cloth covering and have some items which inspire me including pictures of Jesus and Paramhansa Yogananda, the Bible, a candle, and some fresh flowers. I usually sit on a pillow designed for meditation on the floor.

Carve out a regular time to meditate every day. Make it a top priority in your life. Firmly resolve that you will meditate on a regular schedule, suggests Roy E. Davis in his wonderful book, *A Master Guide to Meditation & Spiritual Growth.* "Consider your meditation session as your daily appointment with the Infinite," he says, "and keep that appointment without fail." I devote the early morning before sunrise to meditation and well as the early evening. This disciplined practice helps me to start and end the day on a positive, uplifting note. Whenever you choose to meditate, pick a quiet time of day, if you can. Ear plugs are sometimes helpful.

If you aren't comfortable sitting on the floor, find a chair where you can sit with your spine straight—posture is important. Avoid sitting with your back supported by the chair's back. Maybe tilt the chair forward slightly so the seat is at least parallel to the ground. Sitting with your back and neck straight will make the energy flow more easily through your spine. Find a fairly comfortable position to sit in. Lying down is not recommended because it encourages falling asleep.

As in physical activity, it is better to start small and develop a regular practice than to sit in meditation for hours a day, then give up in frustration. I recommend starting with ten to 15 minutes once a day. In the beginning it is most important to establish a regular time for meditation and to stick with it. Later you may want to sit more frequently or for greater lengths of time.

Regardless of the technique you use, you'll find the mind wanders and the body experiences unusual sensations. Most traditions suggest you should avoid *trying* to stop thinking or being distracted. Rather, when you realize you are distracted, gently bring your mind back to the object of concentration. In fact, each time the mind wanders and is brought back, your ability to concentrate has been strengthened. In other words, your mind is being trained to respond to you rather than you responding to the whims of the mind.

Let's say that you have chosen to focus on your breath as you slowly and deeply inhale and exhale. As soon as you're aware that you're not focusing on your breath, gently but strongly refocus on it. Eventually, by this process of focusing and refocusing on one point, your internal noise is lessened, your head is quieter, and your energy higher.

Deeper levels of meditation begin after the initial noise and distracting thoughts have been cleared away. Usually, periods of quiet—when it's easy to focus—alternate with periods of random thinking. As you continue to meditate, times of easier focus, greater clarity and inner quiet lengthen. These times of quiet joyfulness are the first goal of meditation. There is no limit to the depth, energy, and peacefulness that can be achieved in meditation.

Meditation should be continued until a quiet mental state is reached. Don't stop when it's difficult to concentrate, in the midst of a lot of thoughts. Stop when you are quiet. These periods of noise and quiet will alternate as your meditation breaks through layers of thought and tension. Stop whenever a more stable place is reached. You don't have to reach samadhi to have a great meditation.

Start your meditations with your energy as high as possible. It's nice to have showered first. Feel awake. The higher your energy is, the more awake and alert you feel, the easier it will be to focus and meditate. It's also best to meditate on an empty stomach or at least before eating a heavy meal.

Don't be too rigid in your practice. On occasion, find other special places to meditate. For example, I often become immersed in meditation in nature—at the beach, in the mountains, out in the desert, in the local park, etc. I enjoy the sounds of nature when I meditate outdoors. Being out in nature helps you to see things more clearly and become one with your surroundings.

Nature Meditation

Joseph Cornell's wonderful book, *Listening to Nature*, is a treasure trove of beautiful photographs, quotes and writings on how to deepen your relationship with nature. I keep it on my coffee table for all to see. In it I learned about a nature meditation he refers to as "Stillness Meditation." Here's the technique, which I usually do while out in nature. It helps to quiet restless thoughts and sometimes brings wonderful calmness.

First, relax the body. Do this by inhaling and tensing all over: feet, legs, back, arms, neck, face—as much as you possibly can. Then throw the breath out and relax completely. Repeat this several times.

To practice the technique itself: Observe the natural flow of your breath. Do not control the breath in any way! Simply follow it with your attention. Each time you inhale, think *Still*. Each time you exhale, think *Ness*. Repeating *Still . . . Ness* with each complete breath helps focus the mind and prevents your attention from wandering from the present moment.

During the pauses between inhalation and exhalation: stay in the present moment, calmly observing whatever is in front of you. If thoughts of the past or future disturb your mind, just calmly, patiently bring your attention back to what is before you, and to repeating "Still . . . Ness" with your breathing.

Stillness meditation, explains Cornell, "will help you to become absorbed in natural settings for longer and longer periods. Use it when you want to feel this calmness, indoors or outdoors, with eyes open or closed."

White Light Meditation

The following meditation is one that can be done anywhere and is easy for beginners as well as advanced students of meditation.

1. Sit in a straight backed chair with spine erect and feet flat on the floor. (You can also sit cross-legged.) Fold your hands together in your lap, or hold them in prayer position. Eyes may be opened or closed.

2. Feel yourself relaxing as you take several long, slow deep breaths. Imagine a beautiful white light completely surrounding you. This is your protection as you open sensitive energy centers. In fact you can do this with any of your meditations.

3. For about ten minutes, gently concentrate on a single idea, picture or word. Select something that is meaningful, uplift-

312 • MAIN INGREDIENTS

ing and spiritual to you. You could even focus on some peaceful music (refer to Chapter 12 on "Music: Medicine for Mind, Body & Soul").

4. If your mind wanders from your object of focus, gently bring it back to your awareness.

5. After ten minutes, separate your hands and turn them palms up in your lap. Close your eyes if opened.

6. Relax your hold on the object of concentration and shift your mind into neutral. Remain passive, yet alert, for ten more minutes. Gently observe any thoughts and images as they may float by. Just be still, detached and be with whatever you are experiencing.

7. Open your eyes after ten minutes, close your palms and again imagine that you are surrounded completely by a white light. This is your continued protection as you go about your daily activities with peace and joyfulness.

This 20-minute meditation recharges your energy field and nourishes creativity and tranquillity. At other times during the day, allow a sense of light and love to flow from within your being, and let it fill your entire body. It's very easy to do, and puts you into a meditative state.

How Meditation Improves Athletic Ability

One of the most difficult things to do in sports is to stay totally focused on the task at hand. Through meditation you develop a method and the ability to do just that. Meditation for athletes systematically harnesses untapped mental powers. If you apply it correctly, you can improve your athletic abilities by gaining access to "the zone," that legendary mental state in which an athlete—strictly through the powers of the mind—can exceed his or her capabilities. Keen, laserlike concentration is a trait common to great athletes. Inner dialogue is detrimental to concentration. You cannot concentrate on doing something and simultaneously hold an unrelated conversation with yourself. The optimal athletic mind-set is clear and alert.

In the world of martial arts, meditation has a 1,000-year-old track record as a performance aid. T'ai chi ch'uan, karate, kendo, aikido and judo are just a few of the martial arts that use meditation before practice and competition. Martial artists meditate because they perform better as a result.

The first step in accessing the zone is to put your inner voice to work so it won't wander. Do this by having your inner voice count breaths. Use your breath technique, and upon the complete exhalation of each breath, count it. Go from one through ten, then repeat it over and over. Simultaneously watch your posture and pay attention to your hand mudra, or hand position. Apply total concentration, paying strict attention to the process.

This mental imaging, when run again and again, establishes a positive psychological base for the upcoming athletic event. Scientific testing has verified that athletes can actually improve their technical skills through this detailed mental rehearsing. Additionally, sports psychiatrists and psychologists have determined that intense visualization reduces stress and virtually eliminates the psychological trauma associated with serious competition.

Spiritual Blessings from Meditation

The longer an individual practices meditation, the greater the likelihood that his or her goals and efforts will shift toward personal and spiritual growth. As I travel around the country giving talks and meeting people, it delights me to learn how many people are taking responsibility for their health and lives and are embracing a wholistic program including meditation. It's not uncommon for me to hear something like this: "I began meditating to decrease my stress and to feel a sense of control in my life. But as my practice deepens, not only do I feel more relaxed, I also am developing a more open heart—more sensitivity, greater compassion, and less negative judgment toward others."

Many individuals who initially learn meditation for its self-regulatory aspects find that as their practice deepens they are drawn more and more into the realm of the "spiritual." Meditation is all about breaking through the everyday world of tension and thoughts to create greater inner peace, calm, insight, and enlightenment. It will change your life because it changes you. Find the method or methods which suit you best.

The goal is to truly integrate spirituality into every area of our lives. It takes discipline, courage and a warrior's strength. It's not for the faint of heart or the weak minded. Writes Jack Kornfield: "To open deeply, as genuine spiritual life requires, we need tremendous courage and strength, a kind of warrior spirit. But the place for this warrior strength is in the heart. We need energy, commitment, and courage not to run from our life nor to cover it over with any philosophy—material or spiritual. We need a warrior's heart that lets us face our lives directly, our pains and limitations, our joys and possibilities. This courage allows us to include every aspect of life in our spiritual practice: our bodies, our families, our society, politics, the earth's ecology, art, education. Only then can spirituality be truly integrated into our lives."

In her work with many cancer and AIDS patients, Dr. Borysenko has observed that many people are most interested in meditation as a way of becoming more attuned to the spiritual dimension of life. She reports that many die "healed," in a state of compassionate self-awareness and self-acceptance.

Quiet your mind in meditation to experience the perfect rhythm of the universe. When you go within and allow yourself the freedom to be at peace without judgment, simply meditating and experiencing the oneness of it all, you soon start to find that energy which is blissful and enlightening. That quiet mind state, if practiced enough, will convince you of the oneness and perfection of it all.

We are all one in spirit with God and with each other. Although we may look different on the outside, we are still one with God, one with each other, and share the same innate spirituality. It's easy to forget this truth in today's tumultuous world. When we watch the news or read the newspaper, it's easy to forget that we're all children of God. By meditating and following God's guidance, we naturally live together in peace and harmony. If we are faced with or are witnessing intolerance from others, meditation can give the strength to bless the situation and acknowledge that there is a divine power in charge. Although others may seem worlds apart from us, the peace gained in meditation reminds us that we all look at the same sky, bask in the glow of the same sun, and are blessed by the same all-knowing, innate power that is God. Meditation helps keep our heart connected to God and our eyes focused on our vision. Obstacles are what you see when you take your eyes off the vision and separate yourself from God.

Ralph Waldo Emerson said, "Nothing can bring you peace but yourself." Meditation helps you to find the self.

The Divine Surrender

During my meditation period, I often incorporate prayer, visualization and affirmations. Most often, my prayer involves surrender to the Divine. A prayer of surrender can be one of the most powerful and blessed aspects of meditation.

What is it that we surrender? Our negative feelings, negative thoughts, fears, resentments, addictions and resistance. Resistance to change is nothing more than hardening of the attitudes. Most people are addicted to stress-producing stimuli. We become needy, neurotic people when we look to the world for what the world cannot give us. When we have lost our peace, we look for it everywhere. In fact, we seek desperately. Until we remember that our own capacity to love and be connected to God is what we truly seek, we are doomed to endless compulsion to look for happiness where there is none and for satisfaction where there is only more longing. Life's difficult situations force us to be more conscious of our dependence on God and the need to deepen our connection with Him—to perfect our faith and trust and love.

By surrender I mean to trust in the forces and principles that are always at work in the universe. With surrender, an inner knowingness and contentment overtakes us. With surrender we trust the perfection and beauty of it all, and at the same time know the paradox that all of the suffering that seems to go on all over our planet is a part of that perfection, as is our own strong desire to help end it.

The best way to surrender is to make a personal commitment to forgive every single person that we have ever had any conflict with.

The inevitable result of surrender is to draw closer to God. When we surrender to the Divine our compulsive negative thoughts, fears, addictions and resistance—our lives—will be transformed. Through regular meditation I've come to realize that no part of our lives is unimportant to God. Whatever our need—whether it deals with health, finances, or human relations—nothing is beyond God's presence and power. There is nothing we cannot turn over to God.

To surrender all to God—letting go and letting God—brings out the gifts of love and peace that are within us. Strength and understanding may not come all at once, but as we prove our desire is real, as we are willing to follow and trust, God shows the way. In everything, trust God. That's true surrender.

A prayer of surrender might be, "Lord, no matter what I'm going through, I love You. I am your child; You are with me always." In that prayer of perfect surrender, we feel our life to be in God's divine embrace, and know that everything is well.

Take time to become quiet, to listen within, and to place all in the hands of the One who created and loves you. God knows what is best for you and sees the good that you may not see. God will help you and show you the way. Be open to the lessons you need to learn. Life is a persistent teacher. It keeps repeating lessons until we learn them. Trust that everything that's happening can be for your highest good. As you keep remembering, "I trust God in everything," give thanks for the special relationship you have with the One presence and power.

I find that surrender brings with it the emotion of gratitude. Gratitude, an overflowing feeling of thanksgiving, is the instant response of the soul touched by the awareness of the Divine. With even a momentary awakening to God's presence, such joyous freedom bathes our consciousness—a blessed release from all the tensions and fears and anxieties that weigh us down in this world—that in wordless praise our whole being pours forth a ceaseless "Thank you! Thank you! Thank you!"

The Power of Affirmation

Too often we fail to see God's beauty and goodness right around us. We can overcome this careless forgetfulness by training the mind through repetition of a simple thought-affirmation: "Lord, Thou art in me: I am in Thee."

I usually repeat spiritual affirmations like this one loudly at first, then softly, then in a whisper. I repeat them mentally, again and again, until they become automatic. At that point it has reached my subconscious mind, which will keep it going on its own. And if I keep affirming with even deeper concentration, it reaches the superconscious mind—"the magic storehouse of miraculous powers," as Yogananda said.

Affirmations can—and should—be used for spiritual success. One very simple affirmation I repeat often is: *"I am a child of God."* When we repeat that to ourselves often enough and with deep enough concentration, it reaches the superconscious mind and we realize, through direct experience: "I *am* a child of God!" Then everything in our lives is transformed—our attitudes, our abilities, the way we go about our daily lives.

Let the mind dwell on these positive affirmations when it is not otherwise occupied. With continuous repetition, feel the truth of what you are affirming. By repetition, the reality of His sustaining presence becomes ingrained in our consciousness. A profound certainty grows within us that in every way we are being provided for. Gratitude and joyous praise then flow naturally. Begin now to celebrate this inner thanksgiving, whether you're meditating or not.

I sometimes end my meditations with what I call a "Meditation Prayer." I also say these before I fall asleep, so that the positive, uplifting thoughts can be carried into my subconscious and superconscious mind during the night. Write some of your own and keep them with you to read whenever you have extra time. I keep different ones in my purse, briefcase and car. These can be recited out loud or silently, but make sure you say them with feeling. Here are two of my favorites.

Positive Meditation Prayer

Every day, each and every moment is a new opportunity to begin again, to celebrate the gift of life. There is no past or future. There is only now, a blessed moment filled with unlimited opportunities for good. I live every moment to the fullest by releasing memories that are no longer useful, by letting go of things that can limit me, and by opening my mind and heart to experiences that will uplift me and encourage me to stretch and grow. The past has no power to control me. With God, I can live fully and freely in each moment of my life.

Every thought of not being valuable, of being afraid, of uncertainty and doubt is now cast out of my mind. My memory goes back to God alone, in whom I live, move, and have my being. A complete sense of happiness, peace, certainty and love floods me with light. I have confidence in myself because I have confidence in God. I am sure of myself because I am sure of God.

The Spirit of Love within me knows the answer to any problem which confronts me. I know that the answer is here and now. It is within my own mind because God is right where I am. I now turn from the problem to the Spirit, accepting the answer. In calm confidence, in perfect trust, in abiding faith, and with complete peace I let go of the problem and receive the answer.

I know exactly what to do in every situation. Every idea necessary to successful living is brought to my attention. The doorway to ever increasing opportunities for self-expression is open before me. I am continuously meeting new and larger experiences. Every day brings some greater good. I prosper in everything I do. There is no deferment, no delay, no obstruction or obstacle, nothing to impede the progress of right action, of Divine order in every area of my life, now.

I identify myself with abundance. I surrender all fear and doubt. I let go of all uncertainty. I know there is no confusion, no lack of confidence. I know that what is mine will claim me, know me, rush to me. The Presence of God, of Love, is with me. The Mind of God is my mind. The thoughts of God are my thoughts.

Today I bestow the essence of love upon everything. Everyone I meet shall be loving to me. My soul meets the Soul of the Universe in everyone. This love is a healing power touching everything into wholeness. I am one with the rhythm of life. There is nothing to be afraid of. There is nothing to be uncertain about. God is over all, in all and through all. God is right where I am. I am at peace with the world in which I live. I am at home with the divine Spirit in which I am immersed. I am in love with God and with life itself.

Spirit of Love within me, thank you for this precious gift of life. Today, and always, I choose to honor and serve you by loving myself and everyone else unconditionally and by acknowledging your Presence in everything I think, feel, say and do.

AMEN

Peace Meditation Prayer

Love is here. God is here. Truth is here. Peace, the wonderful peace of God, is right here where I am.

In this beautiful moment of eternity, I turn my attention within. I feel the peace of God that is in me always; the peace that transcends all fear, all concern, all sense of anxiety; the peace that is everlasting. I am a center of perfect peace. Let there be peace on earth and let it begin with me.

Dear Lord, let me be an instrument of peace in my world. Open me to the realization that peace in the world begins with peaceful hearts. I open my heart, my mind and all that I am to Your peace. In this moment, nothing can disturb the calm peace of my soul.

Every atom, cell, tissue and fiber of my being is filled to overflowing with the peace of God. I allow that peace of God within me to come forth and bless my family, my loved ones, my friends and my co-workers. I see and experience the peace of God in my neighborhood, my community, my city, my state and my country. I use my God-given power of visioning to see and to feel the peace of God flooding the hearts and souls of all the citizens of this country.

I affirm and I speak with power the word of peace. Peace is made manifest in my world. The peace of God moves through the hearts and minds of all people everywhere in all countries: all world leaders and world citizens. I take this moment, now, to bring that vision closer to reality. I recommit myself to my own inner peace and to peace in the world in a moment of silence.

Let peace radiate in me, O God. Let Your light of peace within me shine forth so brightly that all darkness and doubt are dispelled. For this power, this realization of peace in my heart and in my world, I am eternally grateful. I give thanks for this precious gift of life.
AMEN

Practicing the Presence

Just imagine your days filled with nothing less than peace, contentment, and happiness. These things are natural when you are constantly aware of and give thinks for God's love and presence in your life. Our only problem is that we're disconnected from the power of our soul.

To see God's presence everywhere, we must see through all forms of illusion or *maya* (an Eastern term for the illusion of the material world). We must ask God to help us see more clearly by seeing with God's eyes. Ask God to open your heart, quiet your mind, and experience a richer, happier, transformed life. God is your source of instant, constant peace.

I don't quite understand why we feel more peaceful when we turn our attention to God, but that doesn't matter. I don't know all about electricity, but I can still flip a switch and get light. I know from experience that when I tap into the peace of God within, I get tranquillity. When I face the challenge of giving a lecture, making a presentation, writing an article or book, or when anything seems to be testing me, I remind myself to flip that switch. We can all learn to be peace-filled people, for no matter what is going on around us, God is there.

Make meditation and prayer a top priority in your life. In time, and with disciplined practice, your life will become a moving meditation and prayer devoted to God. Meditation and prayer are the medium of miracles. When you meditate and pray, you can't *not* change. By living a meditative, prayerful life, the joy you receive from sharing with God can be continuous.

Some of the prayers I say to God each day include:

• God, may my mind be filled with thoughts of You.

- Make me an instrument of peace and harmlessness, through the grace of God.
- God, give me a new heart to see everyone in my life as an innocent child of God.
- I am the peace of God.
- God, guide my thoughts, feelings, words, and actions to reflect your love and light.
- God, show me how I can best serve You today.

Be willing to live a God-surrendered life and to love more. It's in the willingness that lives are changed. The more you can love everything and everyone, and possess an attitude of gratitude, the healthier and happier you will be. If you are all wrapped up in yourself, you are overdressed!

The Gift

I'd like to share one of my favorite stories which appeared over a decade ago in Integral Yoga Magazine. It's written by Krishna Carmen and beautifully encourages us to turn within and accept the ever-present gift of God's Light of Love.

Once upon a time, long ago, God decided to give a special gift to the human beings, for they were very dear to Him. He decided to make a dwelling place in each human heart where He would live forever. In this special place God's children would know Him as He truly is and be one with Him. Here they would be happy and filled with peace. It was surely the most precious gift ever given.

But God thought, "What is a gift without some beautiful wrapping?" So He veiled His wonderful gift with a most enchanting and attractive covering called Maya. Just a glimpse of this paper was enough to make the human race aware of their freedom of choice, aware of their individual uniqueness, aware of their senses so that they could touch and be touched by the world around them. This wrapping was laced with clear mountain streams, beautiful green valleys, life-long friendships and wonderful romances. It bore the fragrance of exotic fruits, deep secret forests and delicate flowers. It was so magnificent that it almost had the appearance of life itself. Truly, any wrapping less beautiful wouldn't have done justice to God's precious gift.

So, with great joy, He carefully folded and secured the paper of Maya around each gift and gave one to each of His children. Needless to say, they were all very pleased with the gifts—they cherished and loved them. To receive a gift is wonderful, but to receive one from God is more than that—it is divine!

But . . . the story doesn't end here. You see, the human race was so excited to get such beautifully wrapped presents, that they didn't think to look inside. In fact, they didn't know there was anything except the enchanting wrapping. For a long time they just sat and gazed at it.

God smiled and waited. But everyone still sat looking at their presents and feeling the paper. A few people would lift their heads for a few seconds to thank God and then quickly look down at them again. Most of them were so engrossed that they didn't even realize anyone else was around—nor did they care!

God gave those who thanked Him a little nudge. "Please look inside," He said. "There's much more." But they didn't understand what He was saying. "Look inside? Inside of what?"

God chuckled, "Here, let me show you," and He very gently tore at a few people's presents. When they saw the rips they were broken-hearted. They cried and wailed. In between sobs and sniffles they said things to God like, "You Meany! You ruined my whole life," and "You're supposed to be kind and loving! Why did You rip my gift?"

The sound of the wailing was almost deafening. And it all seemed sort of silly to God. Here they were crying over the wrapping paper. How could they expect to find the true gift without removing the wrapping? Still, God felt great compassion; they were so young and inexperienced. He knew the crying would stop when they discovered their true gifts. But how long would that take?

After awhile, God noticed a small child who wasn't crying like everyone else. "You don't seem so upset; why not?"

"Well," she answered, "I don't understand why You ripped my package, but I figure You gave it to me, so You must know what You're doing."

God smiled, "I'll show you the real gift." He picked up her package and gently tore it open. It was painful for the child to see her beautiful wrapping fall to the floor, but when she looked up, a smile came to her face, and her eyes filled with a warm golden glow. Tears of joy rolled down her cheeks as she tried to thank God for the inner gifts.

And upon looking down at herself she saw she had been transformed from a young child into a radiant woman—a mature being who shone with the pure light of love. Her light was so bright that it made a few humans look up from their Maya-covered gifts. When they saw her, they knew something miraculous had taken place. Some couldn't understand how she could possibly be happy without the wrapping paper. Others called out, "Mother, come teach us what you know!"

She looked at them and smiled. "You call me Mother, but I am no different from you. I have merely uncovered the gift we all have." A small group gathered around her. "How can we also find this gift? Must we travel far?"

"No," she replied. "You don't need to go a step. Just don't be afraid when troubles beset you and your life seems to be coming apart. This is only the outer layer falling away—don't cling or try to wrap the tattered remains around you. Instead, give yourself over to God so He may hasten the unwrapping of your gift. For once the paper is gone, you will see that God is your very own."

On that day She helped many souls realize their precious inner gift and they in turn helped others. And the Ones who have uncovered God's gift still remain with us, eager and willing to help us search our way through the Maya paper for that place where we are all joined with God.

*"The Bible says, 'Be still, and know that I am God.' This is yoga. 'Be still' means to withdraw one's consciousness from the little ego and the body, from all desires and habits that pull the mind down. . . . We have to throw off identification with the body in order to recognize that it is God who sustains us, whose energy pours through our bodies, whose intelligence works through our consciousness. That is what meditation is—forgetting our mortal consciousness and remembering that we are immortal souls. In soul consciousness is the strength and the ability to accomplish anything in life that we want." —Sri **Daya Mata***

TWENTY

Self-Mastery
The Power to Be Your Best

W*e become experts at preparing to live, but have a difficult time fully enjoying the process of being alive, right now.*
—**Barbara De Angelis, Ph.D.**

"No man is free who is not master of himself." —**Epictetus**

Just for a moment, close your eyes, breathe slowly and deeply a few times, and imagine yourself as a master of the universe. As a master you have the ability to create anything you want, even something that has never existed before. Be outrageous in your thinking and envision what you most want now.

You have this power within you—it is the birthright and potentiality of every human being. The only real limitation to all possibility is your thought, belief and imagination. Once you have a clear vision of what you want, focusing on the result and not just the means, then the natural play of universal forces lead you to the accomplishment of that goal. Og Mandino says, "Use wisely your power of choice." How true that is! And it was Henry Ford who encouraged us to believe in ourselves when he wrote, "Whether you think you can or not, you are right."

When you compromise your dreams and values and instead live a life that's expected of you rather than what your heart asks of you, you give your power away. It takes courage to embrace the unfamiliar and allow miracles to occur. It takes boldness to go after our dreams even though we're navigating uncharted territory. Don't give up. "It takes a lot of courage to release the familiar and seemingly secure, to embrace the new," says my friend, author and motivational speaker Alan Cohen. "But there is no real security in what is no longer meaningful. There is more security in the adventurous and exciting, for in movement there is life, and in change there is power."

You and only you have the ability to create miracles in your mind and life. The choice is always with you. It has nothing to do with luck, and everything to do with believing in yourself as a part of the divine force that suffuses everything in the universe. The great rule of thumb is this: if you can conceive it in your mind, then it can be brought into the physical world.

Living in such a fast-paced world, as most of us do, constantly conspires against inner peace. The intense pace and stress of our daily lives can very easily put our peace, happiness and health, not to mention our spiritual lives, at risk. It's easy to get caught up in the whirl of today's hectic lifestyle—especially if we've forgotten the truth of our potential. This leaves us less time for self-fulfillment. Deteriorating standards and values lead to low self-esteem and rob many of us of our dignity.

If we feel an inner emptiness, we may be tempted by the quick fix, the easy solution, since life is hard and learning to live fully takes more time. But the fact is that we *can* slow things down; we *can* face our own challenges, however large or small, with aplomb and equanimity, on terms that are our own, our heart's guidance. We *can* choose to experience aliveness and become masters of our lives.

In the 1960s, Abraham Maslow wrote his famous *Toward a Psychology of Being,* which helped turn around the emphasis of psychology. Psychology was my undergraduate major at UCLA, and I was drawn to Maslow's work. He chose to study high-functioning people—those living their highest potential—rather than people with problems as was usually the case in psychology. Maslow developed a "psychology of being," not of striving but arriving; not of trying to get someplace, but living fully. He found a common denominator among all his high-functioning subjects.

They all had a vision, were committed to it, were self-motivated and believed they had the power to master life. Do you believe you have the power to master life?

If It's to Be, It's Up to Me

Self-mastery begins by taking inventory of your life. According to Socrates, "The unexamined life is not worth living." Mastery involves taking responsibility for our lives and what we've created rather than blaming other people and circumstances for our lot in life. Blame is a convenient excuse for why our life is not exactly what we would like it to be. Mastery also involves being self-disciplined, being courageous, moving through fear and recognizing our inherent divine power—using it to bring our vision to life.

Why do so many of us only get motivated through fear and loss? Why do we put off living the way we want to live, as if we have all the time in the world? Consider this statement by Raymond B. Fosdick: "The only life worth living is the adventurous life. Of such a life, the dominant characteristic is that it is unafraid. It is unafraid of what other people think . . . . It does not adapt either its pace or its objectives to the pace and objectives of its neighbors. It thinks its own thoughts, reads its own books, it develops its own hopes, and it is governed by its own conscience. The herd may graze where it pleases or stampede where it pleases, but he who lives the adventurous life will remain unafraid when he finds himself alone."

Millions of masters in the making like you are awakening to the concepts of self-responsibility and choice. Its proof is in the success of teachers such as Dr. Deepak Chopra, Marianne Williamson, Dr. Barbara DeAngelis, Dr. Wayne Dyer, Dr. Larry Dossey, Dr. Bernie Siegel, Norman Vincent Peale, Sir John Marks Templeton, John Bradshaw, Tony Robbins and others who help people bring spirituality and wholeness into everyday life. Once introduced to these empowering ideas, people are giving up being victims in favor of being masters. Self-mastery is true heroism in action.

When you have the tendency to blame another person or circumstances for how you feel or for what you are experiencing, stop, check yourself and remember: *What you feel is up to you.* Your feelings are governed by your mind. You can't think one thing and feel something else. Feelings and experiences always correspond to thoughts. The habit of blaming others or circumstances has to stop if you are to become master of your life and live your highest potential. The circumstances and conditions are only tests.

Instead of whining "why?" and pointing the finger of blame, masters say: "This is the situation. I take responsibility for it. I realize I created this emotional 'stuff.' I know I have the power to make new choices about how I view any event and my reactions to it. I am powerful enough to uncreate this situation and re-create something healthy and joyful. I now choose to see everything through the eyes of love."

Love empowers you to higher levels. Nothing will make life better than the consistent experience of love. Let others know that you love them. Tell them and show them, often. Don't wait until it's too late, for you don't know if they will still be here tomorrow. My spiritual teacher, Paramhansa Yogananda, used to say that if we want to live our highest potential, all we have to do is teach the mind how to think differently—how to be gentle, calm, loving and centered on God. Seeing through the eyes of love is the same as seeing through the eyes of God. When you know that you are a spiritual being in a physical body, and you live from that awareness moment-to-moment, your life will be transformed. It's simply an internal shift—an 18-inch journey from your mind to your heart. You will find yourself more certain, fulfilled, successful, content and peaceful than ever before. You will be living in a state of grace.

Anyone who goes about his or her own life with a sense of serenity, contentment, and grace has no need to manipulate others. A well-adjusted person who's master of his or her life doesn't try to control others or circumstances. It is rare for a person who is reasonably satisfied with his or her life to try to run someone else's. Such a person continues to grow through a living process of discovery and renewal.

As paradoxical as it sounds, this is the mind-set for self-mastery: to surrender, trust, turn away from habits of accumulation, outer achievement and quick fixes, and to allow yourself to be purposeful through inward guidance.

"You can never solve a problem on the same level as the problem," claims author Emmet Fox. The more you live from inner guidance—that peaceful, loving center within you—the more you'll find that everything you need to meet your wants and desires will be provided. The essence is knowing that you are already complete, already whole, and that nothing external to yourself in the physical world can make you any more complete.

Your Reality Reflects Your Thoughts & Intentions

You create your thoughts, your thoughts create your intentions, and your intentions create your reality. Intention is *directional energy*. Intentional living, with understanding and skill, is one of the most useful ways to achieve happiness, health and wholeness and to banish obstacles to spiritual growth. When life is lived with conscious intention, insights unfold more easily and life is lived more gracefully. What you see around you, whom you associate with, how you function daily, what your relationships are like, how much money you make, how you get along with others, the shape of your physical body, and virtually everything about you, is the result of your intention.

It is usually fairly easy to be happy and peaceful and to feel somewhat saintlike when removed from social circumstances and relationships; but to always be happy, peaceful and soul-centered, regardless of personal and environmental conditions, is evidence of real spiritual growth. Your personal and environmental condition tends to adjust toward harmony as you become more soul-centered.

Your values and higher spiritual Self reflect your intentions. If you view the world as a giving place, you are probably optimistic about other people being kind and considerate and you see goodness in others and in all situations. You experience much gratitude and are teaching others to be loving. You usually find yourself surrounded by others with similar values.

In your relationship with others, what really matters is the heart-to-heart or love connection. At the level of the heart, we are all connected by love. Your educational background, age, skin color, shape, size, occupation, where you live—none of that matters. That's just your gift wrapping, a special covering, unique to each of us. The essence of who you are is spirit. Spirit makes us all equally special and precious.

Our main job while here on earth is to take our focus and attention off judging others, criticizing, blaming, finding fault, and instead find ways to serve others, share the peace and joy of our hearts and let others know we appreciate them. When we continually find fault and criticize another, he or she withers up like a flower without water. Show love, respect and appreciation to another and they will blossom. Isn't that what we all want—simply to be loved and appreciated? Give this a try: for a day or two, treat others as if the fullness of God resided within them. Imagine that their physical-world attributes are nonexistent.

Being a master of my life means that I put God first before everything. In other words, I choose to live in the presence of God (or love) and allow God's thoughts to direct my thoughts, intentions, words, and actions. This requires that I live my highest and best at all times and in all circumstances. I know the loving presence will give me the strength and courage to follow through on my commitments. Being centered on God also means that I give up any dependency on people, circumstances and material things as my source of happiness and fulfillment. Rather, I'm putting God first in my life, trusting that my life's higher purpose is being revealed to me. Knowing my connection to God, I choose to put my faith in God and in my inner guidance, or intuition.

Success Is an Inside Job

For years, I've done research on what makes people successful. In the process, I came across Daniel Isenberg, a business professor at Harvard Business School. He's a very popular teacher there. He said that for years, his former students would come back to him and say, "We really like your courses, but now that we're out in the real world, what they teach us in the Harvard Business School doesn't make much sense."

This bothered Isenberg because he wanted to teach his students something useful. So he got the names of the 25 most successful executives in the country, and got permission to follow each of them around for a week to try to find out what it was they did that made them successful. Isenberg followed each one for a week, listened to their phone conversations, listened to them talk to their friends and family—and came to the conclusion that what made these people successful had nothing to do with what they teach at the Business School. He discovered two important characteristics shared by all the successful people he observed.

One thing these successful achievers had in common was *a commitment to putting their values first.* There come times in our lives where our goals are in conflict with our values: a time when we want to do something in business, with children, with friends, in a relationship, but we know it's a little unethical or a little judgmental, so we're in conflict between what we want to do at the moment and what we feel or know is right. What these most successful people had in common is loyalty to their values. Without commitment to your values, either you don't achieve your goals, or if you do, they're not really worth achieving after all.

The second thing these highly successful achievers had in common was *an incredible faith in their intuition.* They all exhibited spiritual sensibility. Some of them were churchgoers, some were not, but they all had a sense of a deeper intelligence in the universe that operated through them. They all made their decisions based on their intuitive feelings about what was going on with their businesses or professional lives. How in tune are you with your intuition—God's whisperings?

The Role of the Body in Self-Mastery

Because we live, move and have our being in God, being centered on God also means appreciating and respecting our magnificent bodies. Your body is the temple of the living, loving Spirit and therefore deserves reverence. Treat yourself with dignity. Don't wait until you're sick to appreciate the miracle of your body. Honor the love inside you and the love you are. If you want to become healthier and be the best you can be, begin with how you feel about yourself and, at the same time, recognize your body as God's temple. Heaven on earth is inside each one of us at this moment. "In this life," says Meister Eckhart, "we are to become heaven so that God might find a home here."

We are all composed of a body, mind and spirit and already have everything we need to be the best we can be, to become masters of our lives simply because we are divine beings. So it starts with taking loving care of yourself. Cherish and respect your body temple unconditionally—no matter what its current shape.

Advertisers spend millions of dollars each year suggesting that our shapes and sizes are not right, giving us what seem like impossible examples of what we are supposed to look like. These ads try to make us feel guilty about our bodies. The unspoken implication is that we are not "okay," that we are not pretty enough, slim enough, sexy enough or athletic enough, and that by getting upset at our condition we will then do something positive. The opposite is the case.

I believe that we need to learn to be a friend to our bodies. Every body needs tender, loving care. Getting mad at our bodies only makes matters worse. Although our bodies are but temporary homes for our spiritual being, we must still take care of them because they are sacred vehicles for this earth journey. So love your body and be committed to being fit for your life journey.

Start today by tuning in more to your body. It is a fantastic feedback machine. If you listen, you will discover that it actually talks to you. When you get a headache, for instance, your body is trying to tell you something. Listen to your body's signals. The key is your willingness to listen and act. If you feel a pain, what is your body trying to tell you? It may be telling you that you're eating too much, or eating the wrong kinds of food, or smoking or drinking too much, or not sleeping enough, or not drinking enough water or getting enough exercise. It could be telling you that there's too much emotional congestion in your life.

Typically, instead of listening to the body, we get the messages all twisted and run for something to make the message go away. Many people think the way to handle a headache is to reach for the bottle of aspirin and that it's normal to have a headache. Collectively, this country has been making some poor choices. Just look at all the commercials on TV and advertisements in magazines. We're told that here's what we can do for a headache, fatigue, constipation, irregularity, those sleepless nights, indigestion, or underarm odor. My gosh, take a shower! Why don't they just tell us that? We've come to depend on things outside of ourselves for a quick fix. We've become a self-medicating society because we don't really understand how beautifully robust the human body truly is and how efficiently and effectively equipped we are to meet our problems.

It's normal to be healthy. It's our divine birthright to be well. We just have to get out of our own way. Listen to your body. Respect and appreciate it. Take loving care of it. Choose your doctor carefully—one who practices a wellness lifestyle and who listens to you. There is a tendency today for doctors to turn to technology and all kinds of elaborate testing first before listening to you or their own intuition. I don't think that's a good trend. Ask both of these questions: what the doctor can do for me? And, how can I help myself?

Love, a Main Ingredient to Be Master of Your Health

One of the best things you can do is to love yourself unconditionally. Have you remembered to love yourself today? To love and honor your own inner Self, and to treat yourself with respect and dignity, is the simplest way to experience peace and the joy of living.

Love yourself. Remind yourself to do that all day. Put notes up on the refrigerator and mirrors around your home if you need the reminder. Erich Fromm said, "Our highest calling in life is precisely to take loving care of ourselves." When you change your attitude about yourself from negative to positive, everything else in your life will change for the better.

One of the extraordinary secrets of this world is that life flows outward. It originates inside and is projected outward where it is perceived as the external world. We are not affected by other people or by situations and circumstances in the way we normally think we are. We are affected only by what happens inside us. We are affected by our own feelings, our own thoughts. Nothing outside us has the power to affect us.

Most people denigrate and belittle themselves all the time. In this way you create your own problems. If you think that somebody else hurts you or somebody else makes you happy or feel good or bad about yourself, then that is delusion. Nobody else is responsible for your pain or pleasure. Nobody else is responsible for your sorrow or joy. Eleanor Roosevelt would have probably agreed. She said, "No one can make you feel inferior without your consent."

If you don't know your own Self, then you are lost, confused, everything goes wrong and you have a gnawing sense of failure. When we feel disconnected from our source, we look for the quick fixes. To numb ourselves or to feel temporarily satisfied, we take drugs, stimulants (like caffeinated beverages), overeat or eat junk foods, drink alcohol, work incessantly, and watch too much television.

When you get in touch with your innermost Self and you come in contact with that infinite invisible intelligence that is always a part of you and your daily life, then you know what you should think, do and say. Embrace your feelings—all of them. Defrost the ice around your heart so you can heal your emotional wounds. Don't be afraid of the darkness for it is the harbinger of light. "The dark night of the soul," says Joseph Campbell, "comes just before revelation. When everything is lost, and all seems darkness, then comes the new life and all that is needed." Turn everything in your life over to the divinity within you. That divine Self, that light and love within you, exists within everybody, but is being wasted by those who don't take the time to turn within.

Make it a personal policy never to put yourself down. Never debase yourself or think negatively about yourself. Tune in to the inner guidance that is with you 24 hours a day. We need to become more dependent on God. The reason we are dependent on external things is that we do not have the knowledge of our own Higher Self, the power within us. And to have this knowledge, you have to practice.

Divinity, Another Main Ingredient

Start the day with remembrance of God. Live the day in relationship with God. End the day absorbed in awareness of the presence of God. This is not a naive, simplistic approach to living life well. It is, when natural and sustained, the culmination of spiritual practice.

The end result of spiritual endeavor is God-consciousness. Why not nurture God-consciousness all of the time until it is permanently realized? The alternative is to remain self-centered, with God imagined to be other than around, within, and as us— thus removed from awareness of God only because of our unwillingness or inability to acknowledge the truth of what God is.

A most useful way to begin each day is with prayer and meditation. This not only affirms our understanding that our most important relationship is with the Infinite, it establishes us in the ideal relationship with God—that of knowing that God is our higher True Self and we are in this world to learn to let God's will be done through us.

Make meditation a top priority in your life. The process of meditation is nothing more than quietly going within and discovering that higher component of yourself. Meditation allows you to empty yourself of the endless activity of your mind, and to attain a calmness. Regular meditation is a natural process to attain peace of mind, strengthen the body's immune system, slow biologic aging processes, awaken regenerative energies, enliven the nervous system, and nurture enhanced creative abilities. Meditation will enable you to be more peaceful, soul-centered and God-conscious. With progressive spiritual growth, your understanding of your relationship with the Infinite will improve. You will be more insightful: more intellectually and intuitively capable of discerning the difference between truth and untruth. Ultimately, when you adopt meditation as a way of life, you'll be able to go to that peaceful place anytime and bring that peace and joy to all circumstances in your life.

You need not change your religious affiliation in order to practice meditation. You won't have to become a monk or resign from your daily life. You won't have to give up your job or travel to India. You can bring practical spirituality into your daily life simply by meditating regularly, loving yourself, living from inner guidance and honoring the divinity within you.

Listen to the genius of Franz Kafka: "You do not need to leave your room. Remain sitting at your table and listen. Do not even listen, simply wait. Do not even wait, be quiet, still and solitary. The world will freely offer itself to you to be unmasked, it has no choice, it will roll in ecstasy at your feet."

A daily spiritual practice routine is most helpful. But how we live every waking moment is the proof of its value. It is in the arena of everyday circumstances and relationships that we are provided ample opportunity to the depth and clarity of our understanding. If you are not living well—that is, freely and productively—you are not growing spiritually. How you experience life is in direct relationship to your inner condition: to your psychological health, maturity, your understanding of your purpose for living, and your willingness to do what it takes to live your life successfully.

Therefore, avoid becoming addicted to your spiritual practice routines or indulging yourself in inner work to the exclusion of meaningful activities and relationships. Balance your regular sessions of meditation, inner reflection and prayer with worthwhile involvements in your outer life. In this way you fulfill yourself and your purpose in life.

It doesn't matter what your level of health or spirituality is right now. Regardless of how unspiritual, unhealthy a lifestyle you've chosen, you can, at any moment, choose differently. You can use your past mistakes or poor choices and learn from them. For some people, it takes being at the bottom before they awaken to the fact that they can choose something else. This is exactly what happened to a friend of mine whom I'll refer to as Melissa.

Melissa Transforms Her Life

About two years ago I was giving a talk in Los Angeles on "The Power to Be Your Best." I shared my thoughts about our power and ability to become masters of our lives and create health, success, peace and happiness beyond our highest visions when we surrender our lives to God. I said that surrendering is an act of the heart and is the equivalent of putting inspiration into your life. When you are inspired, you feel purposeful. When you trust in the invisible intelligence of the universe, you feel empowered and guided. This process is natural, not something that requires mastery of an esoteric curriculum. It can happen in a moment and it often occurs just that quickly. In Zen, this process is called *satori*, which translates roughly to "instant awakening."

After my presentation was over and most people had left, I went into the ladies' room and noticed a woman crying. I remembered her because she sat in the front row and cried through much of my talk. Since I had no plans for dinner, I asked Melissa to join me. Surprised, she gratefully accepted.

This is what I learned. Melissa's husband recently left her for a woman half Melissa's age. Her two children had been taken away and given to a relative to care for until Melissa got her life together. She was almost 100 pounds overweight, had no job, was depressed, afraid, and considering suicide. That morning when she felt like giving up and was at her lowest, she took a walk and, as providence would have it, saw a flier for my talk that afternoon in the window of a health food store. Something inside her told her she must attend—even though she had never gone to a health or motivational talk before. She arrived about 30 minutes early and I watched her as I set up. I went over and introduced myself and told her I was grateful she took the time to come and hear my presentation. I could sense her sadness and gave her a hug. That was the initial contact until I met her in the ladies' room after the talk.

Melissa believed in the ideas I discussed but didn't know how to implement them in her life. Everything seemed to be going downhill for her and she didn't know how to climb out. She wanted more than anything to turn her life around—find a job, get her children back, lose weight and get in shape as she used to be just a couple of years before.

I told Melissa that if she was willing to make a commitment with every fiber of her being and was willing to do whatever it took to live her highest vision, then I'd be happy to work with her and guide her. She was delighted. For most of that evening, I had her share with me her highest vision and write down answers to questions. If she couldn't fail and if she were living her best self right now, what would that look like? I also gave her all my books and tapes and told her to peruse everything over the next week. Finally, I wrote out a walking program I wanted her to start the very next morning.

Over the following week, I became her daily health and fitness trainer. We went over a new nutrition program and cleaned out her refrigerator and cupboards of all junk and unhealthy foods. I took her to a few natural food stores and showed her how to shop for health. I trained her at the gym with aerobics, weight training and stretching. I also taught her how to meditate and visualize her goals and dreams. She was an inspiration to me—dedicated and committed. Within three weeks, she found a part-time job which eventually led to full-time employment at a florist shop. Melissa missed working in her garden; since her husband had left she was living in a studio apartment. Within four months she had saved enough money to move into a new apartment and, happily, she got her children back.

Today, Melissa is down to her ideal weight, works out, frequents health food stores regularly, is managing the florist shop, is engaged to be married and is feeling empowered and divinely guided. Last month, her ex-husband even wanted to get back together with her—which she knew wouldn't be for her highest good. Melissa has learned, firsthand, that breakthroughs and miracles occur when she is willing to live her vision and commitment, with her life surrendered to God.

The Power of Commitment

There is power in commitment. When you're committed, you allow nothing to deter you from reaching your goal. If you're committed, you are disciplined even when you are not feeling motivated. Discipline is the ability to carry out a resolution long after the mood has left. There were times when Melissa didn't feel like exercising but she exercised anyway. Sure, there were some slips when she indulged in unhealthy foods from the "avoid" list such as cheese, ice cream, meat, processed foods and creamy sauces. But instead of beating herself up with guilt and anger for doing something "bad," she came to see that these were choices from which she could learn and, perhaps, make better ones the next time. She admitted that splurges on unhealthy food made her feel very enervated the following few days and she quickly came to realize that the momentary taste pleasure wasn't worth hours and days of feeling sluggish and fatigued.

When you make a commitment you are willing to put all of your resources on the line and take responsibility for the outcome. Commitment—to a project, a relationship, a health and fitness program—lends stability to the chaotic whirl of everyday life. Daily acts that reaffirm your commitment will increase your feelings of empowerment and self-esteem. The better Melissa felt about herself, the more easily and effortlessly she would make choices that were for her highest good, like going to the gym earlier than usual some mornings because of a busy schedule, or like choosing to eat more fresh raw fruits and vegetables even when she felt like eating something unhealthy.

It's through everyday behavior that we learn what really counts. Commitment must be woven through all of life: our thoughts, our emotions, our words, and our actions. Often I hear people say they are committed to being healthy, yet they continually let excuses get in the way. They say they'll have to wait "until next Monday or the day after" to exercise because they're "just too busy now," even though they've made a commitment to exercise each day. Or they won't be able to eat nutritious meals for the next two weeks because of birthdays, anniversaries, travels, or because they are "just too stressed out" to make a major change right now.

Commitment means that you get past your excuses and follow through on what you said you were going to do. Make your word count. How do you ever expect someone to make a commitment to you, or how will they ever expect you to follow through on a commitment to them, unless you first show a commitment to yourself?

If you are committed, you will immediately arrange your personal circumstances so that your lifestyle totally supports your commitment. You will do whatever it takes, whatever you need to do to put your life in order, let go of excess baggage and superfluous non-essentials, and consciously focus on what is important.

Lack of commitment is near epidemic proportions in our society. Just look around. People say they're committed to creating a healthier, more harmonious planet; yet they continue to litter, don't recycle or drive cars that pollute. They say they're committed to their relationships, yet they lie, are unfaithful, are unwilling to be vulnerable, or walk out at the first sign of difficulty or challenge. People say they're committed to aligning with the spiritual side of their natures, but they make no time for meditation, solitude, or communion with God.

Many people wish they felt more committed, wish they had something really big to commit to. These people don't realize that *you can't be committed to anything if you aren't first committed to yourself.* By really committing to yourself, by following through on your convictions and decisions and allowing nothing to stand in the way of your becoming master of your life, you will gain tremendous power.

Turning Adversity to Advantage

In my life and the lives of most people I know, the most growth, the greatest lessons and the most rewarding transformations occur from the greatest adversities and challenges, just as Melissa found out. Life has a way of making certain past misfortunes—if we have worked through them—pay extra dividends in the future. On the other hand, if we haven't worked through or learned from them, they have a way of reappearing in worse form. Have you noticed the same negative things or patterns recurring in your life, and only the people change?

Blaming, complaining and taking no action will keep you in a rut. You must have the vision to see beyond the appearances of your life. You must choose to look at your life from a higher perspective. Practice seeing all life around you as an aspect of yourself. In this way, you shatter the illusion of separation and with it, the need to blame and complain.

In quiet and solitude, ask this question: *What is it I need to learn to finish this business so I can move on in my life?* You can choose to turn adversity into opportunity. This transformation begins with taking responsibility for everything you've created in your life. To take responsibility is to accept the consequences of your choices, both good and bad. When you are responsible, you don't transfer blame to other people or circumstances. You must be willing to own everything that happens.

When I began taking responsibility for everything I was or wasn't creating in my life, I was scared. If my life wasn't working, I could blame nobody but myself, and yet, at the same time, I realized that taking responsibility can be very empowering and freeing. This is what living is all about—mastering our lives by becoming all that we were created to be. Spinoza put it this way: "To be who we truly are and to become all that we are truly capable of becoming is the only end in life." Henry David Thoreau recognized that most people don't choose to live fully when he said that "most men lead lives of quiet desperation."

Avoid making routine matters and everyday relationships complicated. Your life, well lived, is your gift to yourself and your thoughtful service to others. Unfailingly and enthusiastically welcome each day with joy and thankfulness because of the limitless opportunities it provides to learn, grow, flourish, and be truly happy and fulfilled. If this approach to each new day has not been your habitual response to life, make it first in order of priorities from now on. And practice the presence of God.

Our challenge is to trust and love ourselves as much as we are loved by God. We live in a friendly universe that is always saying "yes" to us. Our responsibility is to identify and transform those beliefs that have been sabotaging us from accepting and receiving that goodness. When you remove the blockages to God's presence and align with the love that you are, then abundance, prosperity, peace, health, success and happiness will be yours.

There is synchronicity all around us orchestrating our lives even though we might not be able to see it, but it works best when you trust God, believe in yourself, and have faith that nothing is impossible. In *Love Is Letting Go of Fear*, Gerald Jampolsky writes that coincidence is when God decides to do something but prefers to stay anonymous. And in *You'll See It When You Believe It*, Wayne Dyer says: "We have been taught not to believe something until we see it with our own eyes. Since we cannot see synchronicity or experience it directly with our own senses, we become skeptical of it. Our Western culture teaches that all of the mysterious connections are really only random happenstance, and it is easier to believe in these coincidences than in something which eludes our senses."

My Marathon Mystery

The following is a true story. I ran my first marathon in Culver City (Los Angeles area) the first week of December, 1975. I had devoted a year to training. When race day arrived, my emotions were mixed. On the one hand, I was eager and excited to run, although not quite sure what to expect since I had never done this before. On the other hand, I was feeling sad. The day of the race was the one-year anniversary of my grandmother Fritzie's death. Fritzie had been instrumental in teaching me about my own spirituality, about self-reliance, simplicity and living fully. As I was driving to Culver City the morning of the race, I felt a tremendous longing to visit with her. I missed her so much. In the car, I was actually talking with her out loud as a way to soothe the ache in my heart. I even said to her that I was open to her spirit and energy. I asked her to let me know somehow if she could hear me. I asked her to help me through the marathon.

When I arrived at the race site, there were lots of people getting ready. I was wishing I knew someone so I wouldn't have to run alone. The gun went off and so did a few thousand runners. For the first three miles I was alone and felt great—confident, relaxed and energetic. Around the fourth mile, a man who looked to be in his mid-twenties ran up next to me and we began talking. Before we knew it, we were at mile ten, then fifteen, then twenty. It's amazing the things you'll tell someone you've never met before when you're running together. I think it has something to do with the release of certain chemicals in the body and a change in the electrical activity of the brain during aerobic exercise. We talked about our lives, families, interests, dreams and goals. I was feeling extremely grateful to him because our conversation made the miles sail by.

Before we knew it, we were at mile 25. At this point in our conversation, we started talking about where we lived. I told him I live in Brentwood and he told me he lived in Studio City. "That's interesting," I said. "My grandmother used to live in Studio City. What street do you live on?" When we told me the street, I gasped, for it was the same street as Fritzie's. At this point, we were close to the finish line. I had just enough time to inquire about his exact location. We were crossing the finish line when he told me had moved into an apartment eleven months earlier, that the lady who lived there before him had passed away. I could hardly breathe, not because I was tired but because of what he was telling me. He had moved into Fritzie's apartment.

Out of all the thousands of people in the race, I ended up running with the person who lived in my grandmother's apartment, only a few hours after I had asked Fritzie to give me some sign that she was receiving my communication. Coincidence you say? I don't think so. Only believe. Have faith. Trust your inner guidance.

The key to mastery and living fully lies in turning within and asking God to take charge of every aspect of life. Look deep within to get in touch with the truth of your being and the unlimited possibility that awaits you. (See especially Chapters 17 and 19 on Solitude and Meditation.) To assist in the process, you may also want to ponder and answer these thoughts and questions, as I had Melissa do at the start of her commitment program.

Personal Commitment Statement

Answer the following:

• What would my life be like if I were now living my highest vision?
• I commit to do the following in support of my vision:
• These are the ways I will now rearrange my lifestyle to totally support my commitments:
• The non-useful behaviors I will discontinue are:
• The new constructive behaviors I will implement are:
• Since I am a spiritual being living in a physical body, I will now nurture my spiritual self by:

Write out the following Personal Commitment Statement at the bottom of your answers and read it out loud (preferably) with feeling, sign your name and date it. Reread it often. This is your personal commitment. From time to time, as you achieve your goals and live your vision at higher levels, you will want to re-write and refine your Personal Commitment Statement.

I am passionately, unshakably devoted to my vision of how I want my life to be. I am committed to making my vision a reality for I know I have the power and ability to live my vision. Everything unlike my vision is dissipating, easily and effortlessly. With God as my ever-present help, I agree and affirm that I will do my best to help myself to total wellness and spiritual growth, and share my increasing radiance with my world. What I sincerely desire for myself, I also see and allow for others. Thank you for this precious gift of life. Today, as always, I honor and serve God by loving myself and everyone else unconditionally and by acknowledging God's presence in everything I think, feel, say and do.

You Are Not Separate

You can make a profound difference in other people's lives by how you choose to live yours. I'm reminded of the story of a young boy walking down the beach picking up starfish and throwing them back into the sea. A man observed this and finally caught up with the youth. He asked him, "What are you doing this for?"

The boy answered that the stranded starfish would die if left in the morning sun.

"But the beach goes on for miles and there are millions of starfish," countered the man. "How can your effort make any difference?"

The boy looked at the starfish in his hand, threw it to the safety of the waves, and replied, "It made a difference to that one!"

It makes a difference for those around you when you are loving, peaceful, happy, and healthy. It makes a difference every place you go when you are master of your life. You make a difference.

Our bodies are made up of billions of cells. In order to maintain optimum health, each of these cells must operate at peak performance. When we have sick or weak cells, the healthy or stronger ones must work harder so that our body as a whole will be healthy.

Our planet is like a body, and we are all its individual cells—we are all cells in the body of humanity. Ultimately, we are not separate from others. There is no room for negative thinking, unforgiveness, bitterness towards others, or selfishness. It is your responsibility to this body that we call our planet to be a healthy, happy, peaceful, loving cell that radiates only goodness, positiveness, and joy. In this way, you can help make the world harmonious.

The separation and division that has so long colored our thoughts and beliefs regarding our lives on this planet must now be examined and corrected. To create peace on earth, we must stop dividing the world, the nations, the races, the religions, the sexes, the ages, the families, and the resources, and know that it's time to come together and live in harmony, forgiveness and love. Awareness of our oneness must precede our thoughts and actions as a part of our belief system. We are all connected to this living, breathing planet. It's our choice. We can choose to make a difference with the way we live our lives.

In his insightful book, *The Hundredth Monkey*, Ken Keyes, Jr., tells of a phenomenon observed by scientists. The eating habits of macaque monkeys were studied on several islands. One monkey discovered that sweet potatoes tasted better when washed before eating them. That monkey taught her mother and friends until one day a certain number (say 99) of the monkeys knew to wash their sweet potatoes. The next day, when the hundredth monkey learned how to wash sweet potatoes, an amazing thing happened: the rest of the colony miraculously knew how to wash their potatoes too! Not only that, but the monkeys on other islands started washing their potatoes also.

Keyes applies this "hundredth monkey" phenomenon to humanity. When more of us individually choose to make a difference with our lives—when human beings realize we each make a difference and start acting like it, more and more of us will learn this truth until we reach the "millionth person" and peace and harmony spread across the globe.

Where it starts is right here where we are. I believe that we can't change the world, but we can choose to know and change ourselves and, as we do that, the world will be different. But it takes all of us together, committing to being healthy, happy, powerful, peaceful, and pure in heart. We must choose to do the things that make a difference—that support wellness, that serve humanity, and that serve all creation.

We're here on earth not to see through one another, but to see one another through. We are here to experience the fullness of life. To be fulfilled, to be happy and peaceful, to be joyful, healthy, successful and fully alive is our destiny. We are here to become the best we can be. We owe it to ourselves. When we change ourselves, we'll change the world. Says Eric Butterworth, "It is not so much ours to set the world right, rather it is ours to see it rightly."

We are, indeed, powerful human beings, a concept which is often associated with authority and influence over others—rather than an understanding of ourselves. Self-knowledge and self-mastery are a lifelong quest, a process of learning and growing and following our hearts. We must do what we believe in our hearts instead of what we are told to do or are expected to do. Kierkegaard, the philosopher, expressed the idea as the title of one of his books: *Purity of Heart Is to Will One Thing*. The exercise of will toward purity of heart is self-mastery.

"The seventy or eighty years of life that we experience is but a wink of eternity; and relatively speaking, everything happens to us just as fast

as it happens to the bacteria: with every wink of God, a hundred years pass away. So do not waste your time. Do not be controlled by desires. Do not allow yourself to do anything that your conscience does not want you to do. Be master of yourself. If you know within that you are master—of your thoughts, feelings, and actions—nothing else matters. Every minute is a potential link between you and God, so you should not waste your time here on earth, but learn now to be master of yourself."

—*Paramhansa Yogananda*

TWENTY-ONE

Questions & Answers

T*he goal is for you to be truly healthy and happy in every dimension of your being, and to be free from any kind of compulsion. —John Robbins*

Through the years I've been asked countless questions at lectures and workshops, television and radio interviews, or when consulting and counseling. I've noticed that there are several questions that, although worded a little differently each time, come up most often. You may have similar questions, or find these further reflections on attaining health and happiness helpful. My answers will be more than a summary of the book's content. They'll go a little deeper for those who are seriously looking to change their lives.

Q: Susan, you are a proponent of slowing down to smell the flowers. Yet it appears that you live an extremely busy, high-pressure life. How do you keep yourself balanced?

A: Although I am busy, I still keep a peaceful mind in everything I'm doing. I truly believe that we have a choice, and I make certain choices. What I do every morning is to arise before dawn to begin my day with meditation. That sets a tone of peace, joy and enthusiasm for the day. I have learned that my quiet times in the silence with God can be the most revealing and inspiring times of my life. Realizing that God is not remote but an integral part of me, I understand the need to be quiet and listen within. Worries fade away and insignificant matters take their rightful place. A gentle whisper or a certain knowing reveals the truth to me. Silence and meditation are the best way I know to stay balanced. At the very heart of the silence, I realize the presence of God. Wrapped in the safe, protective mantle of God's presence, I feel rested, refreshed, and renewed. God alone is sufficient, for in Him lies all love, all life, all happiness, all joy, all peace—everything that even in your wildest dreams you could not imagine. Cultivate a relationship with Him.

Practice the presence of God every day, and never go to bed at night until you have practiced meditation and are filled with that joy. When you feel that eternal peace and balance within, then whoever comes to you shall feel your peace, be uplifted by it, and feel more balanced themselves. Within your being, you carry all the conditions of happiness by meditating and attuning your consciousness to the ever-present joy which is God. Don't allow your happiness to be subject to any outside influence. Whatever your environment is, refuse to allow your inner peace to be touched by it. That's how you stay balanced.

Then, of course, I also exercise regularly and practice sound nutrition, both of which help keep me in balance. Another choice is how much or how little I attempt to accomplish. You don't have to go faster just because everybody else is. When we push beyond our natural rhythm we grow insensitive to our body's needs and the needs of those around us.

Q: Do you believe in coincidence?

A: It's been said that God orchestrates a coincidence but chooses to remain anonymous. Throughout our lives, coincidences lead us toward the attainment of our life's purpose. By increasing our awareness and remaining connected to our Source, we see that coincidences are happening all around us when we ask the right questions. The answers are easy; it's the questions that are sometimes difficult. We must keep our energy at maximum level to be receptive to the messages that come to us through intuitive thoughts, daydreams and night dreams, and especially from people who show up on our path.

Q: How do you develop intuition?

A: The best way is just to sit still and listen. Turn within and pay attention. Too often we run away from ourselves, filling up our lives with constant activity. We don't take time to be still.

Intuition can be nurtured in a variety of ways which I have written about in Chapter 19 on meditation. The more you act on your intuitive hunches, the stronger and more readily available they become. As you become more sensitive to your oneness with God and life, you will become more intuitive. Receiving those inner messages clearly comes when you learn to give up the analyzing, reasoning, doubting and limiting part of your mind.

Meditation also increases awareness. It restores calmness to the mind so we can perceive God's reflection in our souls. In meditation you turn down the volume on the outer world and relax in the silence. In this haven of peace, you realize you are in the presence of God. As you linger in this divine cocoon, you become more and more relaxed. Listening to God you discover that the answers you seek—guidance, health, wisdom, and more—are available to you just for the asking. Silence is your buffer against the world. When you feel the world beginning to pull you off center, still your thoughts, and become one with the peace and power of God—in the silence.

In prayer, I *talk* to God. In meditation, I *listen* to God. It is not a passive exercise; I remain alert since I am in meditation for inspiration and spiritual unfoldment. I rise in consciousness into an atmosphere of receptivity, into a consciousness where I feel God and all life become one.

James Redfield, author of *The Celestine Prophecy*, advises that you can keep your energy at maximum level by focusing on the beauty of nature or even a beautiful object. As you focus, note the glow encircling everything within your sight. Breathe slowly, deeply and consciously. Feel love entering and exiting your body with each breath. Imagine yourself surrounded by light. Feel its warmth and healing. Perceive its mighty intelligence and power. Discover that you are a radiant being, able to inhale and exhale energy from the universe. The supply is unlimited. You have access to all the energy you will ever need. Quiet your mind; be still. What messages come through to you? What questions are you meant to ask now? What is the next step on your path? Trust and be willing to listen.

Q: Do you have a particular meditation and spiritual practice?

A: Yes. My meditation practice is based on *Kriya Yoga* as I mentioned in Chapter 19. For years I have been studying the lessons from Paramhansa Yogananda's Self-Realization Fellowship. Those lessons are invaluable and truly help me look at all the aspects of my life from a new perspective. The essence of the lessons is that we need to live more in the presence of God, and to look inwardly for the answers to life rather than outside of ourselves. I have always had those beliefs on my own, but the lessons were very practical in terms of reminding me that I can live a more spiritual life in a physical world.

Self-Realization means "to know the Self as soul, made in the image of God." *Fellowship* stands for "fellowship with God, first, and through Him, fellowship with humankind." The Self-Realization Fellowship techniques provide practical step-by-step methods to enable one to recharge the body with cosmic energy; awaken the unlimited power of the mind by concentration; and expand the consciousness by Kriya Yoga meditation, to receive the omnipresent love and joy of God. These are definite scientific techniques that have been used for centuries. When Yogananda was alive he always emphasized "plain living and high thinking." That's how I choose to live. I want my life to radiate my devotion to God and my loving reverence and concern for all fellow beings, creatures and life itself.

Q: When you say "God" and "spiritual," what do those terms mean to you?

A: My concept of God is the essence of life . . . love . . . the universal force that both surrounds us and is within us, and which connects us all to each other. For me spirituality is more than performance of sacraments, prayers and songs. I express my faith by the way I live and by my belief and faith in a Creator—by my reverence for nature and my desire to nurture humankind. Being spiritual also means being honest with myself and practicing self-discipline in every aspect of life. Henry David Thoreau expressed it well when he said, "Our religion is where our love is." I am deeply in love with all people, all creation, and with life itself. Life is sacred and every step we take is on holy ground.

Q: Do you feel that today's busy world can put one's spirituality at risk?

A: The intense pace and stress of our daily lives can very easily put our sense of living a spiritual life at risk. It's easy to get caught up in the whirl of today's hectic lifestyle—especially if you've forgotten the truth of your being. We all need a strong foundation of practical spirituality based on the realization that we are co-creators with the ultimate source of power and creativity. With that type of partnership, anything and everything is possible.

Q: What do you mean by "co-creators," and how do you see that operating in our practical lives?

A: There is a way to accomplish all of our dreams and live up to our highest visions. We all have access to the universal creative power. We are tied directly to it. Our dreams can always be made a reality by taking them seriously, by continuously focusing on what we want. When we do this, the natural pull of the universe will serve as a co-creative force that leads us to any goal we truly want and feel worthy to receive. We must stop judging from the appearances of so-called "reality" and have enough faith to choose a loftier perspective on life. Then we can move toward what we want by taking action.

What I see happen with so many people is that they give up easily when their quest is challenged. Helen Keller wrote that when one door closes another opens. But sometimes we look so long at the closed door, we don't even see the one that is opened. I have found in my own life that stumbling blocks and challenges are just opportunities to learn and grow. Our only real limits are our own thoughts and self-imposed limitations.

Q: What would you say to the person who is struggling to find purpose in his or her life? How can one come to clarity?

A: Several things come to mind. I would ask, "What did you want to do as a young child? What would bring you so much joy and enthusiasm you would do it even if you didn't get paid?" Attaining a clear vision of what you want your life to be should be your number one priority. Thoreau said, "The world is but a canvas to your imagination." It all starts with a mental vision of what you want. You are here to experience and celebrate life and to be enlightened, happy and joyful. This is your true destiny. Take your vision seriously. Why not become the best you can? You owe it to yourself to do that. No one is going to do it for you.

Often we don't begin the one thing we really want to do in life because of fear. The greatest possible growth and personal development is achieved through recognizing and facing our pain and fears. I like what Jack Kornfield says about this in his wonderful book, *A Path With Heart*: "The compartments we create to shield us from what we fear, ignore, and exclude exact their toll later in life. Periods of holiness and spiritual fervor can later alternate with opposite extremes—binging on food, sex, and other things— becoming a kind of spiritual bulimia. Spiritual practice will not save us from suffering and confusion, it only allows us to understand that avoidance of pain does not help."

Q: Do you feel that fear can be empowering?

A: Absolutely. We often just live in the "comfort zone." But you can learn so much about yourself when you look at what creates fear in your life. Then the challenge is to step out beyond your fear, even though you may not have a clear idea of what you want to do.

What I like to tell people in my workshops is that the time you feel least like starting something is precisely the time to forge ahead. Just the physical act of beginning will create the momentum and energy that will allow you to develop beyond your fear and toward your greatest accomplishments. Every step you take is on sacred ground. Everything about your life is sacred. The path to the sacred is your own body, heart, and mind, the history of your life, and the closest relationships and circumstances of your life. If not here, where else could we bring alive joy, compassion, freedom and happiness? Don't place any limitations on your dreams or your Creator by doubting that you can accomplish your soul's desire and live a sacred life. Like Jesus, the Wayshower, you can call on spiritual power and authority that will allow you to overcome whatever it is you need to overcome, achieve whatever you desire to achieve.

Q: How do you recommend we build our goal-seeking muscles?

A: I recommend you start with very easy-to-achieve goals so you can have success and feel empowered. Visualization is a very important part of the process. You must be able to see yourself achieving your goal. Don't push your goal too far out into the future. One thing that I always do when I am visualizing a goal is to accept it and give thanks that it is already part of my reality. Simply put, "act as if." And I always end my visualizations with, "This or something better I now accept in my life." I do that because even though I may be clear on what I want, I am always living in the presence of a Higher Power that has a better sense of what is best for my highest good.

Q: What can we learn from your personal success?

A: I remember as a child I wanted to speak to people about being happy and peaceful. When I was about seven or eight, I had dreams of visiting world leaders of different countries and helping them resolve conflict. I always believed in peace, not war. And I also knew I wanted to be active and do something involving health and fitness. I got in touch with those early visions and made conscious, faith-filled choices based on them.

Another major key to my success in life is discipline. Discipline is the ability to carry out a resolution or commitment long after the mood has left. Plus, part of discipline is to give enthusiasm to whatever you are doing, have faith in yourself, be tenacious, and have high personal standards and integrity. If you do that, your life will blossom.

Pay attention to your feelings and what your body, mind and heart are telling you. You are getting messages all the time. Focus directly on what is right in front of you. Notice what your body and experiences are telling you. When any experience in body, heart, mind or circumstance keeps repeating in consciousness, it is a key that this signal is asking for a deeper and fuller attention.

Another key is regular visualization. Seeing in your mind's eye the end result of what you want to achieve—and feeling the sensation associated with the wish being fulfilled. I spend time each day visualizing. There's a wonderful quote by James Allen, "You think in secret and it comes to pass . . . environment is but your looking glass." It really helps to set aside a few minutes each day to focus on one or more goals that you want to bring into your life.

What happens when you live life with these attitudes is that you resonate at a high frequency. I absolutely mean this literally. Scientific studies have shown that when we are enthusiastic and positive and have faith in ourselves, the frequency of vibration of our molecules is increased at a base cellular level.

Finally, make sure your path has heart. This is essential on any spiritual journey. Be sure that your path is connected with your deepest love. Don Juan, in his teaching to Carlos Castaneda, put it this way: "Look at every path closely and deliberately. Try it as many times as you think necessary. Then ask yourself and yourself alone one question. This question is one that only a very old man asks. My benefactor told me about it once when I was young and my blood was too vigorous for me to understand it. Now I do understand it. I will tell you what it is: Does this path have a heart? If it does, the path is good. If it doesn't, it is of no use."

Q: You are a proponent of on-going personal change. Would you please explain your change concept?

A: Ben Franklin once said that whatever you do for 21 days will become a habit. He is now supported by behavioral scientists. If you meditate or exercise, or perhaps stop smoking or drinking coffee, for 21 consecutive days, your body will accept your new behavior as a habit, or no longer crave what you gave up. This is a wonderful way for a person to begin to take control of life in a non-threatening manner. Most people can commit to a simple 21 days. If you are really committed, then you'll arrange your personal circumstances and lifestyle to support your commitment.

I have done this monthly for over ten years, and I have made twelve beneficial changes every year. I'm not saying this is always easy. Often when you make a commitment to something, things may get worse in your life before they get better. I believe this is so because making a commitment causes everything unlike your goal to surface. Only then can you take responsibility for such things and let them go. Quite often the most rewarding transformations come from our greatest adversities and challenges.

Q: What do you feel are the most basic keys to personal mastery?

A: Six important things immediately come to mind.
  1. Have a very clear vision of what you want in your life.
  2. Be totally committed to that vision.
  3. Live with faith—believing, even when appearances or expected patterns may show you something other than your vision.
  4. Acknowledge that it is in surrender to the co-creative power within that you will find and create everything you are seeking in your life.
  5. Maintain an attitude of gratitude. No matter what's going on in my life, I am grateful for it because I know that I can learn and grow and be a better and stronger person for everything that happens.
  6. Acknowledge the sacredness of your body and life, and walk a path with heart.

Q: Susan, you put a great value on health. Why is this so important to you?

A: The physical, mental, emotional and spiritual are all connected. Lack of physical, mental or emotional health impedes spiritual self-understanding. Superior effort toward physical, mental and emotional health tends to promote superior spiritual self-understanding. Paramhansa Yogananda, writing in *The Divine Romance*, said it this way: "The saints say this is how you must treat the body, as a temporary residence. Don't be attached to it or bound by it. Realize the infinite power of the light, the immortal consciousness of the soul, which is behind this corpse of sensation."

There is really no physical existence except in the universal sense. The body you see is nothing but materialized energy. How could energy be sick? Sickness is a delusion. But simply saying that it is delusion is not enough. Yogananda taught that only by contacting God can one see that God has become the universe, that the human body—and all things—are nothing but a mass of condensed energy, and that energy is "frozen" Cosmic Consciousness, or God. You have the illusion of matter as a solid reality. By meditation you will be able to separate the soul from the illusion of the solid body. You will know that the cosmic golden cord that binds the atoms is the tender consciousness of Spirit. It is with this cord, says Yogananda, that God binds the atoms to become the flower, or the human body. He takes myriad electrons, like a child modeling in clay, and throws them into eternity to become stars or universes. Though we are so very small, yet as souls made in His image we are very big indeed!

Q: How do you find time for your personal health and fitness program?

A: How I find time? I *make* time. I've discovered that if we don't make time for health, then we'll have to eventually make time for sickness. I've made a commitment to health.

Q: What does "commitment" mean to you?

A: You've noticed that I am very much into commitment! It's through our everyday behavior that we know what we've really committed to. If we're committed, then everything we think, feel, say and do is in alignment. Commitment is also an excellent way to free yourself from tension, because then your mind is no longer indecisive.

Lack of commitment seems to be a disease of our generation. Just look around. People say they are committed to a healthier planet, yet they litter, don't recycle and eat lots of animal products—all of which drain our planet's natural resources. People say they're committed to aligning and nurturing the spiritual side of their being, but they make no time in their lives to meditate or commune with their Higher Power. Sometimes a person will get seriously ill or have an accident. That will be their "wake up call." It will force them to get in touch with what is really essential in life. But it's easier just to take time each day to turn within and connect with your Higher Self—to pay attention to what is important, then carry that out into the world.

I'm committed to a practical, self-disciplined, day-to-day spirituality as a way of life—always recognizing the sacredness of our lives.

Q: Susan, the entire world seems to be in one crisis or another. How do you view our times?

A: I believe that everything is a reflection of our consciousness. If I watch the news and get really upset or angry about what's going on then what I'm doing is adding to the turmoil that is already out there. I like to be informed, but I feel that what I can do best is just choose to live my life as peacefully, positively and lovingly as possible. Everything begins in our own hearts. If we can all live more loving and peaceful lives, then we can add those feelings to the mass consciousness and in some small way make a difference. "As we receive God's love and impart it to others, we are given the power to repair the world," says Marianne Williamson in *Illuminata*. Attaining and expressing self-realization is what we're all here to do. It's about loving God, knowing our oneness with Him; and then bringing that love, peace, happiness and realization down into practical application in our daily lives.

Q: What do you feel are the main ingredients for optimum health?

A: Of course nutrition and exercise are essential. But I believe there are also other equally important elements, including deep breathing, fresh air, sunshine, pure water and periodic fasting. And don't forget positive attitude, forgiveness toward yourself and others, and releasing any negative emotions. To this list, I would also add visualization, affirmations, simplifying your life, learning to relax, and becoming more childlike. Then, of course, you want to add meditation, some time for solitude, unconditional love for yourself, and living more from inner guidance.

Q: Why do you recommend eliminating dairy products from our diet?

A: Dairy products cause excess mucus, which in turn causes over-acidity. Cow's milk is a high-fat fluid designed to turn a 45-pound calf into a 400-pound cow in eighteen months. As my friend Dr. Michael Klaper says in his book, *Vegan Nutrition: Pure and Simple*, "It has a 'bovine' mixture of casein protein and saturated fat, and simply is not a natural food for man, woman or child." He continues: "Consider the fat content of these popular dairy foods:

Butter = 80%
Cream = 40%
Ice Cream = 20% - 40%
(Luxury ice creams have the highest content)
Cheese = 25% - 40%
Milk Chocolate = 25% - 40%"

Animal fat from cow's milk clogs the arteries. Dairy products have been conclusively linked with heart attacks, strokes, and cancer growth. (See Chapter 2 on Nutrition.) Dairy products also contain animal proteins, like casein, that can contribute to allergic/inflammatory reaction, such as chronic runny noses, asthmatic bronchitis, and other inflammations of joints, skin and bowels.

Commercials proclaim that dairy products are good sources of calcium, vital for strong bones, and preventatives against osteoporosis. In actuality, milk, cheese, yogurt, and ice cream are not really wholesome sources of calcium. In addition to significant amounts of saturated fat, and allergy-inciting cow protein, these dairy foods contain a large load of phosphate, which can neutralize the benefits of calcium. Studies disclose that dairy products do not prevent osteoporosis. The nations with the highest levels of dairy product consumption are also the nations with the highest rates of osteoporosis. In one study (sponsored by the Dairy Council) women consuming three eight-ounce glasses of cow's milk per day still lost calcium from their bodies, and remained in negative calcium balance, even after a year of consuming almost fifteen hundred milligrams of calcium daily! It is not a diet insufficiently high in calcium, but a diet high in protein, laden with poultry, fish, meat and dairy products that robs the body of calcium. If you are already experiencing osteoporosis, or may be at a risk for it, you can slow the rate of calcium loss by 1) adopting a vegan diet, 2) eliminating caffeine, soft drinks and smoking—all of which leach calcium from the bones, and 3) incorporating weight-bearing exercise (such as lifting weights, climbing stairs or hills, or hiking) outside in the sunshine everyday.

In place of milk, try nut milks or soy beverages (see Chapters 2 and 7 on nutrition and tofu). I also use fresh apple juice (or an apple/berry combination) on my whole grain cereals. Sounds odd but it's really delicious.

While we ourselves are the living graves of murdered beasts, how can we expect any ideal conditions on this earth? —**George Bernard Shaw**

I have no doubt that it is part of the destiny of the human race in its gradual development to leave off the eating of animals, as surely as the savage tribes have left off eating each other when they came into contact with the more civilized. —**Henry David Thoreau**

Q: Who are your greatest teachers or mentors?

A: Five people have made a profound, positive effect in my life. Jesus and Paramhansa Yogananda have both shown me, by example, the importance of practicing love and forgiveness, and living as a spiritual being having a human experience. My highest goal in life is to constantly live in the presence of God and to be a clear vessel to do God's will for me. So I turn to their words often for inspiration. I also encourage everyone to get the Self-Realization

Fellowship home study lessons of Paramhansa Yogananda for daily inspiration and motivation. (See Resources.)

My mom, June, has also been a tremendous inspiration to me in how she lives her life—with joy, enthusiasm, perseverance, and love for everything and everyone. She has a heart of gold and always instilled in me the values of high thinking, living my vision, never giving up and following my heart. She's been a wonderful blessing in my life. My grandmother Fritzie, who I mentioned earlier in this book, I would also add to this list. In many ways, she reminded me of Peace Pilgrim. She was peaceful, happy, independent and self-reliant, traveled the world, ate healthy foods and led a simple life. By example and through her loving words, she helped orchestrate my life and is still navigating with me. I feel her presence often.

And so has Peace Pilgrim inspired me. Peace Pilgrim was a walking, breathing example of living peacefully. For more than twenty-eight years, she traveled the length of North America, all fifty states, the ten provinces of Canada, and parts of Mexico sharing her thoughts about peace. Her journey was on foot, never asking for anything: food, shelter, or transportation. She walked without a penny in her pocket. All she had were the clothes she wore (pants, shirt, tennis shoes and a short, sleeveless tunic lettered boldly on the front "Peace Pilgrim"). Her motto was as simple as her life: "This is the way of peace: overcome evil with good, and falsehood with truth, and hatred with love." There was only one thing that could inspire and support a journey of this extent and provide the strength to see it through for all those years, and that is absolute, uncompromising faith in herself and in God. It's that kind of faith I aspire to daily.

On peace, she said: "When you find peace within yourself, you become the kind of person who can live at peace with others. Inner peace is not found by staying on the surface of life, or by attempting to escape from life through any means. Inner peace is found by facing life squarely, solving its problems, and delving as far beneath its surface as possible to discover its verities and realities." (For a free book or video documentary on Peace Pilgrim, her life and philosophy, see Resources.)

Q: How do your feelings affect your health?

A: Letting your feelings out supports health and expresses love for yourself. Covered-up feelings cause disease. Covering up feelings is another form of lying. And like lying, we do it to protect someone we love or to protect ourselves. *Warning: Covering up feelings—or not being true to your feelings—can be harmful to your health.*

If we examine the word disease, we see that it is composed is DIS and EASE. And when we are not at ease, we get disease. We are all exposed to the same viruses and germs, but the people who get sick are usually those who are under a great deal of stress. Scientists have discovered that one of the characteristics of the cancer patient is a tendency to harbor resentment and an impairment in his ability to express hostility.

In *Love, Medicine & Miracles,* Dr. Bernie Siegel cites the work of Dr. Caroline Bendel Thomas of Johns Hopkins University Medical School, who did a personality profile of 1,337 medical students and surveyed their health every decade throughout their adult lives. She was surprised to find that almost all of those who developed cancer "had throughout their lives been restricted in expressing emotion, especially aggressive emotions related to their own needs." According to Siegel, in order for cancer patients to get well, they need to see "how the needs of others, seen as the only ones that count, are used to cover up one's own." He goes on to say that, for healing to occur, our outer choices have to match our inner desires, so that the energy that was used for these contradictions can now be used for healing.

Q: When asking questions and making important choices in daily living, how do you know if your answer is your inner guidance or merely your ego-guidance?

A: To know how to choose correctly in any given situation, we need to guide our judgments by the power of intuition. We are all endowed with this "sixth" sense, but most people don't use it and, instead, use their other five senses. These senses usually interpret things according to their own likes and dislikes rather than according to what is true and ultimately beneficial for the soul.

In learning to make right decisions, the most important thing you can do is make meditation a regular part of your daily life. In the Bible we read, "Be still and know that I am God." Few understand what that really means: the more still you become, the more you tune in with the omnipresence of God. When a question arises like, "Is this the right thing to do?" you can stand back and impartially ask yourself, "Is this something I want, or is this something God wants for me?" When you have felt peace in meditation, then you will recognize that same peace which is the intuitive indicator of divine inner guidance. Say to God, "Lord, guide me." Keep on saying it—deeply and sincerely throughout the day. Continually think of God and say: "Guide me, bless me." That keeps your mind receptive and open to inspiration, the silent guidance of God.

Yogananda said that "intuition is perceived mostly through the heart." I have found this to be true in my life. When something is not right, I get feelings in my heart. There is an uneasiness that makes me think, "Oh, there is something wrong with that individual, or with that situation." It does not make me uncomfortable, but I am conscious of a little disturbance in my heart. This is what Yogananda referred to when he said: "Whenever you are concerned about something, or trying to find the right course to pursue, calmly concentrate on the heart. Don't try to analyze the problem; just remain watching the heart . . . . Remain calm, and then suddenly a great feeling will come over you and your intuition will point you to the right step you should take at that time. If your mind and emotions are calm and attuned to the voice of intuition within, you will be rightly guided. In your everyday life, you will meet the right people who will bring some solution to your problems, or who will help you in some way—or through their contact and counsel, you will find the right way."

Here is the great truth I encourage you to put into practice. If you persist, you will learn to recognize and be led by the "still small voice" within. However, it doesn't happen overnight. "Through your persistent prayers for guidance and your calm receptivity," says Yogananda, "an inner sense will prompt you as to the best way to proceed. When that happens, go forward with full faith; but all the while remain flexible." Yogananda recommends to affirm: "It seems to me that this is the right way to go. But if at any time, Lord, You show me that I have made the wrong choice, I can step back; I can accept correction."

Q: Is there a message you would like to leave us with?

A: Yes, several points. First I would like to remind you that life is to be enjoyed—to be celebrated. Know what it is that you want in life and commit to your vision. Commit and apply yourself only to things that have your heart—that create the passion and enthusiasm in your life.

If you don't like what's going on in your life and want to change it, you must first change your thoughts. Then your life will change. In other words, to bring something into your life, you must first imagine that it's already there. Be it! If you want to have more peace in your life, for example, you must first be peaceful. If you want more joy, you must first be joyful.

Live more in the present moment rather than thinking about your past or worrying about your future. Be mindful and put your full attention with a loving heart to everything you do.

I encourage you to love, honor and forgive yourself and to open up to the Higher Power, whatever you wish to call it, that is within you. We are spiritual beings in a physical body.

Finally, I encourage you not to take yourself and your life too seriously. Laughter is the lubricant and elixir of life. Laughing at yourself and the incongruities of your daily situation is the best way to quell stress. Lighten up and celebrate life!

Nothing is more powerful than an individual acting out of his conscience, thus helping to bring the collective conscience to life.

—Norman Cousins

Acknowledgments

Andrew Carnegie said his success was due to picking the right helpers. That is certainly true for me regarding this book.

My heartfelt thanks to all my friends at DAWN Publications: Bob Rinzler, for his belief in this book, great insight and loving patience; my editor, Glenn Hovemann, for standing behind my vision and lovingly and gently guiding me every step of the way; and all my other friends at DAWN including Irene Sowton, Paul Kelly, Nancy Raynes, Pat Warner and Denice Skillman for their commitment to excellence, hard work, encouragement, and countless contributions to the birth of this book.

To my special friends and family who have all been a steady source of support, inspiration and love: June B. Smith, Jamie and Tony Carr, Reid Smith, June and Ad Brugger, Kathy Martelli, Helen Guppy, George Marks, Ralph Nelson, Rev. John Strickland, Nancy S. Phelps, Pamela Davis, Dejla Asli, Mary A. Tomlinson, Mary and Wayne Bianchin, Gene Forget, Hilma Flores, Rose Marie Stack, Jim Lennon, Dianne Warren, Don Genhart, George Tsutsuse, Bramachari Terence, Tahayra Manjra, Peter Zschalig, Kathleen Hook, Sal Glynn and Jimmy Langkop.

To all my friends in Coos Bay, Oregon who helped make my vision of a peaceful sanctuary a reality: Dee and Arch Wilkie, Gloria and Wally Hill, Alice and Tom Gayewski, Arlene and Del Atkins, John Chambers, Carole Coffman, Russ and Alex Turman, Lynn Carroll, Lucy Varoujan, Mahendra Prasad, Sue Watkins, Karen McGuire, Bev and Doug Beath, Jean and Bob Macy, Bill Carnahan and Gary Brink.

To Rees Moreman for his scientific expertise and help editing the chapters on flaxseed, fats, and tofu.

And to my two precious nephews, Bryce and Tyler Carr, for bringing such joy and delight to my life.

About the Author

Susan Smith Jones is a leading voice for wellness in America today. She not only teaches wellness, she lives it—dynamically. In 1985, Susan was selected as one of ten *Healthy American Fitness Leaders* by The President's Council on Physical Fitness and Sports,* and in 1988, the President's Council designated Susan as National Master in weight training. Susan enjoys hiking, ocean-swimming, jogging, weight training, cycling, doing yoga, in-line skating and walking. Looking for more of a challenge, she completed a 100-mile run from Santa Barbara to Los Angeles and has participated in several triathlons.

Susan speaks with authority. Her credentials include a doctorate in health sciences, a master's degree in kinesiology and a bachelor's in psychology. She has been a fitness instructor to students, staff and faculty at UCLA for over 20 years. But she is probably best known as an advocate of healthy living and positive thinking. She is the author of eight books, appears regularly on radio and television talk shows, and has written more than 500 magazine and journal articles, many of them award-winning.

Susan also travels internationally as a health and fitness consultant and motivational speaker for community, corporate and church groups. Her inspiring keynote presentations and workshops/retreats are often scheduled one to two years in advance. As a health and fitness trainer, she develops personalized wellness programs for individuals and families.

Susan is founder and president of Health Unlimited, a Los Angeles-based consulting firm dedicated to the advancement of human potential, health education, and peaceful living. She has acquired the nickname of "Sunny" and lives in Brentwood, Los Angeles.

*Other honorees have included Jack La Lanne, Richard Simmons, Coach John Wooden, Senator Richard Lugar, Gold-medalist John Nabers, George Allen, Astronaut James Lovell, Jr., Kathy Smith, Denise Austin, and Ronald Reagan.

Other Products
by Susan Smith Jones

Books

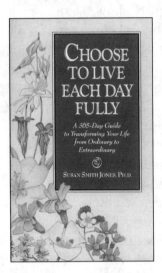

Choose to Live Each Day Fully

This inspring book is a daily guide of 365 affirmations, exercises and lessons to help transform our lives from the ordinary to the extraordinary. Susan, by her uplifting guidance, shows us how to discover and live up to our highest personal potential. This motivational collection shines brightly as a daily companion to all wanting to live an empowered, balanced life. Read one day at a time or several pages at once. You can also select a specific topic of interest from the index. Live your highest vision with this practical, motivating book.

PAPER COVER $13.00

Choose to Be Healthy

Every day we make choices about the way we eat, exercise, think, play and rest. Our experience of health and happiness is a direct result of those choices. In this inspiring book, Susan Smith Jones, shares her powerful insights on how to achieve a healthy balance between the physical, mental and spiritual aspects of daily life. She offers practical advice on topics ranging from nutrition and fitness to the importance of maintaining a peaceful, positive attitude.

PAPER COVER $12.00

Add $4.00 S.+ H. for 1 to 3 books.

Choose to Live Peacefully

Many of us share a vision of world peace, a wish for harmony among all living creatures. By nurturing our inner selves and living in personal peace, we can help to bring about global change. In this Pulitzer Prize nominated book, Susan Smith Jones explores the many aspects of a peaceful, satisfying life—including exercise, nutrition, solitude, meditation, relationships, restoring youthfulness, forgiveness and environmental awareness—and shows how they are linked to world peace.

PAPER COVER $13.00

Other Products
by Susan Smith Jones

Audio Cassettes

Celebrate Life!

This seven cassette series will empower you to create the life you desire and deserve: The seven programs include discussions on: Nutrition for Aliveness, Celebrate Your Magnificence, Make Your Exercise Program A Great Adventure and The Main Ingredients of Positive Thinking and Relaxation. Six of the seven cassettes also include one of Susan's popular guided meditations. Each tape sold separately as well.

SEVEN-CASSETTE SERIES: $80.00 / SINGLE TAPE: $15.00

Learn To Live A Balanced Life
A Fresh Start: Rejuvenate Your Body
Making Your Life A Great Adventure

Here are three of Susan Smith Jones' most popular workshops recorded live. Each program includes two audio tapes offering a complete approach on how to integrate the physical, mental, emotional and spiritual aspects of life. You'll feel like you've participated in one of her dynamic, empowering workshops.

EACH SET: $24.00 / THREE SETS: $60.00

How To Achieve Any Goal—
The Magic of Creative Visualizaiton

A 90-minute audio cassette which includes a twenty-minute meditation you can use very day to help you realize your goals and dreams. An excellent tape to use as a daily companion.

$15.00

TO ORDER ALL PRODUCTS CALL ANYTIME: 1-800-374-5505 OR WRITE: HEALTH UNLIMITED, P.O. BOX 49396, LOS ANGELES, CA 90049. Send check or money order (U.S. funds only). Please allow three weeks for delivery. For more information on any of the products, send a business size self-addressed stampled envelope to the above address.

Resource Directory

Aloe Falls, Yerba Prima, Inc., 740 Jefferson Avenue, Ashland, OR 97520-3743

Aloe Falls by Yerba Prima is preservative-free, great tasting and Certified Active, which means that Aloe Falls is lab verified to provide the health benefits of aloe. Found in your health food store, their Aloe Juice Formula contains 50% aloe vera and a powerful herbal blend of peppermint, chamomile and parsley to boost its soothing properties in your digestive system. They also have Hawaiian Ginger Aloe, and light and refreshing teas and juices. Write for more information.

American Natural Hygiene Society, *Health Science* Magazine, James M. Lennon, P.O. Box 30630, Tampa, FL 33630 (813) 855-6607

This wonderful organization publishes the award-winning *Health Science* magazine. Annual membership dues are $25.00 which includes a subscription to *Health Science*. Members also receive discounts on health books, videos, and cassette programs, seminars, lectures, and more. Write and become a member.

Bastyr University, Seattle, WA (206) 523-9585

With over 600 students enrolled, Bastyr University is an interdisciplinary institution with programs in midwifery, nutrition, acupuncture and Oriental medicine, and applied behavior sciences. They offer B.S. and M.S. degrees through the department of nutrition, with a whole foods emphasis. Graduates can also receive B.S., M.S. degrees and certificates in traditional Chinese herbal medicine through the acupuncture and Oriental medicine department. For more information about the University, call the above number.

Bienenfeld, Joel, D.C., 15247 Sunset Blvd., Suite 206, Pacific Palisades, CA 90272 (310) 459-7636.

Dr. Joel Bienenfeld is a Diplomate of the American Board of Chiropractic Orthopedists and he is a Certified Chiropractic Sports Physician. He is renouned in his work with various athletic teams, including the Chinese Olympic Team, the U.S. Olympic Team and the elite runners of the Los Angeles Marathon. He comes highly recommended as he's been my chiropractor for years and has made a positive difference in my life.

Bionic Products, 466 Central Ave., Suite 20, Northfield, IL 60093 (708) 441-6000, (800) 634-4667

Bionic Products markets a top quality ionizer called the Elanra which I've used for years and highly recommend. I wrote about the benefit of negative ions to health in Chapter 15 on clothing. I highly recommend that you call or write for more information.

BodySlant & Body Lift, P.O. Box 1667, Newport Beach, CA 92663 (800) 443-3917

BodySlant is a superb slant board that also functions as a bed and ottoman. I recommend using it daily. The Body Lift is a simple and comfortable way to stand your body upside down so that your shoulders rest on a thick cushion, your head dangles off the floor, and your neck stretches naturally. I use the BodySlant and Body Lift daily and highly recommend them for better health, vitality, and rejuvenation. For more information or to order, write or call them.

Canadian Natural Health Association, 439 Wellington Street West, Suite #5, Toronto, Canada M5V 1E7 (416) 977-2642

Formerly the Canadian Natural Hygiene Society, they are dedicated to teaching healthful living and natural hygiene as described in Chapter 2. Write or call for more information and a complimentary newsletter.

Cascade Institute of Massage & Body Therapies, 1250 Charnelton Street, Eugene, OR 97401 (503) 587-8101

Cascade Institute is a licensed vocational school preparing adults for a career as a Massage Therapist. The 565-hour program is taught evenings only over one year. Send for a free catalog.

Catalist, (800) 374-5505

Published by Red Rose Collection, *Catalist* is a bi-monthly magazine designed to support your personal growth and assist you in creating positive change in your life. It covers topics as diverse as natural healing, creativity, menopause, sex and spirituality, transformative travel, and angel encounters, and readers are invited to share their experiences for future articles. A one-year subscription (6 issues) is only $10.00. To order, simply call the number above.

Center for Chiropractic and Conservative Therapy, Inc., 4310 Lichau Road, Penngrove, CA 94951 (707) 792-2325

Co-founded by Dr. Alan Goldhamer and Dr. Jennifer Marano, this center offers an alternative approach to the restoration and maintenance of optimum health.

The focus is on helping people make diet and lifestyle changes and on certified supervising fasting.

Center for Spiritual Awareness, Roy Eugene Davis, P.O. Box 7, Lake Rabun Road, Lakemont, GA 30552 (404) 782-4723

To find out about the retreat center, their programs for spiritual growth, all of Davis's inspiring books and related material, write to the above.

DeSouza Chlorophyll Products, P.O. Box 395, Dept. SJ, Beaumont, CA 92220 (800) 373-5171

DeSouza's liquid chlorophyll (also in tablets and capsules) and other personal care products are very beneficial for enhancing health. I highly recommend their entire line of products. For additional information, a catalog, or to order, please write or call the company.

EarthSave, 706 Frederick Street, Santa Cruz, CA 95062-2205 (408) 423-4069

Founded by John Robbins, author of *Diet for a New America* and *May All Be Fed*, EarthSave is a nonprofit organization providing educational materials and leadership for transition to more healthful and environmentally sound food choices, nonpolluting energy supplies and a wiser use of natural resources. Write for their catalog of books, audio and videotapes, and other products.

E•Force, CSA, Inc., Consumer Sales, 14 Norfolk Avenue, South Easton, MA 02375 (800) CSA-0136

I highly recommended the E•Force in Chapter 11 on Exeircse as the perfect all-around piece of fitness equipment. It combines aerobic exercise with user friendly resistance training to help you achieve a total body workout. It features a unique design that allows you to roll it away and store your E•Force vertically when not in use. To order or to receive more information on the E•Force and a variety of other gym/fitness equipment and accessories, call the number above.

Ester-C, Inter-Cal Corporation, 533 Madison Avenue, Prescott, AZ 86301 (520) 445-8063

Inter-Cal is the manufacturer of Ester-C calcium ascorbate. Ester-C is formulated in a wide variety of nutritional supplements by many different distributors and can be found on the shelves of health food stores, drug, stores, and supermarkets. Look for labels with the Ester-C logo (a small "e" enclosed in a big "C"). If you can't find a source, call or write Inter-Cal.

The Expanding Light Retreat Center, 14618 Tyler Foote Road, Nevada City, CA 95959 (800) 346-5350

The Expanding Light is the spiritual retreat center of Ananda Village for people from around the world, and from every spiritual background. It is located near Nevada City, CA in the scenic foothills of the Sierra Nevada Mountains. Programs at The Expanding Light are based on the teachings of Paramhansa Yogananda. The retreat experience includes meditation, classes, free time, programs and three delicious, vegetarian meals each day. Write or call for more information.

The Felix Letter, P.O. Box 7094, Berkeley, CA 94707

Berkeley nutritionist Clara Felix's independent newsletter is four pages of highly informative, alternative suggestions to improve health and diet, with major emphasis on the right fats. One year (6 issues) is $12; two years (12 issues) is $22. Sample and back issue list $1.

Fortified Flax, Omega-Life, Inc. P.O. Box 208, Brookfield, WI 53008-0208 (414) 786-2070, (800) 328-3529

Fortified Flax is one of the best sources of Omega-3 fatty acids and lignans, along with soluble and insoluble fiber. This brand is fortified with the proper vitamins and minerals to help the essential fatty acids in flax metabolize properly and to keep the ground seed fresh. Write for more information.

Gayelord Hauser Seasonings, Modern Products, P.O. Box 09398, Milwaukee, WI 53209 (800) 877-8935

As I mentioned in Chapter 9, these are delicious seasonings. They include Spike (Original and new Salt Free), Herbal Bouquet, Garlic Magic, Onion Magic, and very low sodium Vegit. They are available in health food stores as well as supermarkets. For free samples and a recipe booklet, call the number above.

Good Medicine, Physicians Committee for Responsible Medicine, 5100 Wisconsin Avenue NW, Suite 404, Washington, D.C. 20016

An excellent quarterly newsletter. A year's subscription and annual membership costs $20.00 and is tax deductible.

Juiceman Juicer, Salton Maxim Housewares, 550 Business Center Drive, Mt. Prospect, IL 60056 (800) 233-9054

As I described in Chapter 10 on juicing, this is my favorite juicer. I highly recommend that juicing become a part of your health program. To inquire or to order the juicer, or to receive information on juicing, call the number above.

Kyo-Chrome, Kyo-Green, Kyolic Aged Garlic Extract, and Acidophilase, Wakunaga of America Co., Ltd., 23501 Madero, Mission Viejo, CA 92691 (800) 825-7888

Kyo-Green is an excellent product I wrote about in Chapter 9 on Greens. Kyolic Aged Garlic Extract, Acidophilase and Kyo-Chrome were mentioned in Chapters 2 and 3. For more information or free samples of these products, write or call.

Let's Live Magazine, (800) 676-4333

This is an excellent magazine if you want to learn more about, or the latest on, being healthy—physically, mentally, emotionally and spiritually. I have been writing for this magazine for over 20 years. It's one of the few I read cover-to-cover every month. Call to subscribe.

Mori-Nu Silken "Lite" Tofu, Mori-Nu, 2050 West 190th Street, Suite 110, Torrance, CA 90504

This is a very healthy source of low fat protein which I wrote about in the Chapter 7. For more information and delicious recipes, send a self-addressed, stamped envelope.

Nightingale-Conant's, "Insight," (800) 323-5552.

Hosted by Brian Tracy, *Insight* is an inspiring, motivational monthly audiocassette program by Nightingale-Conant which I've enjoyed for years. It features messages by Brian Tracy, Earl Nightingale and two other leaders in the field of personal development. Call to order or for more information.

Nutrition Action Health Letter, Center for Science in the Public Interest, 1875 Connecticut Avenue NW, Washington, DC 20009

This is an excellent newsletter. Subscriptions are available for $24.00 for one year (ten issues).

Nutrition Advocate, 95 Brown Road, Box 4716, Ithaca, NY 14852 (800) 841-0444.

Get the latest on health, nutrition, and breaking news from the China study (discussed in Chapter 2 on Nutrition). This newsletter includes reviews of new research from the medical literature, with critiques and responses from the original investigators. It's published six times per year, for both professionals and lay readers. An annual subscription is $30.

Peace Pilgrim, Friends of Peace Pilgrim, 43480 Cedar Avenue, Hemet, CA 92544 (909) 927-7678

To receive a free thirty-two page booklet, *Steps Toward Inner Peace,* a free 216-page book, *Peace Pilgrim,* a free marvelous video documentary titled "The Spirit of Peace," or an inspiring newsletter, write to the above address. Friends of Peace Pilgrim is a nonprofit, tax-exempt, all-volunteer organization.

PowerBar, 1442 A Walnut Street, Berkeley, CA 94709 (800) 444-5154

The PowerBar is a delicious sustained-energy bar for endurance athletes and active people. It combines healthful ingredients and important nutrients. It comes in a variety of flavors and is low in fat. For more information or a free newsletter, call the above number.

PMRI Residential Retreats, 900 Bridgeway, Suite One, Sausalito, CA 94965 (800) 775-PMRI, Ext. 221

PMRI stands for Preventive Medicine Research Institute. This non-profit public institute offers Dr. Dean Ornish's week-long residential retreats to teach comprehensive lifestyle changes to individuals. Dr. Ornish attends each of the retreats giving lectures and answering questions about his program. Gourmet low-fat, low cholesterol meals and cooking instruction are also provided.

Red Rose Collection, 42 Adrian Court, Burlingame, CA 94010 (800) 374-5505

This is my favorite catalog which offers magical gifts to inspire and delight, including clothing, jewelry, and decorative accessories for the home and garden. You can also order the *Antioxidant Plus* and *Foundation* I wrote about in Chapter 2 from this company.

Reviva Cosmetics Labs, 705 Hopkins Road, Haddonfield, NJ 08033 (800) 257-7774

I've used Reviva skin products for years and highly recommend them, especially their skin line which includes a special form of glycclic acid, one of the alpha hydroxy acids (AHAs). President and owner, Stephen Strassler was one of the first authorities to tell us that eliminating dead cells is important for radiant skin. Over 23 years ago, Reviva introduced *Light Skin Peel,* America's first exfoliant. Their latest breakthrough is a cream that delivers oxygen directly into the skin via stabilized hydrogen peroxide. Reviva products are available in health food stores. For more information, please call the number above.

Self-Realization Fellowship, 3880 San Rafael Avenue, Los Angeles, CA 90065 (213) 255-2471

Write for more information on Paramhansa Yogananda, his books, meditation, home study lessons, the locations of the Self-Realization Fellowship centers, or a catalog of their books, tapes, quarterly magazine and other products.

Sound R$_X$, 524 San Anselmo Ave., Suite 700, San Anselmo, CA 94960-2614 (800) 909-0707

As I wrote about in Chapter 12 on healing music, Steven Halpern has a variety of wonderful tapes and CDs. His music is very healing and relaxing. I highly recommend that you call for a brochure. In Chapter 12, I listed some of my favorites CDs.

Spectrum Naturals, Inc., 133 Copeland Street, Petaluma, CA 94952 (800) 995-2705

Producers of Veg Omega-3 Organic Flax Seed Oil, Spectrum Spread, Wheat Germ Oil, natural vegetable oils pure pressed without chemicals, and a variety of natural, delicious condiments. Write for their information and consumer education series on healthy oils.

Stronglite, Inc., 255 Davidson Street, Cottage Grove, OR 97424 (800) 289-5487

Manufacturer of high quality massage equipment offering the best value. Portable massage tables available in do-it-yourself kit form (at great savings) or factory assembled. Call for a free color catalog.

Super Blue Green Algae, Cell Tech, 1300 Main Street, Klamath Falls, OR 97601-5914 (800) 883-8848

Founded in 1982 by Daryl and Marta Kollman, Cell Tech produces the best blue green algae, which is grown in Upper Klamath Lake, OR. This lake is known for its pure water which provides a unique growth medium for blue-green microalgae. As I described in chapter 9, their super blue green algae is a rich source of natural nutrition which helps heal and rejuvenate the body. It's an important part of my "whole foods" nutrition program and I highly recommend it. The Cell Tech Network is composed of thousands of men and women, throughout the United States and Canada, who are committed to making positive changes in themselves and in the world. Cell Tech is a company with heart, redefining what it means to be in business. Please call the above number for more information on the company, how to order, or how to become a distributor.

Tree of Life Seminars & Rejuvenation Center, P.O. Box 1080, Patagonia, AZ 85624 (520) 394-2520

Tree of Life is a metaphor for a way of being in the world which supports one's own spiritual evolution in an integrated, balanced, and harmonious way. There are a variety of seminars (including rejuvenation retreats) conducted by Nora and Gabriel Cousens, M.D. Write for a brochure.

Westbrae Natural/Westsoy, 1065 E. Walnut Avenue, Carson, CA 90746 (310) 886-8200, (800) SOY-MILK

Westbrae makes a complete line of delicious non-dairy, all-vegetarian, all natural, organic milk replacements made from rice and soy, in addition to a variety of health food items (nut butters, soups, sauces, condiments, etc.) available in health food stores. For more information on their soy beverages and other products, or for samples or product coupons, call (310) 886-8200, ext. 124.

The Windstar Foundation, 2317 Snowmass Creek Road, Snow-mass, CO 81654-9198 (970) 927-4777

Windstar is a nonprofit organization in Colorado, co-founded by John Denver and Thomas Crum to create a sustainable future for the planet. Windstar has many impressive programs, including their excellent annual symposium, *Choices for the Future*. Hosted by John Denver, this inspiring, empowering symposium is held every Summer in Aspen, Colorado. I spoke on "Wellness" at the first symposium in 1985. Windstar also sponsors a variety of educational programs, including children's workshops in music and science, volunteers for peace, international exchanges, Global Games and other programs geared toward living at one's highest potential. Write or call to request being on Windstar's mailing list.

Y.S. HoneyBee Farms, RR1, Sheridan, IL 60551 (800) 654-4593

I wrote about this company's top quality bee products in Chapter 6. Their bee pollen, propolis, and royal jelly help to increase energy, boost the immune system, rejuvenate and detoxify the body, promote longevity and reverse the aging process. Their products are pure, harvested by healthy bees, are quality controlled and are organic—meaning pesticide, herbicide and pollutant-free. Y.S. Bee Farms bee products are available at your local health food store but I encourage you to call for more information.

Index

A

abdominal strengthening, 190–193
accomplishment. *See* success
Acidophilase, 35–36
acne: treating, 173
actions. *See* behavior
acupressure, 219
addictions: alcoholism, 107–108; drug
addiction, 103; and stress reduction,
201–202; surrendering, 315–316
adrenaline: and energy levels, 181
adventure: life as, x–xvi; as security, 325;
spirit of, 326
adversity: turning to advantage, 339–342.
See also challenges
aerobic exercise: equipment, 189–190; and
metabolism, 58–59; routines, 185–186
affirmations, 252; making, 244–245, 315.
See also visualization
aging, 7; antioxidants and, 37; and bone
mass, 182; enzymes and, 34; garlic and,
43; isoflavones and, 126; meditation
and, 303; and muscle loss/fat gain, 57;
in the sea, 155–156
Agricultural University (Netherlands):
trans-fats research, 78
airport ticket story, 284–285
alcohol: and body fat, 66
alcoholism: and stress reduction, 201–202;
treating, 107–108, 315–316
Alcott, Louisa May: and Emerson, 265
alfalfa, 150
alfalfa sprouts: juice from, 170
algae, 154–157
algin: benefits of, 152
Ali, Mohammed: bee pollen use, 116
Allen, James: on cherishing visions, x; on
man and choice, 1; on thoughts coming
to pass, 9, 354
allergies: flax seed meal and, 108; LNA
and, 103, 104; pollen and, 117–118
almond milk: recipe, 25
Aloe Falls aloe juices, 161
aloe vera: benefits, 160–161; juices, 161
alone: term derivation, 9

alone time: finding, 9–10, 267–272; as
suspect, 267. *See also* solitude
alpha brainwaves: frequency range, 201,
210; New Age music and, 203
alpha-linolenic acid. *See* LNA
altars: for meditation, 308–309
aluminum: and Alzheimer's disease, 152
Alzheimer's disease, 43, 152
American College of Sports Medicine:
exercise recommendations, 59, 186
American Heart Association: dietary
recommendations, 23
American Journal of Surgery: chlorophyll
report, 142
American Public Radio (APR): "Everyday
Healing Food", 31–33
amino acids: in flax seed, 93; in tofu, 123n
amylase, 35
Anderson, Richard: on chromium, 68
Anderson, Robert: *Stretching*, 195–196
anemia: healing, 175
anger: effects of, 3, 8; releasing, 248–249,
315–316. *See also* negative feelings
angina: love and, 293
animal fat: from dairy products, 358
animal products: antioxidants in, 82;
eliminating from diets, 22–23, 26–27;
free radicals in, 82; toxic concentrations
in, 24, 45; trans-fats in, 79. *See also*
animal protein
animal protein, 20–25; and cancer rates,
22; and cholesterol levels, 21–22;
consumption in China and the U.S., 21;
meat protein vs. tofu protein, 130–132;
and osteoporosis, 24–25
animals: strong vegetarians, 168; and
vitamin C, 38–39, 40–41
Annals of Epidemiology: WHR study, 54
antibiotics: in bee products, 111, 112–113
Anti-Oxidant Plus (nutritional supplement), 38
antioxidants: benefits, 37–38, 90;
nutritional supplements, 38; sources,
37–38, 90, 162. *See also* beta-carotene;
vitamin C; vitamin E

Voluntary Simplicity (Elgin), 276
Vosnjak, Mitja: on propolis and stomach
cancer, 114

W

Waist/Hip Ratio (WHR), 54–56; calculat-
ing, 54; health problems associated
with, 54–55; and heart disease, 54;
highs for men and women, 55; ideal, 55
waitress stories, 263–264, 287
wakefulness meditation, 307
Walden (Thoreau), 267
Walker, Norman: on slanting, 228
walking: blind trust walks, 297; as
exercise, 58–59; in solitude, 268; and
stress reduction, 181–182, 268; tips on,
187–188
Wallace, Keith R.: meditation research,
302–303
Walpole, Sir Hugh: on friendship, 295
Walters, J. Donald: on spiritual work, 302
warrior spirit: in spiritual practice, 314
water consumption. *See* drinking water
water retention. *See* edema
watercress, 160; juice from, 176
Watson, Bernard: on relieving asthma, 237
Wattenberg, Lee: phytochemical research,
124
weight, 50–71; body toxicity and, 64;
ideal, 51–52; overweight, 55. *See also*
obesity; weight loss
weight lifting. *See* strength training
weight loss: benefits of, 51; diet and, 63–
65; dieting and, 56–57, 61–63; exercise
and, 57, 184, 190–191; goals, 70;
increasing metabolism, 56–71; keys to
success, 69–70; nutritional supplements,
67–69; positive actions and, 249; program expenditures, 50; spot reducing,
190–191; strength training and, 58,
182, 190–191; subconscious beliefs and,
243
weight tables (MetLife): lenience of, 51–52
wellness. *See* health
wheat germ oil, 84–85
wheat grass: benefits, 153–154; juice from,
176; sources, 157
Wheeler, Virginia: on chicken and cancer,
130
Wherever You Go There You Are
(Kabat-Zinn), 306–307
white blood cells: garlic and, 43;
neuroreceptor sites, 3–4
white light meditation, 311–312

Whitman, Walt: kindness of, 291; on the
secret of making the best persons, 189
WHR. *See* Waist/Hip Ratio
widower story, 297
Willet, Walter: on margarine and heart
disease, 80
Williams, Stanley: on honey, 111
Williamson, Marianne: on repairing the
world, 357
Willstatter, Richard: chlorophyll structure
discovery, 140–141
Wilson, Roberta: on cellulite, 67
winds: as a source of positive ions, 235
Winfrey, Oprah, 282
wisdom: as inner truth, 272–273
Wise, Ruth: on clothing and massage, 222;
on foot massage, 223
Wise, Tracy: on massage tables, 220–221
woman in the restaurant story, 289–290
women's health: exercise and, 24–25, 127,
183; hot flashes; 96, 126; menstrual
bleeding, 146–147; menstrual cycles,
126. *See also* osteoporosis
wool clothing: efficiency of, 233
words: controlling speech, 244–245, 256–
259; keeping your word, 257–258; the
power of brevity, 270–271; practicing
honesty, 13; saying what you want, 247,
253–254; speaking accurately, 257
world: creating harmony in, 344, 357
The World of Bees (Murray), 115
wounds: chlorophyll and, 142

Y

yoga: kriya yoga, 306, 350
Yogananda, Paramhansa: on the body, 356;
on calmness, 266; dietary recommendations, 30–31; on finding the wellspring
of wisdom, 265; on intuition, 362–363;
on living our highest potential, 327; on
self-mastery, 345–346; on service, 278,
279; on simplifying life, 274; on
solitude, 266; SRF lessons, 350
You'll See It When You Believe It (Dyer), 249
Young, Vernon: on soy protein quality, 132
Your Body Doesn't Lie (Diamond), 205
Y.S. Bee Farms: bee products, 121
yuba tofu, 134

Z

Zen mudra, 306
zinc: juice sources, 177
zone therapy, 219

Dawn Publications

Fitness Resources

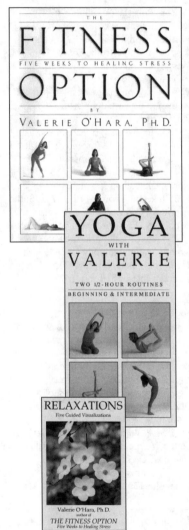

The Fitness Option:
5 Weeks to Healing Stress
Valerie O'Hara, Ph.D.

Here is an easy-to-follow, holistic program that effectively brings a sense of calmness, balance, and health to the modern lifestyle. The comprehensive approach covers physical, emotional, and mental perspectives including: stretching and relaxing exercises, nutritional analysis, breathing techniques, affirmations, and guided imagery.

• Fitness and relaxation exercises you can do on the job
• Over 300 charts, photographs, and drawings

PAPER $13.95

Yoga With Valerie
Valerie O'Hara, Ph.D.

On this video, Dr. O'Hara presents two 1/2-hour routines amidst serene garden and ocean settings. Beginning and intermediate levels.

VIDEO $29.95

Relaxations:
5 Guided Visualizations
Valerie O'Hara, Ph.D.

Against a background of soothing harp music the listener is guided through peaceful images of water, light and flowers.

AUDIO CASSETTE $9.95

Dawn Publications

Cookbook

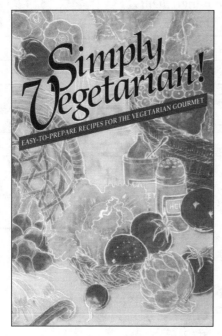

•Over 80,000 sold!
•A classic in its field

Simply Vegetarian
by Nancy Mair & Susan Rinzler

For this age of greater awareness about the need for more balance in our diet, *Simply Vegetarian!* offers a complete variety of soups, salads, side dishes, main entrees, sauces, desserts, and beverages. Easy-to-find ingredients and reasonable preparation times accommodate the schedules of the busiest cooks.

The dishes are rich in taste and texture and will please even the most sophisticated palate. Those new to a vegetarian cuisine will find recipes like Ratatouille, Manicotti, and Chile Rellenos to help smooth the transition to a healthier diet.

PAPER $9.95

• "**Simply Vegetarian**! *is practical and helpful, and deserves daily use in anyone's kitchen."* —VEGETARIAN JOURNAL

• *"It's not just for vegetarians; it's loaded with some new flavor combinations and just plain good food."* —LAS VEGAS REVIEW-JOURNAL

• "[**Simply Vegetarian**!] *proves that health food doesn't have to take days to prepare. More than 150 of the 250 recipies take less than 45 minutes."*

—THE DAILY NEWS, MORFREESBORO, TN

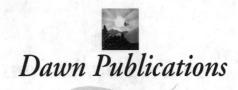

Dawn Publications

QUANTITY	ITEM	PRICE
_____	*The Main Ingredients*	$14.95
_____	_____	_____
_____	_____	_____
_____	_____	_____
_____	_____	_____
_____	_____	_____
_____	_____	_____

7.25 % TAX IN CALIFORNIA _____

SHIPPING: $4.25 FOR 1 OR 2 ITEMS; $5.25 FOR MORE _____

TOTAL _____

Please send payment and order to:
DAWN Publications
14618 Tyler Foote Road
Nevada City, CA 95959
Or Call Toll Free 1.800.545.7475
For a complete listing of our products, please ask for a
DAWN Publications Catalog

NAME————————————————————————

ADDRESS—————————————————————————

CITY/STATE/ZIP—————————————————————

PHONE——————————————————————————

Please charge to my credit card #——————————————

❑ Visa ❑ MasterCard   Expiration Date——————————

Order Form